Organizing Principles of
Neural Development

NATO ASI Series

Advanced Science Institutes Series

A series presenting the results of activities sponsored by the NATO Science Committee, which aims at the dissemination of advanced scientific and technological knowledge, with a view to strengthening links between scientific communities.

The series is published by an international board of publishers in conjunction with the NATO Scientific Affairs Division

A	**Life Sciences**	Plenum Publishing Corporation
B	**Physics**	New York and London
C	**Mathematical and Physical Sciences**	D. Reidel Publishing Company Dordrecht, Boston, and Lancaster
D	**Behavioral and Social Sciences**	Martinus Nijhoff Publishers
E	**Engineering and Materials Sciences**	The Hague, Boston, and Lancaster
F	**Computer and Systems Sciences**	Springer-Verlag
G	**Ecological Sciences**	Berlin, Heidelberg, New York, and Tokyo

Recent Volumes in this Series

Volume 72—Principles and Methods in Receptor Binding
edited by F. Cattabeni and S. Nicosia

Volume 73—Targets for the Desing of Antiviral Agents
edited by E. De Clercq and R. T. Walker

Volume 74—Photoreception and Vision in Invertebrates
edited by A. M. Ali

Volume 75—Photoreceptors
edited by A. Borsellino and L. Cervetto

Volume 76—Biomembranes: Dynamics and Biology
edited by Robert M. Burton and Francisco Carvalho Guerra

Volume 77—The Role of Cell Interactions in Early Neurogenesis: *Cargèse 1983*
edited by A.-M. Duprat, A. C. Kato, and M. Weber

Volume 78—Organizing Principles of Neural Development
edited by S. C. Sharma

Volume 79—Regression of Atherosclerotic Lesions
edited by M. Rene Malinow and Victor H. Blaton

Series A: Life Sciences

Organizing Principles of Neural Development

Edited by

S. C. Sharma

New York Medical College
Valhalla, New York

Plenum Press
New York and London
Published in cooperation with NATO Scientific Affairs Division

Proceedings of the NATO Advanced Study Institute on
Organizing Principles of Neural Development,
held June 1–12, 1982,
in Povoa de Varzim, Portugal

Library of Congress Cataloging in Publication Data

NATO Advanced Study Institute on Organizing Principles of Neural Development
    (1982: Póvoa de Varzim, Portugal)
    Organizing principles of neural development.

    (NATO ASI series. Series A, Life sciences; v. 78)
    "Published in cooperation with NATO Scientific Affairs Division."
    Includes bibliographical references and index.
    1. Developmental neurology—Congresses. I. Sharma, S. C. (Sansar C.), 1938–
        . II. North Atlantic Treaty Organization. Scientific Affairs Division. III. Title.
IV. Series.
QP363.5.N44   1982   599′.0188   84-9860
ISBN 0-306-41726-X

©1984 Plenum Press, New York
A Division of Plenum Publishing Corporation
233 Spring Street, New York, N.Y. 10013

Printed in the United States of America

PREFACE

This volume contains summaries of most of the invited presentations
at the NATO Advanced Study Institute "Organizing Principles of
Neural Development", held in Povoa de Varzim, Portugal, from June
1-12, 1982. The meeting was intended to bring together a select
group of investigators to present their views on problems in the
field and to foster extensive discussions in smaller groups. It
was hoped that such communications would pique curiousity and
creativity among the students and thus help in formulating additional
hypotheses regarding the type of interactions which might underlie
neural development.

Despite the wide range of material covered at this institute,
a common theme seemed to emerge: at all stages of their developmental history, the cells of the nervous system interact with
previously generated cells (both neurons and non-neurons) as well
as with other constituents of the developmental milieu. The presentations at this meeting helped in comprehending how a relatively
"simple" series of sequential events might provide the necessary
information needed to generate the diversity, characteristic of the
adult nervous system, without hypothesizing on the existence of
specific genes acting to control each step.

The intensive discussions by both lecturers and students
throughout the meeting, which many times had to be curtailed
because of the limitations of time, were indicative of the levels
of participation. Several topics seemed to generate primary
attention: How does an axon get from the array of its origin to
the target array? Within the target area, what determines which
and how many of the available neurons form synaptic connections
with particular axons? How are the specific features of synaptic
connections between the arrays attained? In their attempt to link
molecular, cellular and morphological events during neural development, the diversity of topics discussed at the institute will, it
is hoped, be evident in this book.

I am deeply indebted to Prof. Antonio Coimbra whose help in arranging the meeting place in Portugal, his role as the resident organizer for both scientific and social events are deeply appreciated. His participation was crucial to the success of the meeting.

Thanks are due to "The Gulbankian Foundation" - Lisbon and The National Science Foundation US for partial funding of the travel expenses. I have had reasons to appreciate the kindness and help of my friends especially Dr. Sandra Fraley, Dr. Ambrose Dunn-Meynell, Margaret Kobylack and Richard Breckwoldt. Janet Sharma provided technical help and crucial moral support during the entire course of this project. Joan Mozayeni typed the manuscript.

S.C. Sharma
New York Medical College
Valhalla, NY, USA
1984

CONTENTS

IN VIVO AND IN VITRO STUDIES ON THE DEVELOPMENT OF THE PERIPHERAL

NERVOUS SYSTEM

Julian Smith and Nicole M. Le Douarin

Institut d'Embryologie du C.N.R.S.
Collège de France
Nogent-sur-Marne   France

The origin of the peripheral nervous system (PNS) is currently attracting considerable attention, both from the embryological and the neurobiological standpoints. The embryologist is fascinated by the problems posed by the differentiation of a variety of distinct cell lines from a unique source - the neural crest - while the neurobiologist is attracted by the relative simplicity of a system the study of which may, in the long term, bear fruit relevant to an understanding of higher brain function. It is not surprising, therefore, that the past few years have witnessed an explosion of interest in this topic, which, accompanied by an increasingly multi-disciplinary approach, has helped to increase significantly our knowledge of the development of sensory and autonomic ganglia during vertebrate embryogenesis. This chapter will be largely concerned with the ontogeny of the PNS in the avian embryo, which has long been the preferred experimental model for a number of obvious practical reasons. At certain points, however, reference will be made to relevant studies performed with mammalian systems.

Origin of Peripheral Ganglion Cells

With the exception of certain sensory cranial ganglia, which arise from the placodal ectoderm, the neural crest is the sole source of precursor cells for the ganglia of the PNS (Hörstadius, 1950; Weston, 1970; Le Douarin, 1982). The neural crest itself arises along the edge of the neural primordium at the neural stage. As the neural tube closes the crest cells leave their site of origin and migrate (often for considerable distances) to specific locations in the developing embryo, where they differentiate into the various

1

constituent cell types of the PNS, and also into many other, non-
neural, categories of cell, such as melanocytes, endocrine cells,
skeletal and mesenchymal tissues.

Unfortunately for the observer, neural crest cells possess no
apparent distinguishing features that differentiate them from the
tissues through which they pass and in which they develop. Studies
on their migration in the embryo have therefore largely relied upon
grafting experiments in which host neural crest is replaced by a
donor crest labelled in some way. Experiments of this kind have been
performed with transplanted crest previously labelled with [3]H-
thymidine (Weston, 1963; Chibon, 1966). However, the development of
a stable marking technique, based on easily recognizable (after suitable cytochemicel treatment) structural differences between chick
and quail nuclei, has proved particularly useful in establishing the
precise sites of origin along the neural axis of the different components of the PNS (Le Douarin, 1969; 1976; 1980). Used in conjunction
with the revelation of other cellular and/or extracellular markers,
this technique has, in addition, provided valuable information
concerning the pathways of migration taken by crest cells from the
neural primordium to their definitive sites of arrest.

Normal Developmental Fate of Crest Cells at Different Levels of the Neural Axis

A broad analysis of the levels of origin along the neural axis
of some of the different ganglia and paraganglia of the PNS was performed by Le Douarin and Teillet (1971, 1973), who replaced fragments
of the neural primordium (neural tube plus neural folds) of chick
embryos by the equivalent fragment from quail donors at the same
stage of development. The operation does not noticeably perturb
embryogenesis and the migration and localization of the grafted crest
cells and their progeny can be followed by examining histological
sections of the host at different times after the transplantation.
In this way, a correspondence can be established between the level
from which the grafts had been taken and the definitive location of
their different derivatives. Thus, the sympathetic chain was shown
to derive from the totality of the neural crest from the level of the
6th somite to the posterior end of the embryo. The chromaffin cells
of the adrenal medulla arise specifically from the level corresponding to somites 18-24. As for the enteric ganglia, most of them
originate from a relatively short (from somites 1-7) length of "vagal"
neural crest. An additional contribution is made by crest at the
lumbosacral level, although the parasympathetic ganglion of Remak is
the major derivative of this region (Teillet, 1978). Finally, the
spinal ganglia are shown to arise at the level of each somite from
the corresponding region of the cervicotruncal crest (Figure 1).

Since then, other workers, using the quail-chick system, have
made important contributions to our knowledge of the site of origin

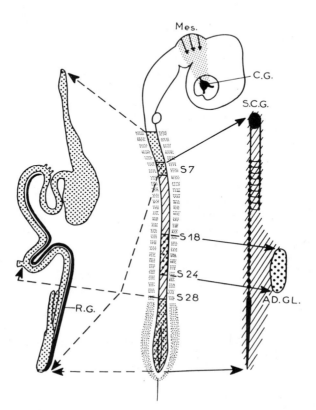

Figure 1:   Axial distribution of neural crest cell precursors of
autonomic ganglia and plexuses. The vagal level (somites 1-7) of
the neural crest gives rise to all the enteric ganglia of the pre-
umbilical gut and contributes to those of the post-umbilical gut.
The lumbo-sacral crest is the source of the ganglion of Remak and of
some post-umbilical enteric ganglion cells. The ciliary ganglion
derives from crest at the mesencephalic level. The sympathetic
chains and plexuses arise from the neural crest posterior to the 5th
somite, the adrenal medulla from the level of somites 18-24. Mes -
mesencephalic crest; CG - ciliary ganglion; SCG - superior cervical
ganglion; S - somite; ADGL - adrenal gland; RG - ganglion of Remak.

of various sensory and autonomic ganglia in the head (Narayanan and Narayanan 1978a, b; 1980; Noden, 1978; Ayer-Le Lièvre and Le Douarin, 1982).

Migration Pathways of Peripheral Ganglion Cell Precursors

To each of the different axial regions of the neural crest mentioned above (vagal, cervicotruncal, lumbosacral) correspond routes of migration leading the crest cells to their appropriate sites of colonization and differentiation. These pathways have been worked out in some detail in a number of cases, partly by means of the quail-chick marker system, partly by immunocytochemical staining of fibronectin, a principal component of the crest cell migration pathway (Newgreen and Thiery, 1980; Thiery et al., 1982; Duband and Thiery, 1982).

The early stages of crest cell migration leading to the formation of sensory and sympathetic ganglia in the trunk have been the object of a detailed study in our laboratory (Thiery et al., 1982). At this level of the embryo, there exist three potential migratory pathways. The first, dorsolateral, is taken by future melanocytes which colonize the skin. Of the two others, which are both dorsoventral, one leads crest cells between the neural tube and the inner face of the somites, while the other conducts them through the space between two consecutive somites.

The first crest cells to migrate dorsoventrally penetrate the space between adjacent somites and rapidly become distributed along the dorsal aorta roots where they condense to produce the primary sympathetic chains. Some hours after the onset of crest cell migration, the pathway between neural tube and somite materializes. This sudden widening of the space may be due to hydration of hyaluronic acid and glycosaminoglycans (Pratt et al., 1975; Derby, 1978). As the crest cells proceed ventrally, the somitic mesenchyme dissociates into dermomyotome and sclerotome. The latter, which surrounds the notochord and neural tube (giving rise to the vertebral primordia), obstructs the pathway, thus blocking the passage to the crest cells which accumulate and form the primordia of the sensory ganglia. It is to be noted that no crest cells from the trunk (except for those that differentiate into Schwann cells or melanoblasts) penetrate the dorsal mesentery and migrate into the gut or the somatopleure.

In contrast, dorsoventral pathways apparently do not play an important part in distributing crest cells originating at the vagal level of the neuraxis. Most of the cells migrate via a pathway situated immediately below the ectoderm whence they reach the pharynx. The precursors of the enteric ganglia then enter the developing mesoderm of the foregut, in which they migrate caudally, colonizing it up to the cloaca and giving rise to the plexuses of Meissner and Auerbach.

Neural crest cells from the lumbosacral region of the embryo follow the dorsoventral pathways characteristic of the trunk level but, in addition, some cells penetrate the mesentery where they form the ganglion of Remak and also contribute to enteric ganglia of the post-umbilical gut. In the hindmost region of the embryo, where the coelomic cavity is absent, the sympathetic ganglia of the pelvic plexus are in close association with the parasympathetic ganglionated nerve of Remak.

Developmental Potentialities of Crest Cells at Different Levels of the Neuraxis

The results described above demonstrated an apparent heterogeneity of the crest cell population along the neural axis in terms of their migratory behavior and ultimate differentiated fate. The latter can be exemplified by a consideration of neurotransmitter function: whereas the sympathetic chains and plexuses and the adrenal medulla are characterized by synthesis, storage and secretion of catecholamines (CA), the parasympathetic and enteric ganglia typically produce and liberate acetylcholine (ACh). Do these divergent chemical specializations reflect the presence in the neural crest of two types of preprogrammed precursor cell, one (cholinergic) in the vagal region, the other (adrenergic) in the remainder of the crest, or are they the result of external influences on an undetermined cell type? By changing the position of the crest cells along the neuraxis prior to their migration, it was possible to provide a tentative reply to this question. Neural primordia were transplanted heterotypically between quail and chick embryos. Analysis of the resulting chimaeras showed that "adrenomedullary" crest cells grafted at the vagal level could colonize the gut and develop into physiologically normal cholinergic ganglia. Similarly, mesen/rhombencephalic neural crest, transplanted to the adrenomedullary level, differentiated into adrenergic sympathetic ganglia and into CA-containing cells in the adrenal medulla of the host (Le Douarin and Teillet, 1974; Le Douarin et al., 1975). Subsequent experiments showed that prosencephalic (the anterior-most level) neural crest, which does not normally produce neurons, can give rise to sensory, sympathetic and parasympathetic neurons if grafted into a suitable heterotopic position (Noden, 1978; Le Douarin et al., 1979; Le Lievre et al., 1980; Ayer-Le Lievre and Le Douarin, 1982). One of the inferences to be drawn from this series of experiments is that the entire length of the neural crest possesses precursor cells both of cholinergic and adrenergic neurons or paraneurons. A similar bipotentiality with respect to neurotransmitter synthesis has been observed in cultured neural crest (see later section).

It has therefore to be concluded that the neural crest is, in fact, a relatively homogeneous structure and that its subsequent phenotypic diversity is a result of the intervention of local environmental factors. In other words, the neural crest as a population is multipotential and able to give rise to all the various cell types of the PNS. This does not necessarily mean that individual cells possess the same abilities. Even at the level of the population, there is evidence that different regions of the neural crest are not exactly equivalent (Le Douarin and Teillet, 1974; Noden, 1978). However, despite these restrictions, it is clear that factors extrinsic to the neural crest play an important role in its subsequent development.

Lability of The Differentiated State in Developing Peripheral Ganglia

Just as transplanting neural crest from one level of the embryo to another can provide clues concerning the developmental capabilities of crest cells, so manipulation of the environment in which differentiating ganglion cells evolve can yield information about the restriction of this potential during embryogenesis. Such experiments, which have been performed both in vivo and in vitro, have revealed that the tissue environment can still exert a profound effect on young neuroblasts, even though gangliogenesis is well under way.

In vivo experiments performed in our laboratory entailed the transplantation of various developing quail peripheral ganglia into the neural crest migration pathways of 2-day chick embryo hosts (Figure 2).

a. Graft of autonomic and dorsal root ganglia. Pieces, comprising approximately 2000 cells, of developing autonomic (ciliary, Remak and sympathetic chain) and sensory (spinal) ganglia were removed from young quail embryos and placed between the somites and neural tube at the adrenomedullary level of a 2-day chick embryo. Donor ganglia were taken from embryos of 4 1/2 to 6 days of incubation, i.e. at a time when chemical differentiation was already significantly advanced. The fate of the transplanted ganglion cells was followed at various times after the operation. Each type of ganglion eventually dissociated into individual cells which became distributed among the neural crest derivatives of the host (Le Douarin et al., 1978; 1979; Le Lièvre et al., 1980) and from 6 days onwards the grafted cells had reached their definitive localization. Their pattern of distribution was characteristic of their origin. Thus, whereas cells from all three kinds of peripheral ganglia (parasympathetic, sympathetic and sensory) colonized sympathetic ganglia and plexuses and the adrenal medulla, developing histochemically demonstrable CA, only the ciliary ganglion provided cells capable of migration to the ganglion of Remak and into Auerbach's and Meissner's plexuses of the mid- and hind-gut. Even more striking was the finding that the host spinal ganglia were colonized only by cells issuing from implanted dorsal root ganglia (DRG) and never from grafts of autonomic ganglia.

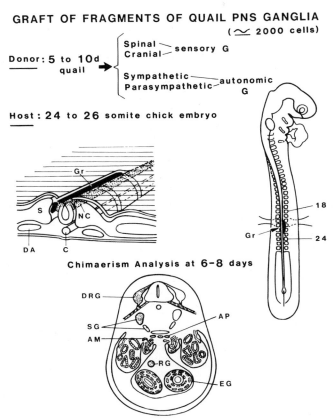

Figure 2: Diagram to show the procedure for back-transplantation of
peripheral ganglion fragments and the final sites of localization of
graft-derived cells in the host embryo. The sites occupied are all
crest-derived, PNS structures. However, the distribution of the
donor cells depends on the nature of the ganglion grafted. Thus,
while both sensory and autonomic ganglia can colonize autonomic
structures of the host, only sensory ganglia provide cells capable
of differentiating in the DRG. Gr - graft; S - somite; NC - neural
crest; C - notochord; DA - dorsal aorta; SG - sympathetic ganglion;
AM - adrenal medulla; AP - aortic plexus; RG - ganglion of Remak; EG
- enteric ganglia.

These results led us to formulate several conclusions. Firstly, the distribution of grafted cells in the host reflects differential affinities of autonomic and sensory ganglion cells for diverse target sites. Thus grafted autonomic neurons and glial cells colonize the autonomic structures, while grafted sensory ganglion cells become localized in the host DRG as well as in the sympathetic ganglia and adrenal medulla. It should be noted, however, that this ability to give rise to sensory neurons after back-transplantation is lost by DRG once their neurons have become post-mitotic, i.e. after 7 days of incubation. Presumably, therefore, segregation of autonomic and sensory cell lines occurs early in development, the sensory precursor cells (which are absent from young autonomic ganglia) having a relatively limited life-span. Finally, developing peripheral ganglion cells are plastic with respect to their chemical differentiation, since cells from ganglia that never synthesize CA under normal developmental conditions are able to express the adrenergic phenotype given the appropriate environment.

Because the experiments described above involved transplantation of a heterogeneous population of cells, it was not clear which of the cell types involved was able to change its (their) fate under the conditions of the graft. One possibility was that the cells responding to new developmental cues were not in fact neurons, but belonged to the small population of small ganglionic cells (the majority of which are probably normally satellite cell precursors), which are abundant in peripheral ganglia at the age when they were taken for grafting. The problem of whether neurons can develop from this class of cell was approached by means of the nodose ganglion.

b. <u>Transplantation of the nodose ganglion</u>. Of dual embryonic origin (the neurons arising from the placodal ectoderm, the glial cells from the neural crest), the nodose ganglion of the vagus nerve lends itself well to studies on the segregation of glial and neuronal cell lines. By grafting a quail rhombencephalic primordium isotopically into a chick host, Ayer-Le Lièvre and Le Douarin (1982) were able to construct chimaeric nodose ganglia in which the satellite cells were of quail origin and the neurons of the chick species. Fragments of such a mosaic nodose ganglion, at 5 1/2 to 9 days of incubation, were grafted into 2-day chick embryo as described above. The fate of the quail cells could thus be followed in the host. At 6-10 days, a certain number were found in the sympathetic ganglia and adrenal medulla and, in some of them, CA stores could be revealed cytochemically. In addition, many quail cells colonized the gut and participated in the formation of the enteric plexuses.

It was also possible to construct a chimaeric nodose ganglion in which the neuronal population was selectively labelled with the quail marker. When this sort of ganglion was transplanted, the neurons rapidly degenerated.

These findings indicate that neuronal potentialities exist within the population of non-neuronal cells of the developing nodose ganglion. It is therefore not unlikely that a similar situation holds in other peripheral ganglia of entirely neural crest origin. The results obtained after their transplantation would not therefore constitute a true example of phenotypic switching, but rather a case of the expression of potentialities hitherto repressed.

c. Phenotypic plasticity in autonomic neurons in vitro. The best documented example of phenotypic lability in developing neurons is provided by the superior cervical ganglion (SCG) of the neonatal rat in vitro (for a review, see Patterson, 1978). The development of the principal neurons (already adrenergic at birth) is highly dependent on the conditions under which the culture is carried out. Thus, when grown in the absence of non-neuronal cells, dissociated SCG neurons pursue their adrenergic differentiation. On the other hand, in the presence of certain types of non-neuronal cells or medium conditioned by them, the neurons become primarily choliner-gic, developing high levels of choline acetyltransferase (CAT) activity and acquiring numerous clear cytoplasmic vesicles at the expense of the dense-core type (Patterson and Chun, 1974; 1977a, b; Johnson et al., 1980; Landis, 1980). By means of biochemical, elec-trophysiological and electron microscopic studies on cultures of single SCG neurons, it was possible to show that the conversion from adrenergic to cholinergic metabolism was due to a true phenotypic change. Under certain "intermediate" conditions, neurons displaying adrenergic and cholinergic properties simultaneously could be detec-ted (Furshpan et al., 1976; Landis, 1976; Reichardt and Patterson, 1977; Potter et al., 1981). The factor responsible for this pheno-typic switch is a protein that has been partially purified from glioma and heart (Weber, 1981).

d. Phenotypic plasticity in autonomic neurons in vivo. That the phenotypic shift observed in SCG neurons in vitro is not merely the reflection of certain artificial culture conditions but may be relevant to plastic changes normally occurring in development, is suggested by the results of recent experiments on the ontogeny of eccrine sweat gland innervation in footpads of the rat (Landis, 1981; 1983). The latter is most probably entirely due to choliner-gic sympathetic nerves. Shortly after birth, numerous fibers con-taining endogenous CA and small, dense-core vesicles can be detected but these adrenergic properties disappear over the next week or so. Concomitantly, acetylcholinesterase staining and VIP-like immunoreac-tivity become pronounced. Although no CA-containing fibers are ever observed in the adult rat, a CA uptake system is present. Interest-ingly, treatment with 6-hydroxydopamine (which causes selective degeneration of adrenergic nerves) during the first postnatal week results in the total loss of the cholinergic sympathetic innervation of the sweat glands. These observations strongly suggest a transi-tion from adrenergic to cholinergic function in vivo.

Other studies in the rat have also provided evidence for the existence of crest-derived cells that possess the adrenergic phenotype only temporarily. These cells, immunoreactive for tyrosine hydroxylase and dopamine β-hydroxylase, are demonstrable in the intestine at about the same time as CA and CA-synthesizing enzymes first appear in developing neurons of the sympathetic chains of the rat embryo (Cochard et al., 1978; 1979; Teitelman et al., 1979). They also possess a CA uptake system (Jonakait et al., 1979) and are responsive to nerve growth factor and glucocorticoids (Kessler et al., 1979; Jonakait et al., 1980). Their adrenergic features, presumably acquired via neural tube-notochord-somite interactions (see following section), cannot be maintained in the gut environment and CA-synthesizing ability is lost within 3-4 days. Although it is tempting to hypothesize that they eventually switch to producing an alternative neurotransmitter, the ultimate fate of these cells has yet to be determined. Apparently they do not die immediately, since a CA uptake system can still be demonstrated after CA enzyme immunoreactivity has disappeared.

Factors Involved in the Chemical Differentiation of Autonomic Neurons

The preceding section underlines the importance of extrinsic factors in peripheral neuron development. It can be concluded that the ultimate fate of neuron precursors, especially with regard to their choice of neurotransmitter (and all the enzymatic machinery that this implies) appears to be largely dependent on the sites in which they settle in the developing embryo prior to gangliogenesis. However, developmental signals could arise, not only from tissues situated at the points of crest cell arrest, but also from those that border the migration routes. As described earlier, a number of crest cell migration pathways have been identified and it is therefore possible to deduce which cell types are potential sources of developmental cues influencing the chemical differentiation of peripheral neuron precursors. Their effects can then be studied in experimental associations in vivo or in vitro.

This kind of approach has, in particular, led to a better understanding of the interactions involved in the development of adrenergic sympathetic neuron precursors. A number of studies have shown that the first detectable signs of the catecholaminergic phenotype (CA fluorescence or tyrosine hydroxylase immunoreactivity) appear after the trunk crest cells have undergone a phase of migration and have aggregated to form the primary sympathetic chains (Enemar et al., 1965; Cohen, 1972; Allan and Newgreen, 1977; Cochard et al., 1978; Teitelman et al., 1979). This differentiation occurs in the vicinity of the notochord and the neural tube, within the environment constituted by the sclerotomal moiety of the somitic mesenchyme. All these tissues are therefore candidates for a role in symphatho-blast differentiation in a variety of experimental systems. Thus in in vivo grafts on the chorioallantoic membrane, CA-containing cells were found to develop from neural crest provided that neural tube and somites were also present (Cohen, 1972). In a detailed examination of the tissue interactions involved, Norr (1973) showed that both neural tube (plus notochord) and somitic mesenchyme were also required for the development of crest-derived adrenergic cells in organ culture. The effect of the neural tube was apparently indirect, via a "conditioning" of the somitic tissue. The action of the notochord on adrenergic cell differentiation has been demonstrated in artificial association in ovo of neural primordium and aneural hindgut. Crest cells were found to migrate into the gut, forming myenteric and submucous ganglionic plexuses that never contained adrenergic cells unless the notochord was also present. In this case, CA-containing cells could be seen in groups along the developing muscular layer as early as 2 days after the beginning of the experiment (Teillet et al., 1978). The extent to which adrenergic differentiation occurred was a function of the number of fragments of notochord added (Cochard and Le Douarin, 1982).

The inter-relationships between crest, neural tube, notochord and somite are undoubtedly complex and have been highlighted by the results of recent experiments in which the effects of surgical removal of the neural tube and/or the notochord on peripheral neurogenesis in vivo were examined (Teillet and Le Douarin, 1983). In the absence of both axial structures, somitic cells rapidly degenerated, as did the neural crest cells associated with the somitic mesenchyme at that time. If either the neural tube or the notochord was left in situ, most of the somitic cells survived and adrenergic structures developed.

Analysis of cholinergic neuron development is rendered difficult by the absence to date of a universally applicable, specific histo- or immunochemical method for detecting CAT activity. By means of radiochemical techniques, it has been shown that ACh synthesis can be measured as soon as parasympathetic or enteric ganglioblasts have assembled at the appropriate sites of ganglion formation (Chiappinelli et al., 1976; Smith et al., 1977; Le Douarin et al., 1978). Later studies showed that neural crest itself, excised by microsurgery from the mesencephalic region of 5- to 12- somite quail embryos, was capable of converting ^{3}H-choline to ACh by a CAT-mediated reaction (Smith et al., 1979). Taken together with the demonstration that 90% of neural crest cells contain another cholinergic marker, the catabolic enzyme acetylcholinesterase (Drews, 1975; Cochard and Coltey, 1983), these observations strongly suggest that key constituents of the cholinergic system are present in the neural crest as soon as it is formed. There is therefore no need to invoke exogenous influences during or after crest cell migration to explain the initial emergence of the cholinergic phenotype. However, target-derived factors undoubtedly play an important role in the subsequent maturation of cholinergic neurons (Smith et al., 1977).

Neuronal Differentiation in Cultured Neural Crest

Cultures of neural crest are being increasingly used to study various aspects of early differentiation of peripheral neurons. Theoretically, in vitro techniques provide unique opportunities for analyzing the developmental responses of neural crest cells to changes in their external environment. In practice, the large number of unknown variables in such experiments does not facilitate the interpretation of the results obtained. Furthermore, extrapolation of in vitro observations to the situation in the intact embryo should be made with caution. Nevertheless, a number of interesting findings have resulted from studies with cultured crest.

It was found several years ago that neurotransmitter-related phenotypes appeared in cultures of avian neural crest. Cholinergic and adrenergic cells developed in vitro from crest taken at the cephalic and trunk levels of the embryo respectively (Greenberg and Schrier, 1977; Cohen, 1977). Subsequently it has been shown that both regions of the neural crest can give rise to cholinergic and adrenergic cells, so confirming the bipotentiality revealed by in vivo transplantation experiments (Kahn et al., 1980; Fauquet et al., 1981; Maxwell et al., 1982). The appearance of CA-containing cells in the absence of notochord or somite (Cohen, 1977) was, at first view, surprising. Although the neural tube, present during the first 24-48 hours of culture, may have played a part in this apparently spontaneous adrenergic differentiation, the fact that a similar phenomenon occurs in secondary cultures of crest cells grown at clonal density (Sieber-Blum and Cohen, 1980) does show that continuous cell-cell interactions are not necessarily required for the catecholaminergic phenotype to emerge.

Using a somewhat different experimental system, however, we found that very little CA was produced by cultures of surgically isolated neural crest unless cells of non-crest origin were also present (Fauquet et al., 1981). Of the different embryonic tissues tested, somitic mesenchyme and notochord were, together, quantitatively the most effective inducers of adrenergic differentiation, although even aneural hind-gut stimulated CA production. However, the results of these experiments, which combined radiochemical assay with cytological examination, revealed that chemical differentiation and the appearance of characteristic neuronal morphology are not necessarily coupled. Even cocultures synthesizing significant amounts of CA contained very few cytologically identifiable neuron-like cells and virtually none that possessed CA stores of sufficient size to be visualized by cytofluorescence. In contrast, excellent biochemical and cytological differentiation of adrenergic nerve cells occurred in cocultures of sclerotomal mesenchyme, isolated together with migrating trunk neural crest from 3-day embryos (i.e. 24 hours older than the crest and somites used for the cocultures described above). Under our experimental conditions, therefore, a certain "primitive" degree of adrenergic differentiation could occur in cultures of young crest cells that were associated with a variety of non-neural tissues, but complete maturation of sympathetic neuron precursors in vitro was dependent on a developmental event occurring in vivo between embryonic days 2 and 3. This event is apparently difficult to reproduce in culture. The discrepancies between our observations and the published descriptions of catecholaminergic differentiation in vitro in the absence of non-crest cells may be at least partly accounted for by differences in the developmental stages of the embryos used or in the techniques employed for isolating the crest. It should also be pointed out that extracellular material has been reported to have a stimulatory effect on CA production (Sieber-Blum and Cohen, 1980; Sieber-Blum et al., 1981; Loring et al., 1982). The variable presence of such substances in serum or embryo extract could also be a possible source of conflicting results.

In order to eliminate the inconstancy caused by the presence of the complex components of the culture media, we grew neural crest in a chemically defined medium lacking serum and embryo extract (Ziller et al., 1981; 1983). Under these conditions, a number of mesence-phalic crest cells rapidly differentiated into neurons without under-going cell division. Within 24 hours, neurite outgrowth was readily apparent and, at 3 days, the cells had developed long processes (up to 2 mm) and had a typical neuronal appearance, possessing character-istic neuronal markers such as neurofilament proteins and tetanus toxin binding sites. Cytologically, neuronal differentiation was incomparably superior to that occurring in serum-supplemented medium. On the other hand, no detectable neurotransmitters, other than a small amount of ACh (3-10 times less than that produced by an equivalent number of crest cells in complex medium), were produced by these neurons.

As far as the maturation of the cholinergic phenotype is con-cerned, little is known of the events involved in the consolidation of the ACh-related properties that are apparently already associated with early neuroblast precursors. Every culture of neural crest ex-amined was found to synthesize ACh (Fauquet et al., 1981) and the absolute and relative amounts of this neurotransmitter could be sti-mulated by coculturing with various young embryonic tissues. The ex-tent to which ACh production was increased depended on the nature of the cocultured tissue and, to a certain degree, on the source of the serum employed and the axial level from which the crest was taken.

Although the nature of the agents that stimulate cholinergic properties in immature crest derivatives are unknown, they are per-haps analagous (or even identical) to the soluble factors present in a variety of tissues that have been shown to stimulate CAT acti-vity in cultures of various types of central and peripheral neurons (Giller et al., 1973; Godfrey et al., 1980; McLennan and Hendry, 1980; Nishi and Berg, 1981; Kato and Rey, 1982).

Concluding Remarks

Although our comprehension of the ways in which the PNS is constructed is still inadequate, it is nevertheless possible to draw a number of general conclusions as much to stimulate further progress as to summarize current achievement.

It has been amply demonstrated that, in normal development, the fate of peripheral neuron precursors in the neural crest depends on their initial position along the neuraxis and on their migratory behavior once they leave it. External cues play an important role in their orientation along specific developmental pathways and, even when they have terminated their migration and begun to differentiate, crest cell derivatives remain responsive to extrinsic signals for some time.

Whether the influence of non-neural tissues on neuronal development is instructive (i.e. acts on pluripotent precursors) or permissive (selecting one particular class of cells from a heterogeneous population) remains to be determined.

The results obtained after transplantation of diverse peripheral ganglia have brought new light to bear on the problem of the progressive restriction of the developmental capabilities of neural crest cell derivatives during ontogeny (i.e. the segregation of cell lines). The available evidence suggests that sensory and autonomic cell lineages diverge early in development. Even so, both types of ganglion contain cells with a broader range of developmental potentialities than those expressed in normal embryogenesis.

The study of specific aspects of chemical differentiation in autonomic neuron precursors has demonstrated a plasticity in the choice of neurotransmitter in cultured neurons and has suggested that a similar phenomenon can occur in vivo. These observations lend weight to the idea that cholinergic and adrenergic neurons arise via a common, bipotential precursor. Furthermore, it is becoming apparent that neuronal differentiation is a multi-step process and that the factors responsible for the initial expression of a particular neuronal phenotype are not necessarily the same as those required for its stabilization and maturation. The molecular mechanisms underlying these developmental events remain obscure.

REFERENCES

Allan, I.J. and Newgreen, D.F. 1977, Catecholamine accumulation in
    neural crest cells and the primary sympathetic chain, Am.J.
    Anat., 149:413-421.

Ayer-Le Lièvre, C.S. and Le Douarin, N.M., 1982, The early develop-
    ment of cranial sensory ganglia and the potentialities of their
    component cells studied in quail-chick chimaeras, Dev. Biol.,
    94:291-310.
Chiappinelli, V., Giacobini, E., Pilar, G. and Uchimara, H., 1976,
    Induction of cholinergic enzymes in chick ciliary ganglion and
    in muscle cells during synapse formation, J. Physiol.,
    257:749-766.
Chibon, P., 1966, Analyse expérimentale de la régionalisation et des
    capcités morphogénétiques de la crête neurale chez l'Amphibien
    Urodèle Pleurodeles waltlii (Michah). Mem. Soc. Zool. Fr.,
    36:1-107.
Cochard, P. and Coltey, P., 1983, Cholinergic traits in the neural
    crest: acetylcholinesterase in crest cells of the chick embryo,
    Dev. Biol., in press.
Cochard, P. and Le Douarin, N., 1982, Development of intrinsic
    innervation of the gut, Scand. J. Gastroenterol., 17:suppl.
    71:1-14.
Cochard, P., Goldstein, M. and Black, I.B., 1978, Ontogenetic
    appearance and disappearance of tyrosine hydroxylase and cate-
    cholamines in the rat embryo, Proc. Natl. Acad. Sci. USA,
    75:2986-2990.
Cochard, P., Goldstein, M. and Black, I.B., 1979, Initial develop-
    ment of the noradrenergic phenotype in autonomic neuroblasts of
    the rat embryo in vivo, Dev. Biol., 71:100-114.
Cohen, A.M., 1972, Factors directing the expression of sympathetic
    nerve traits in cells of neural crest origin, J. Exp. Zool.,
    179:167-182.
Cohen, A.M., 1977, Independent expression of the adrenergic pheno-
    type by neural crest cells in vitro, Proc. Natl. Acad. Sci.,
    USA, 74:2899-2903.
Derby, M.A., 1978, Analysis of glycosaminoglycans within the extra-
    cellular environments encountered by migrating neural crest
    cells, Dev. Biol., 66:321-336.
Drews, U., 1975, Cholinesterase in embryonic development, Prog.
    Histochem. Cytochem., 7:1-52.
Duband, J.L. and Thiery, J.P., 1982, Distribution of fibronectin in
    the early phase of avian cephalic neural crest cell migration,
    Dev. Biol., 93:308-323.
Enemar, A., Falck, B. and Hakanson R., 1965, Observations on the
    appearance of norepinephrine in the sympathetic nervous system
    of the chick embryo, Dev. Biol., 11:268-283.
Fauquet, M., Smith, J., Ziller, C. and Le Douarin, N.M., 1981,
    Differentiation of autonomic neuron precursors in vitro:
    cholinergic and adrenergic traits in cultured neural crest
    cells, J. Neurosci., 1:478-492.
Furshpan, E.J., Mac Leish, P.R., O'Lague, P.H. and Potter, D.D.,
    1976, Chemical transmission between rat sympathetic neurons and
    cardiac myocytes developing in microcultures: evidence for
    cholinergic adrenergic and dual-function neurons, Proc. Natl.

Acad. Sci. USA, 73:4225-4229.

Giller, E.L., Schrier, B.K., Shainberg, A., Fisk, H.R., Nelson, P.G., 1973, Choline acetyltransferase activity is increased in combined cultures of spinal cord and muscle cells from mice, Science, 182:588-589.

Godfrey, E.W., Schrier, B.K. and Nelson, P.G., 1980, Source and target cell specificities of a conditioned medium factor that increases choline acetyltransferase activity in cultured spinal cord cells, Dev. Biol., 77:403-418.

Greenberg, J.H. and Schrier, B.K., 1977, Development of choline acetyltransferase activity in chick cranial neural crest cells in culture, Dev. Biol., 61:86-93.

Hörstadius, S., 1950, The Neural Crest:Its properties and derivatives in the light of experimental research, Oxford University Press, London.

Johnson, M.I., Ross, C.D., Meyers, M., Spitznagel, E.L. and Bunge, R.P., 1980, Morphological and biochemical studies on the development of cholinergic properties in cultured sympathetic neurons. I. Correlative changes in choline acetyltransferase and synaptic vesicle cytochemistry, J. Cell Biol., 84:680-691.

Jonakait, G.M., Wolf, J., Cochard, P., Goldstein, M. and Black, I., 1979, Selective loss of noradrenergic phenotype in neuroblasts of the rat embryo, Proc. Natl. Acad. Sci. USA, 76:4683-4686.

Jonakait, G.M., Bohn, M.C. and Black, I.B., 1980, Maternal glucocorticoid hormones influence neurotransmitter phenotypic expression in embryos, Science, 210:551-553.

Kahn, C.R., Coyle, J.T. and Cohen, A.M., 1980, Head and trunk neural crest in vitro: autonomic neuron differentiation, Dev. Biol., 77:340-348.

Kato, A.C. and Rey, M.J., 1982, Chick ciliary ganglion in dissociated cell culture. I. Cholinergic properties, Dev. Biol., 94:121-130.

Kessler, J.A., Cochard, P. and Black, I.B., 1979, Nerve growth factor alters the fate of embryonic neuroblasts, Nature, 280:141-142.

Landis, S.C., 1976, Rat sympathetic neurons and cardiac myocytes developing in microcultures: correlation of the fine structure of endings with neurotransmitter function in single neurons, Proc. Natl. Acad. Sci. USA, 73:4220-4224.

Landis, S.C., 1980, Developmental changes in the neurotransmitter properties of dissociated sympathetic neurons: a cytochemical study of the effects of medium, Dev. Biol., 77:349-361.

Landis, S.C., 1981,. Environmental influences in postnatal development of rat sympathetic neurons, In: Development in the nervous system, British Soc. Dev. Biol. Symp., 5:147-160.

Landis, S.C., 1983, Development of cholinergic sympathetic neurons: evidence for transmitter plasticity in vivo, Federation Proceedings, in press.

Le Douarin, N., 1969, Particularites du noyau interphasique chez la caille japonaise (Coturnix coturnix japonica). Utilisation de ces particularites comme "marquage biologique" dans les recherches sur les interactions tissulaires et les migrations cellulaires au cours de l'ontogenese, Bull. Biol. Fr. Belg., 103:435-452.

Le Douarin, N.M., 1976, Cell Migration in early vertebrate development studied in interspecific chimaeras. In "Embryogenesis in Mammals", Ciba Foundation Symposium, Elsevier-Excerpta Medica-North-Holland, Amsterdam, p. 71-101.

Le Douarin, N., 1980, The ontogeny of the neural crest in avian embryo chimaeras, Nature, 286:663-669.

Le Douarin, N.M., 1982, The neural crest. Cambridge University Press.

Le Douarin, N.M. and Teillet, M.A., 1971, Localisation par la methode des greffes interspecifiques, du territoire neural dont derivent les cellules adrenales surrenaliennes chez l'embroyon d'oiseau, C.R. Acad. Sci., 272:481-484.

Le Douarin, N.M. and Teillet, M.A., 1973, The migration of neural crest cells to the wall of the digestive tract in avian embryo, J. Embryol. Exp. Morphol., 30:31-48.

Le Douarin, N.M. and Teillet, M.A., 1974, Experimental analysis of the migration and differentiation of neuroblasts of the autonomic nervous system and of neurectodermal mesenchymal derivatives, using a biological cell marking technique, Dev. Biol., 41:162-184.

Le Douarin, N.M., Renaud, D., Teillet, M.A. and Le Douarin, G.H., 1975, Cholinergic differentiation of presumptive adrenergic neuroblasts in interspecific chimaeras after heterotopic transplantations, Proc. Nat. Acad. Sci. USA, 72:728-732.

Le Douarin, N., Teillet, M.A., Ziller, C. and Smith, J., 1978, Adrenergic differentiation of cells of the cholinergic ciliary and Remak ganglia in avian embryo after in vivo transplantation, Proc. Natl. Acad. Sci. USA, 75:2030-2034.

Le Douarin, N.M., Le Lievre, C.S., Schweizer, G. and Ziller, C.M., 1979, An analysis of cell line segregation in the neural crest. In:"Cell Lineage, Stem Cells and Cell Determination". INSERM Symp. n° 10, Ed. N. Le Douarin, Elsevier/North Holland Biomedical Press.

Le Lièvre, C.S., Schweizer, G.G., Ziller, C.M. and Le Douarin, N.M., 1980, Restrictions of developmental capabilities in neural crest cell derivatives as tested by in vivo transplantation experiments, Dev. Biol., 77:362-378.

Loring, J., Glimelius, B. and Weston, J.A., 1982, Extracellular matrix materials influence quail neural crest cell differentiation in vitro, Dev. Biol., 90:165-174.

Maxwell, G.D., Sietz, P.D. and Rafford, C.E., 1982, Synthesis and accumulation of putative neurotransmitters by cultured neural crest cells, J. Neurosci., 2:879-888.

McLennan, I.S. and Hendry, I.A., 1980, Influence of cardiac extracts on cultured ciliary ganglia, Dev. Neurosci., 3:1-10.

Narayanan, C.H. and Narayanan, Y., 1978a, Determination of the embryonic origin of the mesencephalic nucleus of the trigeminal nerve in birds, J. Embryol. Exp. Morphol., 43:85-105.

Narayanan, C.H. and Narayanan, Y., 1978b, On the origin of the
    ciliary ganglion in birds studied by the method of interspeci-
    fic transplantation of embryonic brain regions between quail
    and chick, J. Embryol. Exp. Morphol., 47:137-148.
Narayanan, C.H. and Narayanan, Y., 1980, Neural crest and placodal
    contributions in the development of the glosso-pharyngeal vagal
    complex in the chick,Anat. Rec., 196:71-82.
Newgreen, D. and Thiery, J.P., 1980, Fibronectin in early avian
    embryos: synthesis and distribution along the migration
    pathways of neural crest cells.
Nishi, R. and Berg, D.K., 1981, Two components from eye tissue that
    differentially stimulate the growth and development of ciliary
    ganglion neurons in cell culture, J. Neurosci., 1:505-513.
Noden, D.M., 1978, The control of avian cephalic neural crest cyto-
    differentiation. II. Neural tissues. Dev. Biol., 667:313-329.
Norr, S.C., 1973, In vitro analysis of sympathetic neuron dif-
    ferentiation from chick neural crest cells, Dev. Biol., 34:16-
    38.
Patterson, P.H., 1978, Environmental determination of autonomic
    neurotransmitter functions, Ann. Rev. Neurosci., 1:1-17.
Patterson, P.H. and Chun, L.L.Y., 1974, The influence of non-
    neuronal cells on catecholamine and acetylcholine synthesis and
    accumulation in cultures of dissociated neurons, Proc. Natl.
    Acad. Sci. USA, 71:3607-3610.
Patterson, P.H. and Chun, L.L.Y., 1977a, The induction of acetyl-
    choline synthesis in primary cultures of dissociated rat
    sympathetic neurons. I. Effects of conditioned medium,
    Dev. Biol., 56:263-280.
Patterson, P.H. and Chun, L.L.Y., 1977b, The induction of acetylcho-
    line synthesis in primary cultures of dissociated rat sympa-
    thetic neurons. II. Developmental aspects, Dev. Biol.,
    60:473-481.
Potter, D.D., Landis, S.C. and Furshpan, E.J., 1981, Adrenergic-
    cholinergic dual function in cultured sympathetic neurons of
    the rat, CIBA Foundation Symp., 83:123-138.
Pratt, R.M., Larsen, M.A. and Johnston, M.C., 1975, Migration of
    cranial neural crest cells in a cell-free hyaluronate-rich
    matrix, Dev. Biol., 44:298-305.
Reichardt, L.F. and Patterson, P.H., 1977, Neurotransmitter synthe-
    sis and uptake by individual rat sympathetic neurons developing
    in microcultures, Nature, 270:147-151.
Sieber-Blum, M. and Cohen, A.M., 1980, Clonal analysis of quail
    neural crest cells: they are pluripotent and differentiate
    in vitro in the absence of non-crest cells, Dev. Biol.,
    80:96-106.
Sieber-Blum, M., Sieber, F. and Yamada, K.M., 1981, Cellular fibro-
    nectin promotes adrenergic differentiation of quail neural crest
    cells in vitro, Exp. Cell Res., 133:285-295.
Smith, J., Cochard, P. and Le Douarin, N., 1977, Development of
    choline acetyltransferase and cholinesterase activities in

enteric ganglia derived from presumptive adrenergic and
    cholinergic levels of the neural crest, Cell Different.,
    6:199-216.

Smith, J., Fauquet, M., Ziller, C. and Le Douarin, N., 1979, Acetyl-
    choline synthesis by mesencephalic neural crest in the process
    of migration in vivo, Nature, 282:852-855.

Teillet, M.A., 1978, Evolution of the lumbo-sacral neural crest in
    the avian embryo: origin and differentiation of the ganglionated
    nerve of Remak studied in interspecific quail-chick chimaeras,
    W. Roux's Arch. Dev. Biol., 184:251-268.

Teillet, M.A. and Le Douarin, N.M., 1983, Consequences of neural tube
    and notochord excision on the development of the peripheral
    nervous system in the chick embryo, Dev. Biol., in press.

Teillet, M.A., Cochard, P. and Le Douarin, N., 1978, Relative roles
    of the mesenchymal tissues and of the complex neural tube-
    notochord on the expression of adrenergic metabolism in neural
    crest cells, Zoon, 6:115-122.

Teitelman, G., Baker, H., Joh, T.H. and Reis, D.J., 1979, Appearance
    of catecholamine-synthesizing enzymes during development of rat
    sympathetic nervous system: possible role of tissue environment,
    Proc. Natl. Acad. Sci. USA, 76:509-513.

Thiery, J.P., Duband, J.L. and Delouvée, A., 1982, Pathways and
    mechanisms of avian trunk neural crest cell migration and local-
    ization, Dev. Biol., 93:324-343.

Weber, M.J., 1981, A diffusible factor responsible for the determina-
    tion of cholinergic functions in cultured sympathetic neurons,
    J. Biol. Chem., 256:3447-3453.

Weston, J.A., 1963, A radioautographic analysis of the migration and
    localization of trunk neural crest cells in the chick,
    Dev. Biol., 6:279-310.

Weston, J.A., 1970, The migration and differentiation of neural crest
    cells, Adv. Morphog., 8:41-114.

Ziller, C., Le Douarin, N. and Brazeau, P., 1981, Différenciation
    neuronale de cellules de la crête neurale cultivée dans un
    milieu défini, C.R. Acad. Sci. Paris, 292:1215-1219.

Ziller, C., Dupin, E., Brazeau, P., Paulin, D. and Le Douarin, N.M.,
    1983, Early segregation of a neuronal precursor cell line in
    the neural crest as revealed by culture in a chemically defined
    medium, Cell, 32:627-638.

ORGANIZING PRINCIPLES FOR DEVELOPMENT

OF PRIMATE CEREBRAL CORTEX

Pasko Rakic

Section of Neuroanatomy
Yale University School of Medicine
New Haven, USA

If the elegant and detailed experiments presented at this
meeting have taught us any lesson it is that we cannot explain brain
development solely in reductionist terms by dealing with minute
details of its component elements and without giving a proper account
of properties of the system as a whole. In my presentation, I will
emphasize development of the cellular and modular organization of
the primate neocortex where the principle of integrality can readily
be appreciated. The accumulated evidence indicates that precise
neuronal organization of such a complex cellular structure depends,
to a large degree, on epigenetic or intercellular rather than in
rigid genetic 'intracellular' developmental programs. Here I am
using the term epigenesis in Waddington's definition to denote a
process by which "development is brought about through a series of
control interactions between the various parts" (Waddington, 1956).

In the case of cortical ontogeny, the epigenetic history of its
neural components begins with the final cell division that occurs
within the ventricular zone. Following the last division, cells
pass through several successive steps that include migration, differentiation and establishment of synaptic connections with nearby and
distant neurons. During this period, each neuron interacts with
other elements in a local cellular milieu where instructions outside
the cell may determine the character of the next step of its biochemical and morphological differentiation. This principle of cellular
interdependence is particularly evident during genesis of the large
and slowly developing brain and therefore, I will draw factual information from studies of developing rhesus monkey performed in my
laboratory during the last decade. However, it should be emphasized

21

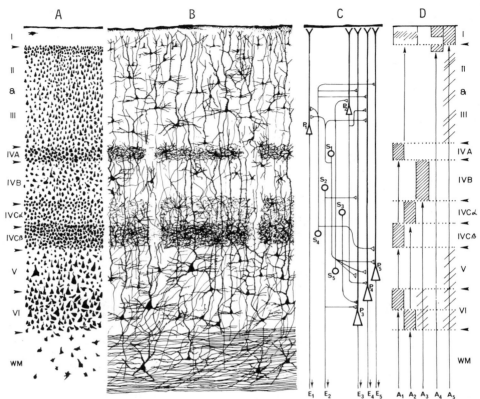

Figure 1. Composite diagram of the laminar and columnar organization of the primary visual cortex of the rhesus monkey which inte-
grates observations derived by many investigators via several
techniques (for recent review see Gilbert and Wiesel, 1981; Hubel
and Wiesel, 1978; Lund, 1981). On the left (A), the cytoarchitectonic appearance of the visual cortex (area 17) in Nissl stain
displays horizontal cell stratification into layers and sublayers.
The adjacent diagram (B) is an appearance of visual cortex in the
Golgi impregnations superimposed with afferent axonal plexules in
sublayers IVA and IVC stained by the reduced silver method. As
verified by the autoradiographic method, these afferents form
stripes or columns that are about 350-400 μm wide. Only one complete column flanked by two half-columns is illustrated. Column C
displays a simplified diagram of the local neuronal circuits.
Thus, stellate cells of sublayers IVC beta (S_4) and IVA (S_1) project predominantly to layer III, where they synapse either directly
upon dendrites of efferent pyramidal cells (P_1 and $P_{2,3,4}$) or

that our work has been made possible by methodological and conceptual advancements from other laboratories studying adult cortical organization in a variety of mammalian species (for recent review see: Schmitt et al., 1981; Rakic and Goldman-Rakic, 1982). The themes chosen here are not all-inclusive, but they may serve as an illustration of basic principles of cortical development as well as background for contemplating future research.

RELATION OF ADULT NEURONAL POSITIONS TO SEQUENCES OF CELL GENESIS

Although the basic organization of the cerebral neocortex had been worked out by Ramon y Cajal by the turn of this century (1899, 1911), the introduction of new methods enabled discoveries of new facts that led to new concepts not entertained at the turn of the century. For example, we have considerable knowledge about the relationship between the cell's position, its origin and phenotype including, in some cases, its biochemical make-up and synaptic connectivity. Although it has been well established that cortical cells differ in their morphology from large pyramidal to small stellate shaped cells, it has only recently been demonstrated that the neurons of different types located at slightly different positions, even when they possess the very same shape, may have considerably different projections. The semischematic diagram of monkey visual cortex in Figure 1C reveals the position-dependent differences in which each cell class receives a specific input and issues a specific output not only to layers of the same cortical column but also to other cortical and subcortical areas. To unravel how this complex synaptic circuitry is constructed, one first has to determine the time of origin of each cell class. To provide this information, we injected a series

---

indirectly through another local circuit neuron (small pyramidal cell P_2). The majority of stellate cells of sublayer IVC alpha (e.g., S_3) probably contact efferent pyramids (P_3) within layer V. Some stellate cells of layer IV beta (S_2) contact nearby neurons within the same layer, but also project to adjacent visual association cortex (E_2). However, most visual efferents are formed by large pyramids (P_{3-5}) of layer V which project to the superior colliculus (E_3); pyramids of upper layers VI (P_4) which project to the parvocellular moiety of the lateral geniculate nucleus (E_4) and pyramids of lower VI (P_5) which project to the magnocellular moiety (E_5). The right hand column (D) displays the relative position of the terminal field originating from five major afferent systems: A_1 (from the parvocellular moiety of LGd), A_2 (from the magnocellular moiety of LGd), A_3 (from the superior temporal cortex), A_4 (from the inferior pulvinar), and A_5 (from area 18); from Rakic (1983).

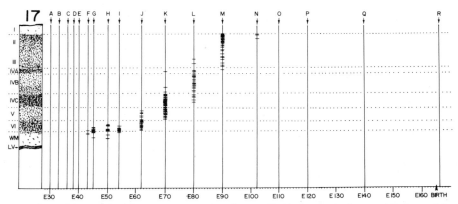

Figure 2. Diagrammatic representation of the positions of heavily
labeled neurons in the primary visual cortex (area 17 of Brodmann in
the depth of clacarine fissure) of juvenile monkeys, each of which
had been injected once with ^{3}H-thymidine at selected embryonic days.
Numerals on the drawing of the cortical dentate layers are according
to classification of Brodmann. Embryonic days (E) are represented
on the horizontal line, starting on the left with the end of the
first fetal month (E28) and ending on the right at term (E165).
Positions of the vertical lines (A to R) indicate the embryonic day
on which each animal received a pulse of ^{3}H-thymidine. Labeled
neurons were found only in animals injected between E43 and E102.
The heavily labeled cells in the cortical laminae were first
located by examination in dark- and bright-field microscopy and
then their exact position within the cortex was plotted by the use
of a Zeiss microscope equipped with a drawing tube. The relative
position of labeled cells within the cortex and their distance from
the pia is marked by a short horizontal bar on the vertical line
that traverses the entire width of the cortex. On each vertical
line (except line N), short horizontal markers indicate positions
of all heavily labeled neurons encountered in one 2.5 mm long strip
of the cortex. Since the number of labeled neurons decreases
towards the end of neurogenesis, the three labeled neurons in area
17 indicated on the vertical line N (E102) were found only after
examination of 80 areas of calcarine cortex, each 2.5 mm wide, in
40 autoradiograms. Abbreviations: LV, obliterated posterior horn
of the lateral ventricle; WM, white matter; (modified from Rakic,
1974).

of pregnant monkeys with DNA precursor ^{3}H-thymidine (^{3}H-TdR) which permanently labels all cells in the last mitotic division (Rakic, 1974, 1976a). Later, we processed the occipital lobe of the offspring produced by these animals for light microscopic autoradiography, and recorded the position of radioactively labeled neurons. Figure 2 shows graphically that the final position of each neuron in the cortex correlates systematically with the time of its origin. Thus, neurons destined for positions in deeper cortical layers are generated earlier and those destined for more superficial layers are generated progressively later.

Comparison of data illustrated in Figure 1 with that of Figure 2 reveals that the first cells generated become mainly large pyramids of the deeper cortical layers which project to subcortical centers. Most cells generated at the middle stages of corticogenesis become local circuit neurons of the granular layer and finally, cells generated at late stages form the major portion of small superficial pyramids, most of which establish cortico-cortical connections. Although the pattern of inside-to-outside gradient of neuron origin had been suspected from histological studies performed by Ramon y Cajal (1911) and has been well documented by ^{3}H-thymidine autoradiography in rodents (reviewed in Caviness and Rakic, 1978; Sidman and Rakic, 1973), this neurogenetic gradient is exceptionally sharp and well defined only in primates (Rakic, 1974). Furthermore, using ^{3}H-TdR autoradiography in rhesus monkey fetuses sacrificed one hour following isotope injection, we found that none of the cortical neurons are generated within the cortical plate itself (Rakic, 1975). Obviously, all cortical neurons have to migrate a considerable distance from the site of their origin near the ventricular surface in order to attain their final positions within the developing cortex.

MODE OF MIGRATION OF POSTMITOTIC CELLS TO THE NEOCORTEX

Perhaps it is pertinent to emphasize that neuroanatomists at the turn of the century recognized that the neocortical plate is formed by cell migration from the germinal layer near the ventricular surface (Ramon y Cajal, 1911). However, although they observed that most mitotic figures are situated at the cerebral ventricular surface, the fraction of cells that eventually migrate and the mode of their movement was a complete mystery. Indeed, little was added to our understanding of cellular mechanisms of neuronal displacement until the advent of electronmicroscopy. Some twelve years ago, I began a series of ultrastructural studies on the cellular aspect of cell migration to the neocortex in rhesus monkey (Rakic, 1971, 1972). In retrospect, the choice of experimental subject was rather fortunate since a large and slowly developing primate brain allowed considerably better resolution of cellular events than the smaller, rapidly growing cortex of subprimate species.

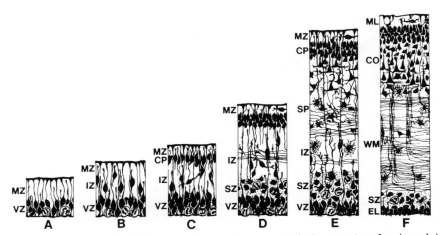

Figure 3. Schematic illustration of sequential events during histogenesis of the cerebral neocortex. This modified version of my
original drawing used by the Boulder Committee (1970) is updated to
include recent findings on gliogenesis, mode of neuronal migration an
formation of the transient subplate zone. Each picture encompasses
the full thickness of the developing cerebral wall so that the ventri
cular surface is at the bottom and the pial surface at the top. In
the cerebrum of every mammal so far examined, one can recognize a
series of transient developmental zones that are essentially without
direct counterpart in the mature brain. Picture A shows the stage at
which the cerebral wall consists only of the proliferative ventricula
(VZ) and acellular marginal (MZ) zones. An additional intermediate
zone (IZ) containing displaced postmitotic cells is present at the
next stage, as shown in B. At this stage, cells of neural lineage and
radial glial cells that stretch across the cerebral wall become dis-
tinguishable by immunohistochemical methods. In picture C, the
incipient cortical plate (CP) is formed by cells that have migrated
from the ventricular zone. In D, another proliferative layer - the
subventricular (SV) zone - is introduced external to the ventricular
zone and horizontally or obliquely disposed axons, originating mostly
from the thalamus, invade the intermediate zone. Picture E displays
the formation of the subplate zone (SP) which consists of horizontally deployed fibers, large and mostly multipolar neurons, as well as
radially oriented bipolar cells migrating externally to the differentiating pyramidal neurons of the deep cortical layers. Picture F
shows the final stage of neocortical development with the ventricular
zone transformed into the ependymal layer (EL) and remnants of proliferation present in the subventricular zone. The subplate zone
disappears while the intermediate and marginal zones become transformed into white matter (WM) and the molecular layer (ML) respective
ly. Further details and appropriate references are given in the text
(from Rakic and Goldman-Rakic, 1982).

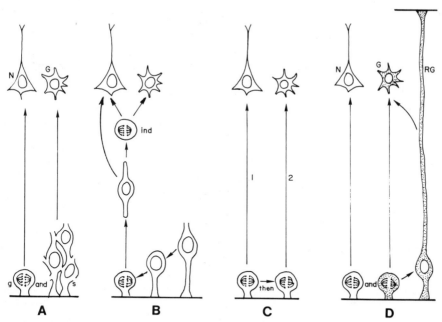

A   **B**   **C**   **D**

Figure 4.   Schematic illustration of previous theories of the origin
of neuronal and glial cell lines (A,B,C) and the current scheme (D).
A.   Almost a century ago, Wilhelm His distinguished two separate cell
lines in the germinal matrix (or ventricular zone) lining the embryonic ventricles: the round "germinal cells" (G) with mitotic nuclei
which lie close to the ventricular surface and give rise to neurons
(N), and the "spongioblasts" (S) whose nuclei lie at various distances from the ventricle. The "spongioblasts", that His thought
formed these two cell types, simply represented different mitotic
phases of a single cell class. B.   Since the first half of this century, it has been generally accepted that cells of the ventricular
zone produce indifferent cells (ind) that migrate into the intermediate (or mantle) zone where they divide further and/or transform
into either neurons or both neurons and glial cells. C.   The results
of ^{3}H-thymidine autoradiography developed in the late fifties led
several investigators to suggest that the dividing cells first give
rise to neurons (1) then, after neurogenesis has ceased, the same
dividing population begins to produce glial cells (2). D.   The localization of glial fibrillary acidic protein (GFA) by electronmicroscopic immunohistochemical technique (Levitt, Cooper and Rakic, 1981)
has demonstrated that both GFA-positive (stippled) and GFA-negative
mitotic cells coexist in the ventricular zone. The GFA-positive
cells initially produce radial glial cells (RG) and later, directly
or indirectly, produce protoplasmic and fibrillary astrocytes or
various specialized astrocyte-related cells (from Rakic, 1981b).

    At early developmental stages, even in the monkey telencephalon,
distances that postmitotic cells have to span are relatively small.
However, the size of primate brain increases considerably during mid-
gestation and consequently the length of migratory pathways must
also increase proportionally. I noticed that migratory neurons in
mouse, monkey and human are the same in both shape and size! As a
consequence, relationships between the cell size and migratory pathway
become most dramatic in the primate cerebral vesicle by the midgesta-
tional period when young bipolar neurons, only a few hundred microns
long, have to traverse a distance twenty to fifty times their total
length (Rakic, 1972). In order to understand the mechanism of this
remarkable cell translocation, it is essential to realize that at
early embryonic ages, the cerebral wall is composed of a sheet of
columnar, pseudostratified epithelial cells that, for the most part,
stretch from the ventricular to pial surface.

    The basic principles of how this apparently simple epithelial
tissue becomes transformed into a complex cerebral hemisphere with
its convoluted cortical mantle were worked out at the turn of the
century (Ramon y Cajal, 1911). However, numerous new details,
important concepts and ideas about cellular mechanisms were introduced during the last decade. As a result, the basic schema and
nomenclature proposed a dozen years ago by the Boulder Committee
(1970) has served its original purpose and needs to include new
findings and concepts introduced through the methods of modern cell
and developmental biology (Rakic and Goldman-Rakic, 1982). As
illustrated in Figure 3 an initially simple mammalian telencephalic
wall develops several well delineated cellular layers or zones.
The sole proliferative centers are the ventricular zone (VZ) and the
subventricular zone (SZ). These two embryonic zones were recognized
and designated by these terms by the Boulder Committee (1970). However, contrary to general understanding twelve years ago, the cellular composition of these proliferative zones is not homogeneous.
The first indication of the intermixing of neuronal and glial cells
comes from combined Golgi and electronmicroscopic analysis in embryonic monkey brain (Rakic, 1971, 1972). This was supported by a
detailed examination of the morphogenesis of radial glial cells in
Golgi preparations (Schmechel and Rakic, 1979b). However, more convincing confirmation came recently by the introduction of an immunohistochemical method using antibodies to glial specific protein
(GFA) as a marker (reviewed in Eng and D'Armond, 1981). Using perox-
idase-antiperoxidase, we demonstrated that both ventricular and
subventricular zones in the rhesus monkey contain at least two
populations of dividing cells, GFA-positive and GFA-negative
(Levitt, Cooper and Rakic, 1981). A diagram provided in Figure 4
summarizes, in a somewhat simplified manner, both the previous and
present theories of the origin of neuronal and glial cell lines in
the primate telencephalic wall. The main point relevant to this
presentation is that from the earliest stages, both glial and

neural cells and their mutual interactions have to be taken into
account in considering cortical development (Rakic, 1981b).

Studies conducted in the developing rhesus monkey in the past
decade (Rakic, 1971, 1972, 1978; Rakic et al., 1974) indicate that
the radial pathways of migrating cells are most probably established
by a guidance mechanism that depends on the cellular interaction
between membranes of the migrating neurons and adjacent radial glial
cells. These transient populations of cells have elongated fibers
that stretch radially across the full thickness of developing telencephalic wall and relatively early they show cytological and biochemical properties of glial cells (Rakic, 1972; Schmechel and Rakic,
1979b; Levitt and Rakic, 1980). Furthermore, immunohistochemical
study at ultrastructural level (Levitt, Cooper and Rakic, 1981) shows
that glial cells are established early as a separate line in the proliferative zones (Figure 4). The radial glial cells which appear to
play a role as scaffolding of the developing cerebral wall, do not
divide for about two months in midgestation (Schmechel and Rakic,
1979a). Eventually they re-enter the cell division cycle and transform into astrocytes. Based on Golgi and electronmicroscopic evidence it appears that the elongated radial fibers of glial cells may
serve as guides along which the young neurons migrate externally
toward and into the developing cortical plate (Rakic, 1971, 1972).
The point of particular interest is that the young neurons migrating
to the monkey neocortex appear to be relatively simple bipolar cells
with a leading process of a length that is usually only a fraction
of the total migration pathway. I have proposed that they find
their way to distant cortex using radially oriented glial fibers as
guides (Figure 5). Such structurally defined guidelines may be essential in the primate telencephalon because the terrain that a post-
mitotic neuron must penetrate consists of a mixture of cellular
elements that include neuronal and glial cells and varieties of
their cytoplasmic processes, as well as blood vessels of various
sizes and orientations. Throughout the course of its migration,
the plasma membrane of a young neuron and its elongated radial guide
remain in contact, suggesting the existence of some kind of recognition and affinity between the surface components of the two cell
types, or between cells and intercellular coating and/or binding
matrix substance. This contact may provide a basis for selective
affinities between these two cell types which may be responsible for
directed cell movement.

POSSIBLE MECHANISM OF CELL DISPLACEMENT

How can one reconcile the apparent contradiction that migrating
neurons and radial glial fibers display a strong affinity for each
other and at the same time permit the movement of the first along
the latter? One of several possibilities that could account for
this phenomenon is that the membranes of two cells become fixed at
any one point along their interface (Rakic, 1981b). According to

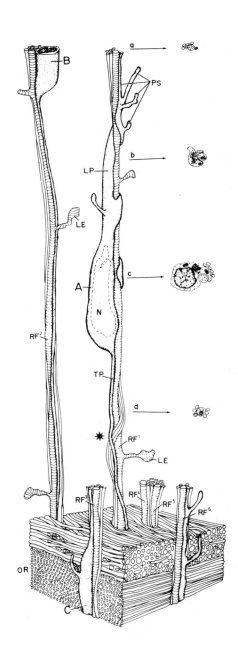

this model, the migrating cell could, nevertheless, move by adding new membrane components to its growing tip and the leading process would progressively extend along the radial glial fiber while the nucleus is subsequently transferred to a new position within the perikaryal cytoplasm (Figure 6B and C). The rate of movement of migrating neurons in the primate telencephalon, which varies between 0.5 and 4.0 μm per hour, is compatible with a capacity for generation and insertion of new membrane along the leading process. Several observations give credence to such a mechanism including the finding of a continuous increase in the surface area of migrating cells as they approach the cortex (Rakic et al., 1974) and the predominant growth of cytoplasmic expansions at their leading tips (Bray, 1973). Since glial and neuronal cell surfaces may contain binding of complementary molecules that attract each other, this model can be tested and one can anticipate the production of an antiserum that could label binding sites or whose application in vivo could interfere with neuronal migration. The two cell classes can be held together by a cell adhesion molecule equal or similar to one described in embryonic chick, mouse and human (McClain and Edelman, 1982). Such a molecule would normally promote cell-to-cell binding and a failure in local surface modulation may result in migratory defects.

⬅

Figure 5. Three-dimensional reconstruction of migrating neurons, based on electron micrographs of semi-serial sections. The reconstruction was made at the level of the intermediate zone. The subventricular zone lies some distance below the reconstructed area, whereas the cortex is more than 1000 μm above it. The lower portion of the diagram contains uniform, paralled fibers of the optic radiation (OR) and the remainder is occupied by more variable and irregularly disposed fiber systems; the border between the two systems is easily recognized. Except at the lower portion of the figure, most of these fibers are deleted from the diagram to expose the radial fibers (striped vertical shafts RF_{1-6}) and their relationships to the migrating cells A, B and C and to other vertical processes. The soma of migrating cell A, with its nucleus (N) and voluminous leading process (LP) is situated within the reconstructed space, except for the terminal part of the attenuated trailing process and the tip of the vertical ascending pseudopodium. Cross-sections of cell A in relation to the several vertical fibers in the fascicle are drawn at levels a-d at the right side of the figure. The perikaryon of cell B is cut off at the top of the reconstructed space, whereas the leading process of cell C is shown just penetrating between fibers of the the optic radiation (OR) on its way across the intermediate zone. Abbreviations: LE, lamellate expansions; PS, pseudopodia (from Rakic, 1972).

A neuron ultimately acquires its permanent position in relation to other cells within the cortical plate itself; however, this final step may be the end product of migratory events, but it can be independent of the preceding process of cell migration (Rakic, 1975; Caviness and Rakic, 1978). At present, we cannot exclude a possibility that the correct position attained by a migrating young neuron may be determined by the interaction of incoming cells and the local milieu that consists of previously generated cells. The examination of the telencephalic wall demonstrates that a group of neurons, originating from the same site in the ventricular zone can migrate along a single radial guide, eventually forming an ontogenetic radial column within the developing cortex (Rakic, 1981a). Under normal conditions each neuron soma within a given ontogenetic column takes a position distal (external) to its predecessor and as a result, cells of each cortical layer originate from inside-outward at a progressively later time (Figures 2 and 3). In a neurological mutant mouse (reeler), cortical cells which appear to migrate normally towards the cortical plate seem to be unable to bypass previously generated cells (Caviness and Rakic, 1978). It has been suggested that faulty interaction between radial glia and migration neurons at the termination of their journey may be the cause of cell malposition (Pinto-Lord et al., 1982; Caviness and Rakic, 1978). On the other hand, it is possible that the leading tip of a migrating cell fails to produce a sufficient amount of proteolytic agents such as plasminogen activator serine proteoses (Moonen et al., 1982) which may be essential for breaking the bond between migrating neurons and glial cells.

ROLE OF GLIAL GRIDS AND ONTOGENETIC RADIAL COLUMNS IN PARCELATION OF CORTICAL AREAS

The pattern of radial glial cell distribution described above may have another implication for the establishment of neocortical organization. In the cerebrum of all mammalian species, but especially in primates, the mature cortical surface is parcelled into cytoarchitectonic areas that are each characterized by explicit cellular constellations, distinctive inputs and outputs, intricate local circuits and specific functional correlates (e.g., Rakic and Goldman-Rakic, 1982). These cytoarchitectonic areas lie in a topographic relation to one another that is consistent from individual to individual and is, to some extent, also preserved across species. Since the migration of each postmitotic cell from the ventricular or subventricular zones to the cortical plate is constrained to the given radial vector by the glial guide, it follows that the proliferative zones that produce those neurons at and near the ventricular surface of the developing cerebrum must also be parcelled as a two-dimensional mosaic structure that consists of ontogenetic radial columns (Rakic, 1978, 1981a).

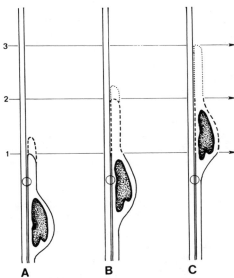

Figure 6. Diagram showing a possible mechanism for the displacement
of migratory cells along the surface of radial glial fibers (vertical
shafts A-C). To traverse the distance between levels 1 and 2, new
plasma membrane may be inserted along the interface of the two cells
(dashed line in A), while the cell nucleus becomes translocated within the cytoplasm of the leading process (B). As the leading tip grows
to reach level 3, additional new membrane is inserted (dotted line in
C) along the interface with the glial surface and the nucleus moves
to a higher position between level 1 and 2, resulting in an overall
displacement of the cell body. This model does not require actual
translocation of the neuronal surface along the surface of glial
fibers, and allows the binding sites (circles) between the two
opposing membranes to remain constant for some time (from Rakic,
1981b).

        The aggregates of neurons aligned along one radial glial fasci-
cle in the developing cortical plate has been referred to as a
"minicolumn" by Mountcastle (1979) and an "ontogenetic column" by
Edelman (1979). Our best approximation is that in fetal monkey
telencephalon, the number of proliferative units in the ventricular zone about equals the number of ontogenetic columns in the
cortical plate (Fig. 7). Thus, each proliferative unit may have a
corresponding ontogenetic radial column. Obviously, ontogenetic
columns widen considerably in the course of subsequent development as individual neurons grow, differentiate, and acquire synaptic connections from local and extrinsic sources. However, we do

not know at present whether any relationship exists between these developmentally defined transient ontogenetic radial columns and the disjunctive terminal fields of afferent fibers systems (e.g., ocular dominance stripes) of the adult cortex. We can only say that the ontogenetic column represents a consequence of the sequential migration of many generations of neurons, all of which have arrived along the same radial glial fascicle from a single proliferative unit. Further, since each proliferative unit may possibly have a matching ontogenetic radial column in the cortical plate (Figure 7), and since the two are connected with elongated glial cords, the relationship between the ventricular zone and expanding cortex remains preserved in spite of considerable morphogenetic changes in the cerebral surface.

Our working hypothesis has been that the existence of glial grids may serve to assure reproduction of the mosaicisms of the proliferative zones on the expanding and curving cortical mantle. Most recently, we found that a similar relationship exists in the early hippocampal region (Nowakowski and Rakic, 1979) including the dentate plate (Eckenhoff and Rakic, 1983). Based on the presently available information it appears that the three-dimensional spatiotemporal gradients in the adult cortical mantle reflect the spatial and temporal organization of the essentially two-dimensional proliferative zones. However, the glial grid concept may explain only how cells acquire proper position; it does not give a clue as to what initiates and governs their differentiation. Each topographic territory acquires its final cytological and synaptic organization by a combination of intrinsic genetic properties of the constituent neurons and uniqueness of axonal inputs from the subcortical structures during the migration or after cell arrival at the cortex (see below). Thus, the final characteristics of cytoarchitectonic fields depends on many factors, but the existence of glial guides and compartmentalization of the telencephalic wall seems to minimize the amount of information needed for initial construction of the neocortex (Rakic, 1978; 1981a).

FORMATION OF AFFERENT CORTICAL CONNECTIONS

Contrary to general understanding and our predictions of one decade ago (e.g., Sidman and Rakic, 1973), specific thalamic afferents enter the developing cortex only after their principle target cells in layer IV complete their migrations and attain appropriate positions within the developing cortical plate (Rakic, 1976b, 1977). This sequence holds true for the primate visual cortex, and most likely applies for the other neocortical areas as well. This sequence of developmental events was revealed only after the advent of two types of autoradiographic methods: one that enables tagging DNA of migrating cells (described earlier) and the other that permits the use of the transneuronal transport method for tracing long fiber tracts. In addition, refinement of prenatal surgery in the mid-seventies enabled us to remove fetal monkeys from the uterus, inject an eye or part of the brain with radioactive tracers and/or extirpate these structures and replace the fetus back in the uterus (Rakic, 1976b; Goldman and Galkin, 1978). In the particular set of experiments that focuses on the visual cortex, monkey fetuses were sacrificed two weeks after unilateral eye injection of radioactive tracers (mixture of ^{3}H-proline and ^{3}H-fucose) and subsequently processed for light microscopic autoradiography. The two week interval that passed between the injection and sacrifice of the fetus was carefully chosen to allow sufficient time for the label to be transported transneuronally and to fill geniculo-cortical axons entering developing cerebral vesicles.

As illustrated semidiagrammatically in Figure 8, the autoradiographic analysis indicated that geniculo-cortical axons enter the occipital lobe at relatively early stages. However, these fibers do not invade the developing cortical plate itself until the beginning of the second half of gestation (Rakic, 1976b, 1977). The autoradiograms clearly display that in the monkey fetus, axons originating in the lateral geniculate (LGd) grow selectively towards prospective area 17, stopping rather abruptly at the border to area 18. In the region subjacent to prospective area 17, they accumulate in the subplate zone (Figure 3). In this zone, the fibers may "wait" for several weeks before they grow to the cortex. Following invasion of the cortex, around mid-gestation (E91 specimen), geniculate axons carrying input from each eye first become distributed uniformly over the entire territory of layer IV (Rakic, 1976b, 1977). Three weeks before birth (E144), afferents begin to segregate vertically into sublayers IVA, and IVC alpha and beta that receive separate input from parvo and magnocellular layers of the LGd (compare Figures 1 and 8). Furthermore, geniculate fibers also begin to sort out horizontally into alternating high and low grain density area indicating emergence of ocular dominance columns (Rakic, 1976b). These columns, initially 250-300 μm wide, subsequently expand and by the second postnatal month reach the normal adult width of 350-400 μm (Hubel et al., 1977).

Although there must be some spillover of radioactivity from retinal axons into extracellular space within the LGd, small leakage does not alter the interpretation of our autoradiographic data in either the thalamic or cortical level. The strongest evidence that geniculo-cortical fibers subserving the left and right eye are intermixed transiently during fetal development comes from the comparison of our experiments with short and long term survival following monocular eye injection at the mid-gestational period. Thus, in a fetus injected at E78 and sacrificed one day later (E79) the entire LGd is uniformly labeled regardless of whether the injection is given to the left or the right eye. However, in another fetus whose eye was injected with the same isotope at about the same time (E77) but was sacrificed fourteen days later (E91), the distribution of radioacti-

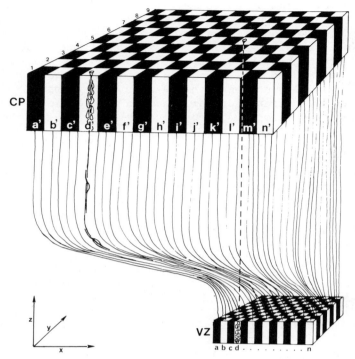

Figure 7. Diagramatic three-dimensional representation of the relationship between the proliferative layer situated around the ventricular surface (VZ, ventricular zone) and the developing cortical
plate (CP) situated at the pial surface of the cerebral wall. Although the cerebral surface in primates expands enormously during
prenatal development, producing a considerable shift between these
two cellular sheets, each point in the cortex remains attached to
the corresponding point in the proliferative zone by the elongated
shafts of radial glial cells (Rakic, 1972, 1978). Since all neurons
produced at a given site in the ventricular zone migrate in succession along the same radial glial guides, they all end up in the single
ontogenetic column (Rakic, 1981a). These columns remain in a consistent sequence because proliferative units a through n in the
ventricular zone are fruitfully reproduced as ontogenetic columns a'
to n' in the cortical plate. On their way, migrating cells bypass
deep, earlier generated neurons of the cortex and assume the most
superficial position. The glial guidance prevents the possibility of
mismatching, e.g., between proliferative unit d and cortical mode

vity shows territories of higher and lower grain densities. If the
diffuse labeling of the LGd in the first case is a result of a
spill-over of radioactivity from one layer to the next, the pattern
of label in the LGd would not change in the intervening fourteen
days, and would remain diffuse at the time of sacrifice. Based on
these findings, we concluded that the uniform label at the early
stages is not an artifact, but rather a result of genuine intermixing of fibers originating from the two eyes.

The interpretation of the autoradiograms of the developing cortex is somewhat more complex, and less direct than for the LGd.
Short survival experiments are not useful for analyzing cortical
afferents since more than one week is required for sufficient transneuronal transport. Here, the specimen injected at E120 and sacrificed at E134 provides the best evidence. At this stage, pathways
subserving the left and right eye are segregated in the LGd, but
remain intermixed in the cortex (Rakic, 1976b). In addition, quantitative and electrophysiological analyses performed on developing
kittens also supports the notion that the intermixing of geniculate
fiber terminals at the cortical level is biologically a real
phenomenon (LeVay et al., 1978). Finally, since the boundary between
radioactive territories and non-radioactive territories is rather
sharp in the vertical direction, and the tangential direction at
later stages of development, the spillover of radioactivity at the
cortical level must be negligible. In conclusion, although detailed
quantitative analysis of grain counts has not been done in the developing monkey cortex, all available data support our previous state-
ment that development of the geniculo-cortical connections in
primates proceeds through two broad phases (Rakic, 1976b, 1983). In
the first phase, LGd axons subserving input from each eye invade the
cortical plate but their endings are distributed over the entire
layer IV in an unmixed manner. In the second phase, terminals subserving the left and right eye sort out horizontally into ocular

J'5, which would occur if the migrating neurons were to take a
direct, straight path, illustrated by the dotted line. As a result
of this developmental mechanism, it appears that the tangential
coordinates (X and Y) of each cortical neuron may be determined by
the relative positon of its precursor cell in the proliferative zones
while the radial (Z) position within the cortex is determined by the
time of its genesis and rate of its migration. Thus, the specification of topography and/or modality (shown as checkered) may be
determined by spatial parameters, while the heirarchical organization of neurons within each radial columnar unit is determined by
temporal factors (from Rakic and Goldman-Rakic, 1982).

dominance stripes while the axons originating from magno- and parvo-cellular layers of the LGd segregate vertically.

The development of extrageniculate projections to the occipital lobe was not pursued with similar vigor due to the lack of suitable anatomical methods. Recently, we took advantage of the transient presence of cholinesterase (ChE) reactivity in developing pulvinar neurons to reveal the development of prestriate visual projections (Kostovic and Rakic, 1983). This type of histochemical study of cortical afferents is possible only because various subdivisions of the developing primate thalamus have different susceptibility and/or different schedules of emergence and disappearance of ChE activity when cortical neurons still stain negatively. Thus, pulvinar neurons and their projections stain positively at the fetal ages when most of the neighboring thalamic nuclei (e.g., LGd) that project to the adjacent cortex are stain-free. Examination of the ChE histochemical material shows that development of pulvinar projections in the monkey occipital lobe basically follow the same developmental sequences and rules that were described for the genesis of the geniculo-cortical axonal system (Rakic, 1976b, 1983). In the first phase that occurs within the first half of gestation (between E50 and E80), pulvinar fibers enter the intermediate zone of the occipital lobe but do not invade the developing cortical plate which still lacks a majority of its neurons. In the next phase, between E80 and E100, pulvinar fibers accumulate within the subplate zone, but their concentration is particularly high in the sectors directly below the prospective prestriate cortex of the occipito-temporo-parietal confluence. As in the case of geniculo-cortical fibers described above, the subplate zone may be considered as a "waiting compartment" of afferent axons (Rakic, 1976b, 1977) where thalamic fibers are stored until all or most of their target neurons are generated and have reached their positions within the cortex. In the final phase which occurs between E100 and E125, pulvinar fibers enter the developing cortical plate at the prestriate areas. There is a clear laminar distribution of pulvinar fibers at the developmental stages when they can be stained with the ChE method; however, one cannot see a horizontal periodicity in the form of alternating stripes that are characteristic of this afferent system in adult monkeys (Ogren and Hendrickson, 1977). Therefore, one can presume that the segregation of pulvinar stripes in the prestriate area may occur at later stages, but in a manner similar to the segregation of ocular dominance stripes in the striate areas (Rakic, 1976b; Hubel et al., 1977). However, the processes of sorting out of the pulvinar input cannot be revealed by the present method since it occurs at later stages when the transient ChE reactivity of the pulvinar axons become extinct.

The precise and clearly targeted development of projections observed in both striate (Rakic, 1976b, 1983) and prestriate (Kostovic and Rakic, 1983) afferents suggests the possibility that these axonal tracts recognize their target areas before any visible sign of cytoarchitectonic differentiation within the cortical plate. However, one can argue that pulvinar axons grow to the "appropriate" cortical area because the adjacent cortex is populated by the fibers that have arrived earlier or simultaneously from the adjacent thalamic LGd nucleus. One can speculate even further that the border between striate and prestriate areas may be created by the competition between geniculate and pulvinar projections for the cortical neurons and that this competition indirectly determines the boundaries of cytoarchitectonic parcelation. This hypothesis seems to be compli-cated by the finding that a small contingent of pulvinar axons does enter the striate area, although these appear to seek different synaptic targets that are situated mostly in layers I and II, rather than in deeper layers, particularly III, IV and VI which are prefer-entially innervated in the prestriate area (Kostovic and Rakic, 1983). Likewise, a small number of LGd fibers that invade pre-striate areas terminate mostly in layer V and avoid layer I, III and VI which are the targets of pulvinar axons in this cytoarchitectonic field. This differential distribution of thalamic fibers between the striate and prestriate cortex occurs before main cytoarchitectonic differences of the occipital lobe become visible in the Nissl stained sections. At present, we cannot distinguish between effects of axonal competition, and the possibility that the cortical plate may contain a heterogenous population of neurons that, although morpho-logically similar, already possess surface properties that are recognizable by the ingrowing fiber tracts.

FORMATION OF EFFERENT CONNECTIONS

The use of prenatal neurosurgery allows us also to inject radio-active tracers or fluorescent dyes into the visual cortex of fetal monkeys and thereby determine timing and mode of emergence of efferent cortical connections to the other cortical areas and/or subcortical centers. In the first series of such studies (Shatz and Rakic, 1981), monkey fetuses were temporarily exteriorized from the uterus and injected with ^{3}H-proline into the posterior pole of the devel-oping occipital lobe. Each fetus was returned to the uterus, sacri-ficed 24 hours later, and its brain processed for light microscopic autoradiography.

The label was first detected in the prospective magnocellular layers of the LGd in the E70 specimen. A considerable amount of radio-activity was also present in the nearby cell-poor zones suggesting the existence of a waiting compartment. At these young fetal ages, topographic order in the cortico-geniculate projection could not be determined due to the large size of the injection sites relative to the small cerebral vesicles. However, by E84, the portion of the prospective parvocellular layers contained label which was charac-teristically wedge-shaped and appropriately located with respect to the site of the cortical injection, suggesting that topographic order

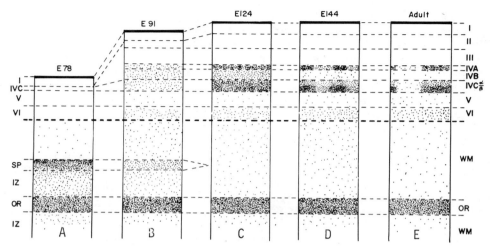

Figure 8. Semidiagrammatic summary of the development of geniculo-
cortical connections and ocular dominance stripes in the visual
cortex of the occipital lobe of the rhesus monkey from the end of the
first half or pregnancy to adulthood. Stripes A through E illustrate
a portion of the lateral cerebral wall in the region of area 17, as
seen in autoradiograms of animals having received unilateral eye
injection of a mixture of ^{3}H-proline and ^{3}H-fucose 14 days earlier.
The age of animals at the moment of sacrifice is provided at the top
of each column in embryonic (E) and postnatal (P) days. Note that at
E78, the cortical plate consists of only layers V, VI and a small
portion of IVC (see Rakic, 1974). Abbreviations: IZ, intermediate
zone; OR, optic radiation; SP, deep portion of subplate layer; WM,
white matter (from Rakic, 1981a).

may be already established at this age. About ten days later (E95),
label in the LGd assumed a configuration similar to that of the adult.

     The projection from the visual cortex also invades the superior
colliculus and pulvinar around E70. In the superior colliculus,
label is initially confined to the stratum opticum, but by E84, it
extended into the superficial gray matter. At the time cortical
efferents invade the superior colliculus, the many retinal axons
are already in their places and have established their synaptic
junctions (Cooper and Rakic, 1983). Thus, unlike the synchronous

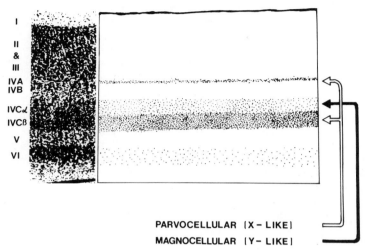

Figure 9. Semidiagrammatic illustration of the distribution of
geniculo-cortical terminals in the visual cortex of a two-month-old
monkey in which one eye was enucleated during the first third of
gestation and the remaining eye injected with radioactive tracers two
weeks before sacrifice (for details see Rakic, 1981c). The distribution of grains is aligned with photograph of cresyl-violet stained
visual cortex to show relative positons of horizontal uniform sheets
of projections without any sign of ocular dominance columns. Note,
however, that vertical segregation of input from the magnocellular
and parvocellular moieties of the LGd into sublayers IVA, IVC alpha
and IVC beta is clearly indicated (from Rakic, 1983).

development of reciprocal thalamo-cortical relations, cortico-
collicular projections appear to follow retino-collicular projections
by a lag of several weeks and thus, cortical axons enter an already
topographically ordered tectum.

     From the above studies, we established that all known classes of
efferent pathways from the visual cortex to subcortical structures in
the rhesus monkey are already present by the middle of the 165 day
gestational period. It may be significant that the development of
the efferent cortico-geniculate pathway proceeds along a remarkably
similar schedule to that of the afferent pathway from the LGd to the
primary visual cortex (Rakic, 1976a, 1977). As described above, by

E78, geniculocortical afferents are gathered within the white matter just below the cortical plate, but it is not until E91 that they are seen clearly within cortical layers IV-VI. Similarly, a substantial cortical projection throughout the LGd is not found until E96; cortico-geniculate efferents have arrived and accumulated in the vicinity of the LGd by E70. Thus, despite large differences in the time of origin of the neurons participating in these connections (Rakic, 1974, 1977), the reciprocal pathways between LGd and visual cortex appear to be established roughly in synchrony during the mid-gestational period.

Another finding from the studies of subcortical-cortical efferents that may be biologically significant is topographical order among corticogeniculate projections in the E84 specimen. Thus, this order is present before the LGd becomes laminated and more importantly, before fibers from the left and right eye segregate in this species (Rakic, 1976b). Therefore, it appears that neither lamination nor segregation is required for establishment of topographical order in cortico-geniculate projections (Shatz and Rakic, 1981). Recently, I obtained evidence for this from examination of animals in which pre-natal binocular enucleation was performed in the first half of gestation, and the animals sacrificed after birth. The LGd was considerably smaller and without layers, but the topography of the cortical projections was preserved.

The development of a given cortical cytoarchitectonic area cannot be understood without taking into account establishment of its connections with other cortical fields. Thus, it may seem paradoxical that in spite of much interest in the visual cortex, we do not have basic information on timing, sequences and developmental mechanisms involved in the genesis of its cortico-cortical connectivity. Although there are some thought provoking studies of the excessive collateralization of long distance ipsilateral and contralateral cortical visual connections in cat (Innocenti, 1981), similar data for primates are still lacking. The method of double labeling of cortical neurons with fluorescent dyes has recently been used successfully to analyze development of other cortical fields in fetal monkeys (Schwartz and Goldman-Rakic,1982). This approach, when applied to animals with prenatally sustained cortical ablations, promises to provide new insight into this important aspect of cortical development. For example, we need to know how axons, originating from the second and third layer pyramids find their proper target areas in ipsi- and contralateral cortex, and whether they, by virtue of their presence and quantity, determine relative size of the cytoarchitectonic cortical fields. One can speculate that their distribution across cerebral cortex depends on the competition between inputs from other cortico-cortical axons as well as from the thalamo-cortical projections. Although the prospect of unraveling such a complex interplay between various inputs seems formidable, the methods of analysis are available and, as discussed below, the answers may be within our reach.

REMODELING OF CORTICAL CONNECTIONS BY PRENATAL SURGICAL LESIONS

The new information on development of cortical connections that
is described above raises several questions about mechanisms underlying formation of territorial distribution of axonal terminals
within the cortex. The most obvious one is whether competition
between two sets of thalamic inputs plays a role in formation of
segregated terminal fields in the cortex. The visual system provides a relatively simple way to study this issue. For example, by
removing one eye at a critical developmental period and then allowing
the operated fetus to be delivered a few months later and examine
its connections autoradiographically, one can study the distribution
of geniculo-cortical input in the absence of competition from the
contralateral eye. Similarly, binocular enucleation performed at
early stages (around E60) results in dramatic diminution of the LGd
and thus reduction in geniculo-cortical input (Rakic, unpublilshed
observation). Would an attenuation of thalamic input result in
changes in parcelation of the occipital lobe?

In a series of experiments in which one eye was unilaterally
enucleated at fetal ages, we found that the distribution of LGd terminals in the primary visual cortex is permanently abnormal (Rakic,
1981c). This was demonstrated by examining the pattern of transneuronally transported radioactive tracers injected into the remaining
eye of the mature monkeys in which the other eye was enucleated
around E60. In such cases, ocular dominance stripes fail to develop
and the LGd axon terminals form two continuous, uniform, and uninter-
rupted horizontal sheets located within layers IVA and IVC (Figure
9). Since, as described in the proceeding section, LGd projections
subserving two eyes initially overlap, these results can be explained, at least in part, by a failure of terminals subserving the
remaining eye to retract from the territory that normally becomes
occupied exclusively by terminals subserving the other (enucleated)
eye. Although the results of these experiments clearly demonstrate
that cortical neurons which normally receive input from the left eye,
now receive input from the right eye, at present, we cannot determine
which LGd neurons issue these projections. For example, it is equally possible that the observed abnormal connectivity is established by
the "right-coded" LGd neurons that project to "left-coded" cortical
neurons, as well as that all "left-coded" LGd neurons remain hooked
to "left-coded" cortical neurons. In the latter case, rearrange-
ment would occur mainly in the LGd, while thalamo-cortical connections remain basically uneffected.

In the monocularly enucleated monkey, the vertical segregation
of the thalamic input into cortical sublayers IVA, IVCA and IVCB proceeds in spite of the absence of visible horizontal segregation into

ocular dominance stripes and transient projection to layers IVB is
eliminated as in the normal monkey (Rakic, 1981c). Since the sublayers IVA and IVC beta in the visual cortex receive input from the
parvocellular moiety of the LGd, while IVCA receives input from magnocellular moieties of the LGd (Hubel and Wiesel, 1977), it seems
reasonable to assume that segregation of X and Y-like systems in the
cortex may have proceeded uneffected by unilateral eye enucleation
(Rakic, 1983).

     Enucleation of both eyes at prenatal ages produces even more
dramatic results. In such cases, as a rule, LGd is much smaller in
size, does not have cellular laminae and therefore, issues only a
fraction of projections to the cortex. For example, in two monkeys
enucleated at E62 and E90 respectively, and examined after birth,
LGd contains less than one quarter of its normal number of neurons
(Rakic, preliminary unpublished observation). Nevertheless, these
axons project to the area 17 and apparently become distributed in
proper layers since the border to area 18 in these cases is sharp
and clear. Implantation of HRP pellets in the occipital lobe of
the monkey enucleated bilaterally at mid-gestation demonstrate that
both the geniculo-cortical input, revealed by the retrograde transport, as well as the cortico-geniculate output, revealed by anterograde transport, are topographically organized. Although the
results of these experiments need to be evaluated quantitatively,
the preliminary observations illustrate the potential for this experimental approach for analysis of cortical development in primates.

CONCLUSIONS

     Available data show that ontogeny of primate neocortex proceeds
through a sequence of well delineated developmental events that
include: region-specific proliferation kinetics, early segregation
of neuronal and glial cell lines, differential rate of neuronal
migration, and orderly formation of afferent, efferent and local
synaptic connections that ultimately result in a specific wiring network. We learned that although major cell classes such as neurons
and glia may be determined relatively early in development, final
position of an individual neuron, its phenotopic expression and
thereby, its specific synaptic connectivity, may depend on extracellular signals that a given cell receives by interacting with nearby cells or with distant cells directly via axonal connections or
indirectly via diffusible substances. Although in recent years an
enormous amount of information has been accumulated on the differentiation of individual nerve cells, formation of their organelles and
synaptic contacts, we are still quite ignorant when we try to understand the meaning of these events in terms of building a complexly
organized neuronal structure such as primate neocortex. There are
many properties of the developing brain that have been overlooked,
especially now when so much can be learned by breaking the tissue
apart and by examining individual neurons or even only its small

components. As neurophysiologists often failed to consider the difficulty of extrapolating the function of a single neuron to the
behavior of a complex neuronal network (Marr and Nishihara, 1978),
some developmental neurobiologists also failed to take into account
that a complex system cannot be understood as a simple extrapolation
of properties of elementary components. Since cell-to-cell interactions are obviously essential for shaping the final structure of
any organ in multicellular organisms, they must be even more crucial
for the development of the primate neocortex, perhaps the most
complex structure in the universe. Here, one should recall a witty
aphorism by Paul Weiss (1971) who paraphrased John Donne's poem in
the title of his paper "A cell is not an island entire of itself".
This aphorism emphasizes that in order to understand brain development, structure and function, especially that of the cerebral
cortex, one has to take into account the interactions among the
entire community of interconnected nerve cells. As shown long ago
in the field of biochemistry, one enzyme produced by a single gene
can change the composition of other proteins produced by different
genes in somas or different cell classes. It can be expected that
one brain cell can induce expression of specific phenotype in other
receptive cells. Using presently available methods, developmental
neurobiologists will be able in the near future to unravel causal
sequences and roles of cell-to-cell interactions that determine
phenotypic expresson of nerve cells and thus indirectly, wiring
arrangements of the neocortex. The presently available evidence,
although still rather crude, nevertheless reveals that epigenetic
sequences rather than rigid intracellular programs, play a major
role in determining fine details of synaptic organization of the
neo-cortex. Disruption, or even delay of one step can cause a
chain reaction that leads to an abnormal organization of the cortex, and ultimately to abnormal function.

REFERENCES

Boulder Committee, 1970, Embryonic vertebrate cental nervous system.
        Revised terminology. Anat. Rec., 166:257-261.
Bray, D., 1973, Branching patterns of individual sympathetic neurons
        in culture, J. Cell Biol., 56:702-712.
Caviness, V.S., Jr. and Rakic, P., 1978, Mechanisms of cortical
        development: a view from mutations in mice, Ann. Rev.
        Neurosci., 1:297-326.
Cooper, M.L. and Rakic, P., 1983, Gradients of cellular maturation
        and synaptogenesis in the superior colliculus of the fetal
        rhesus monkey, J. Comp. Neurol, in press.
Eckenhoff, M. and Rakic, P., 1983, Radial organization of the dentate
        gyrus: A Golgi, ultrastructural and immunohistochemical analysis
        in the developing rhesus monkey, J. Comp. Neurol., submitted.

Edelman, G.M., 1979, Group selection and phasic reentrant signaling:
    A theory of higher brain function. In: F.O. Schmitt and E.G.
    Worden (eds): The Neurosciences: Fourth Study Program. MIT
    Press, Cambridge, pp. 1115-1144.
Eng, L.F. and DeArmond, S.J., 1981, Immunocytochemical studies of
    astrocytes in normal development and disease. In: S. Fedoroff
    and L. Hertz (eds.): Advances in Cellular Neurobiology. Vol. 3.
    Academic Press.
Gibert, C.D. and Wiesel, T.N., 1981, Laminar specialization and intra-
    cortical connections in cat primary visual cortex. In: F.O.
    Schmitt (ed-in-chief): The Organization of the Cerebral Cortex.
    MIT Press, 163-191.
Goldman, P.S. and Galkin, T.W., 1978, Prenatal removal of frontal
    association cortex in the rhesus monkey: anatomical and
    functional consequences in postnatal life, Brain Res.,
    52:451-485.
Hubel, D.H. and Wiesel, T.N., 1977, Functional architecture of
    macaque monkey visual cortex, Proc. R. Soc. Lond. B., 198:1-59.
Hubel, D.H., Wiesel, T.N. and LaVay, S., 1977, Plasticity of ocular
    dominance columns in monkey striate cortex, Phil. Trans. Roy.
    Soc. Lond. B., 278:377-409.
Innocenti, G.M., 1981, Growth and reshaping of axons in the establish-
    ment of visual callosal connections, Science, 212:824-827.
Kostovic, I. and Rakic, P., 1980, Cytology and time of origin of
    interstitial neurons in the white matter in infant and adult
    human and monkey, J. Neurocytol., 9:219-242.
Kostovic, I. and Rakic, P., 1983, Development of prestriate visual
    projections in the monkey and human fetal cerebrum revealed by
    transient cholinesterase activity, J. Neurosci., submitted.
LeVay, S., Stryker, M.P. and Shatz, C.J., 1978, Ocular dominance
    columns and their development in layer IV of the cat's visual
    cortex: A quantitative study, J. Comp. Neurol., 179:223-244.
Levitt, P., M.L. Cooper and Rakic, P., 1981, Coexistence of neuronal
    and glial precursor cells in the cerebral ventricular zone of
    the fetal monkey: An ultrastructural immunoperoxidase analysis,
    J. Neurosci., 1:27-39.
Levitt, P.R. and Rakic, P., 1980, Immunoperoxidase localization of
    glial fibrilary acid protein in radial glial cells and atrocytes
    of the developing rhesus monkey brain, J. Comp. Neuro.,
    193:515-540.
Lund, J.S., 1981, Intrinsic organization of the primary visual
    cortex, area 17, as seen in Golgi preparation. In: F.O. Schmitt
    (ed-in-chief): The Organization of the Cerebral Cortex. MIT
    Press, 106-124.
Marr, D. and Nishihara, H.K., 1978, Visual information processing:
    Artificial intelligence and sensorium of sight. Technol. Rev.,
    81:1-7.
McClain, D.A. and Edelman, G.M., 1982, A neural cell adhesion mole-
    cule from human brain, Proc. Natl. Acad. Sci. USA, 79:6380-6384.

Moonen, G., Grau-Wagemans, M.P. and Selak, I., 1982, Plasminogen
    activator - plasmin system and neuronal migration, Nature,
    298:753-755.
Mountcastle, V.B., 1979, An organizing principle for cerebral
    function: The unit module and the distributed system. In: F.O.
    Schmitt and F.G. Worden (eds): The Neurosciences: Fourth Study
    Program. MIT Press, Cambridge, pp. 21-42.
Nowakowski, R.S. and Rakic, P., 1979, The mode of migration of neu-
    rons in hippocampal region of the rhesus monkey, J. Neurocytol.,
    8:697-718.
Ogren, M.P. and Hendrickson, A.E., 1977, The distribution of pulvinar
    terminals in visual areas 17 and 18 of the monkey, Brain Res.,
    137:334-350.
Peters, A. and Saldanha, J., 1976, The projection of the lateral
    geniculate nucleus to the area 17 of the rat, Brain Res.,
    105:533-537.
Pinto-Lord, C.M., Evrard, E. and Caviness, V.S.,Jr., 1982, Obstructed
    neuronal migration along radial glial fibers in the neocortex of
    the reeler mouse: A Golgi-EM analysis, Dev. Brain Res.,
    4:379-393.
Rakic, P., 1971, Guidance of neurons migrating to the fetal monkey
    neocortex, Brain Res., 33:471-476.
Rakic, P., 1972, Mode of cell migration to the superficial layers of
    fetal monkey neocortex, J. Comp. Neurol., 145:61-84.
Rakic, P., 1974, Neurons in rhesus monkey visual cortex: systematic
    relation between time or origin and eventual disposition,
    Science, 183:425-427.
Rakic, P., 1975, Timing of major ontogenetic events in the visual
    cortex of the rhesus monkey. In: N.A. Buchwald and M. Brazier
    (eds): Brain Mechanisms in Mental Retardation. Academic Press,
    New York, pp. 3-40.
Rakic, P., 1976a, Differences in the time of origin and in eventual
    distribution of neurons in areas 17 and 18 of visual cortex in
    rhesus monkey, Exp. Brain Res. Suppl., 1:244-248.
Rakic, P., 1976b, Prenatal genesis of connections subserving ocular
    dominance in the rhesus monkey, Nature, 261:467-471.
Rakic, P., 1977, Prenatal development of the visual system in the
    rhesus monkey, Phil. Trans. Roy. Soc. Lond. Ser. B.,
    278:245-260.
Rakic, P., 1978, Neuronal migration and contact guidance in primate
    telencephalon, Postgrad. Med. J., 54:25-40.
Rakic, P., 1981a, Developmental events leading to laminar and areal
    organization of the neocortex. In: F.O. Schmitt, S.G. Dennis
    and F.G. Worden (eds): The Cerebral Cortex. MIT Press,
    Cambridge, Mass. 7-28.
Rakic, P., 1981b, Neuronal-glial interaction during brain development,
    TINS, 4:184-187.
Rakic, P., 1981c, Development of visual centers in the primate brain
    depends on binocular competition before birth, Science,
    214:928-931.

Rakic, P., 1983, Geniculo-cortical connections in primates: Normal
     and experimentally altered development, Progess in Brain Res.,
     58:393-404.
Rakic, P. and Goldman-Rakic, P.S., 1982, Development and modifiabil-
     ity of cerebral cortex, Neurosciences Res. Prog. Bull.,
     20:429-611.
Rakic, P., Stensaas, L.J., Sayre, E.P.and Sidman, R.L., 1974,
     Computer-aided three-dimensional reconstruction and quantita-
     tive analysis of cells from serial electron microscopic
     montages of fetal monkey brain, Nature (London), 250:31-34.
Ramon y Cajal, S., 1899, Comparative study of the sensory areas of
     the human brain. In: Clark University 1889-1899 Decimal
     Celebration, Worchester, Mass., pp. 311-381.
Ramon y Cajal, S., 1911, Histologie due systeme nerveux de l'Homme
     et des vertebres. Maloine, Paris. Reprinted by Consejo
     Superior de Investigaciones Cientificas. Madrid. 1955.
Schmechel, D.E. and Rakic, P., 1979a, Arrested proliferation of
     radial glial cells during midgestation in rhesus monkey,
     Nature (London), 2767:303-305.
Schmechel, D.E. and Rakic, P., 1979b, A Golgi study of radial glial
     cells in developing monkey telencephalon: morphogenesis and
     transformation into astrocytes, Anat. Embryol., 156:115-152.
Schmitt, F.O., Worden, F.G., Adelman, G. and Dennis, S.G. The
     organization of the cerebral cortex. MIT Press, Cambridge,
     Mass.
Schwartz, M.L., and Goldman-Rakic, P.S., 1982, Single cortical
     neurons have axon collaterals to ipsilateral and contralateral
     cortex in fetal and adult primates, Nature, 299:154-156.
Sidman, R.L. and Rakic, P., 1973, Neuronal migration, with special
     references to developing human brain: a review. Brain Res.,
     62:1-35.
Shatz, C. and Rakic, P., 1981, The genesis if efferent connections
     from the visual cortex of the fetal monkey, J. Comp. Neurol.,
     196:287-307.
Waddington, C.H., 1956, Principles of Embryology. Allen and
     Unwin, London.
Wiess, P.A., 1971, A cell is not an island entire of itself.
     Perspective in Biology and Medicine, 14:182-205.
Wiesel,T.M., Hubel, D.H. and Lam, D.M.K., 1974, Autoradiographic
     demonstration of ocular dominance columns in the monkey
     striate cortex by means of transneuronal transport,
     Brain Res., 79:273-27.

CELLULAR INTERACTIONS AND THE SURVIVAL AND MAINTENANCE OF

NEURONS DURING DEVELOPMENT

Ronald W. Oppenheim

Department of Anatomy
Bowman Gray School of Medicine
Wake Forest University
Winston Salem, North Carolina

and

Neurobiology Program
University of North Carolina
Chapel Hill, N.C.

INTRODUCTION

Perhaps the most fundamental organizing principle of the developing nervous system is the role of cell and tissue interactions in regulating the countless steps leading from the zygote to the adult. Virtually nothing in the entire field of neuroembryology makes much sense if viewed from a perspective that is devoid of an appreciation of the pervasiveness of cell-to-cell inter-relationships. Starting with the origins of the nervous system during primary induction and continuing up to the final stages of neurobehavioral development no stage or event in neurogenesis is ever entirely independent of the influence of cellular interactions.

Although no one today would deny the correctness of these statements, this has not always been the case. Less than 100 years

----

Portions of this chapter have been published previously
in a slightly different form in a publication available
only to members of the Society for Neuroscience
(cf. Hamburger and Oppenheim, 1982).

49

ago, such statements would have been considered widely speculative
(if not outright heretical), since they were almost entirely unsub-
stantiated by either observations or experiments and because they
lacked a unified conceptual framework (i.e., a modern epigenetic
foundation). When a leading embryologist of the last century
actually suggested that certain morphogenetic events could be
explained by tissue movements and interactions (His, 1884), his
ideas were not only criticized but were derided and ridiculed to
an extent almost unheard of in todays vastly more polite and
permissive scientific milieu (Gould, 1977).

The events that occurred between then and now that were responsible for this changing intellectual climate are familiar to all
students of embryology (Oppenheimer, 1967; Oppenheim, 1982a). Briefly, beginning in the 1890's, biologists such as W. Roux, H. Driesch,
H. Spemann and R. Harrison rejected the static, descriptive comparative embryology that characterized 19th century biology, in favor of
a modern epigenetic and experimental approach. For the first time
in the history of biology, experimental analysis was considered the
preferential means of "communicating" with the embryo. Writing in
1894, Roux attempted to formulate this new approach and in doing so
he managed to capture the vastness of the task that lay ahead:

"By isolating, transposing, destroying, weakening, stimulating, false union, passive deformation, changing the
diet and the functional size of the parts of eggs, embryos
or even of more developed organisms, by the application
of unaccustomed agencies like light, heat, electricity
and by the withdrawal of customary influences, we may be
able to ascertain a great many formative operations in the
parts of the organism" (p.167).

It was within this framework that the study and appreciation of
cellular interactions in the developing nervous system originated.

For the first 2-3 decades of this century, a considerable amount
of the efforts of experimental embryologists was devoted to determining the relative contributions of "intrinsic" vs "extrinsic" factors
to both morphogenetic and histogenetic events. What this meant in
practice for studies of neural development was that specific nuclei,
ganglia, cell columns and even entire brain regions were studied
following the removal of either (or occasionally both) their efferent
targets or their afferent input (for a detailed review see Detwiler,
1936; Jacobson, 1978). It was repeatedly shown that the normal
development of these neuronal "units" depended upon interactions
with their efferent and afferent partners.

It is especially pertinent to the subject matter of this chapter that the recognition that a substantial loss of differentiating
neurons occurs normally during embryonic development arose within

the context of these experiments on the relationship between neurons and their targets and/or their presynaptic afferents (Oppenheim, 1981a). Several early investigators reported that the deletion or enlargement of either the targets of, or the afferent inputs to, a neuronal population altered the number of neurons in the population (Detwiler, 1936). But since regression and cell death had no place in the repertory of mechanisms studied by experimental embryologists, most investigators interpreted their results as a modification of proliferation and/or the recruitment of neurons from a (hypothetical) of undifferentiated precursor cells. The idea that target-induced "hypo-" or "hyperplasia" might be due to increased or decreased cell degeneration was, at the time, not a plausible alternative for embryologists.

Levi-Montalcini and Levi (1942, 1944) being less encumbered by an experimental embryological bias, were the first to interpret hypoplasia correctly in terms of neuron loss. They found that, following leg-bud extirpation in chick embryos, the number of differentiated neurons in lumbar dorsal root ganglion (DRG) declined between 6 and 19 days of incubation. But it took a repetition of this experiment to substantiate this claim by the detection of actually degenerating (pyknotic) neurons, this time in the brachial DRG of 5- to 7-day embryos following wing-bud extirpation (Hamburger and Levi-Montalcini, 1949). Levi-Montalcini discovered an equally severe degeneration process going on simultaneously in the cervical and thoracic DRG of the same embryos, although these ganglia had not been affected by the operation. The fortunate temporal coincidence of natural and experimentally induced neuron death suggested immediately that the two phenomena were closely related. Moreover, the further observation that the degeneration period coincided approximately with the arrival of the axons from the DRG at their target area gave the first clue to the explanation of natural neuronal death; namely, that in early stages the ganglion cells send out more neurites than the periphery can support; the excess neurons would then break down at the stage at which cells are susceptible to environmental conditions. It was not until the discovery of the Nerve Growth Factor (NGF), however, that the nature of this relation was first dimly recognized. The "environmental conditions" were identified as a trophic agent thought to be supplied by the target. Consequently, neuronal death was attributed to unsuccessful competition for a trophic agent; however, it has only been in the last few years that the specific trophic role of NGF in the regulation of natural neuronal death has begun to be elucidated (e.g. Hamburger et al., 1981; Hendry and Campbell, 1976; Oppenheim et al., (1982a).

Despite the fact that both natural and induced neuronal death were first systematically described over 30 years ago by Hamburger and Levi-Montalcini (1949), only following the work of Hughes (1968, review) and Prestige (1967) on motoneuron death in frog spinal cord did a gradual re-awakening of interest in natural neuronal death occur (Cowan, 1973; Oppenheim, 1981a).

Since that time, natural neuronal death has been found to occur not only in motoneurons and sensory and autonomic ganglia, but also in certain interneurons in the central nervous system (Oppenheim, 1981a). Further analyses have been primarily limited to nuclei and ganglia with a manageable population size, and we do not know whether units with very large populations, such as small interneurons with short axons in the cortex or spinal cord also undergo a significant cell loss.

Neuronal death in the developing vertebrate nervous system is composed of several categories, some of which are shared with other developing organ systems, while some are unique to the nervous system (Glucksmann, 1951; Silver, 1978; Jacobson, 1978; Oppenheim, 1981a). This chapter focuses on a category of neuronal death which is unique to neuronal tissue. It is referred to as "histogenetic" or "naturally occurring" neuronal death and is characterized by three critical aspects: a substantial loss of embryonic and/or postnatal neurons amounting in a few cases to as much as 80% of a population; the loss of cells is restricted to a well-defined period; the period of cell loss is characteristic of each population. Neuronal death displays a reproducible pattern in both time and space, and is an important factor in the regulation of the number of neurons in the ganglia and columns.

A basic assumption underlying the following discussion is that (where cell death occurs) neurons are capable of independent initial differentiation, but sooner or later become dependent on a trophic (maintenance) factor which is supplied in a limited quantity; hence, there is a competition resulting in the death of the losers. In other words, neuronal death is considered to be probabilistic in nature and due to extrinsically imposed restrictions, rather than to intrinsic or genetically, preprogrammed constraints.

The fundamental difference between the genetically preprogrammed and probabilistic models of cell death, however, is that whatever genetic differences may exist in the latter, they find their expression in differential capabilities for competition and not in an absolute (preprogrammed) all or none capacity for survival. In fact, a major unresolved question in this field is whether, and if so how, neurons within a population differ in their intrinsic capacity for competition and survival.

Finally, there is the important question of the biological value of the massive loss of differentiating neurons during development. For spinal motoneurons and a few other neuronal populations that have been examined it seems reasonably clear that neuronal death is not acting as an error correction mechanism (Oppenheim, 1981b; Landmesser, 1980); large numbers of neurons die despite having pro-

jected axons to their correct targets (see below). Although it is
conceivable that a greater-than-adult number of neurons are necessary
for some transient embryonic function, the present consensus is that
the overproduction and subsequent loss of neurons is necessary for
the quantitative matching of neurons with their targets.

With the possible exception of the neurons in the chick ciliary
ganglion (Landmesser and Pilar, 1978), the analysis of natural neuronal death of spinal somatic motoneurons in the chick embryo has
been more comprehensive than the analysis of any other class of
neuron. The information discovered (and the questions raised)
during this analysis provides a convenient point of departure for
a discussion of neuronal death and its regulation by cellular
interactions.

2.   Spinal Somatic Motoneurons

Cell death of motoneurons in the lumbar lateral motor column
(LMC) of the chick embryo extends from embryonic day 5 (E5) to E12
and involves a loss of 40-50% of the original population (Hamburger,
1975; Chu-Wang and Oppenheim, 1978a,b; Laing and Prestige, 1978).
This numerical depletion of LMC neurons is accompanied by the appearance of a significant number of dying neurons; the degeneration
process has been characterized in detail at the ultrastructural level
(Chu-Wang and Oppenheim, 1978a,b).

The onset of cell death in this population follows the cessation of proliferation (Hollyday and Hamburger, 1977) and overlaps
only slightly with the migration of postmitotic neurons to the LMC.
Moreover, since these motoneurons initiate differentiation prior
to the onset of cell death, all of the major early events of neurogenesis occur prior to the beginning of degeneration. Since this
is not the case for all neuronal populations, chick spinal motoneurons are especially favorable for the analysis of neuronal death.

A similar cell loss also occurs in the brachial and thoracic
motoneurons of the chick (Oppenheim and Majors-Willard, 1978;
Maderdrut and Oppenheim, 1982) as well as among the electric organ
motoneurons in fish (Fox and Richardson, 1981) and in frog
(Prestige, 1967), mouse (Harris-Flanagan, 1969; Lance-Jones, 1982)
and rat (Nurcombe et al., 1981) spinal motoneurons. Thus, it seems
likely that massive moto-neuron death is a common vertebrate
characteristic.

An analysis of cell size and other aspects of differentiation
among a random sample of LMC neurons in normal embryos prior to the
onset of cell death (on E5-6) has failed to reveal a subpopulation
which display signs of impending degeneration (Chu-Wang and
Oppenheim, 1978a,b). Furthermore, an analysis of the differentiation of moto-neurons prior to the onset of cell death in embryos in

which, owing to unilateral limb-bud removal, virtually all of the peripherally deprived cells will eventually die, has also failed to reveal any obvious differences between the deprived motoneurons and those in normal embryos (Hamburger, 1958; Oppenheim et al., 1978).

In both the normal and the peripherally-deprived situation (i.e., after early limb-bud removal), all motoneurons have sent axons into the ventral root or beyond. Moreover, massive injections of horseradish peroxidase (HRP) into the proximal part of the hindlimb of normal embryos on E5 - i.e., prior to cell death - result in the labelling of approximately 95% of the motoneurons in the related segments of the lumbar spinal cord (Oppenheim and Chu-Wang, 1977; Chu-Wang and Oppenheim, 1978b). Similar results in other populations of neurons such as the chick isthmo-optic nucleus (Clarke and Cowan, 1976) and the mouse (Lance-Jones, 1982) and rat (Nurcombe et al., 1982) spinal motoneurons show that virtually all of the neurons in these populations also send axons to their targets prior to neuronal death. Not only does this provide important evidence for the normal differentiation capacity of neurons which will eventually die, but it also implies that the critical factors involved in the competition process occur at the target site.

The results of the limb-bud removal experiments are also consistent with the important role ascribed to the target, since in this situation, as predicted, motoneuron death is increased from the normal 40-50% to 90% or more. An even more critical observation is that an experimentally induced increase in the size of the target by transplantation of a supernumerary hindlimb reduces the natural death of lumbar motoneurons from 40-50% to 25-35% (Hollyday and Hamburger, 1976). (A greater reduction might have been expected, but because of physical constraints, a majority of lumbar motoneurons were unable to send their axons into the supernumerary leg.) Before we conclude that motoneuron death is exclusively regulated by competitive interactions at the target, however, the role of afferents must be considered.

Natural neuronal death of primary afferent neurons in the chick DRG (Hamburger et al., 1981), overlaps temporally with the period of motoneuron death (see below); limb removal also induces an increased cell loss in the DRG (Hamburger and Levi-Montalcini, 1949). Thus, both natural as well as induced motoneuron death could be controlled, in part, by primary afferents; descending propriospinal and supraspinal fibers could also be involved (e.g., Oppenheim, 1975). Recent experiments, in which both intrinsic (spinal and supraspinal) and extrinsic DRG afferents were surgically removed prior to the onset of motoneuron death, show that natural neuronal death is not affected; deafferented embryos have normal numbers of motoneurons on E10-12, that is, after the cessation of natural cell death (Okado and Oppenheim, 1981). By contrast, the simultaneous removal of both intrinsic and extrinsic sources of motoneuron afferents

results in a significant (i.e. 25-30%) loss of motoneurons by E 10.
These findings indicate that, in addition to target (efferent) related factors, afferents may also be involved in the survival of
motoneurons during the normal period of cell death (Okado and
Oppenheim, 1983). Afferents may also be important in controlling
the natural death of other neuronal units (Cunningham, 1982).

During the stages in which spinal motoneurons are dying in the
chick, the limb muscles are in the process of segregating from the
dorsal and ventral muscle masses. Neuromuscular junctions (NMJ) are
present, but few in number, during the early stages of cell death.
Although a small amount of motoneuron death occurs prior to the onset
of neuromuscular function (as determined by the presence of limb
movements), there is nonetheless a reasonably close correlation
between limb innervation, the onset of limb motility and cell death.

The observation that the natural death of spinal motoneurons
coincides with the onset of neuromuscular function in the limbs led
to an examination of the role of synaptic and/or muscular activity
in this process. Experiments in which neuromuscular activity was
chronically blocked by drugs during the entire cell death period
i.e., from E5 to E10, has shown that motoneuron death can be reduced
or entirely prevented (Pittman and Oppenheim, 1979; Laing and
Prestige, 1978). As long as neuromuscular activity is blocked,
motoneurons fail to degenerate. Following the resumption of neuromuscular activity in the embryo, a delayed cell death ensues.
Recently, however, it has been possible to study four chicks
treated with d-tubocurarine (curare) from E5 to E9 which hatched
and survived for three to four days. Despite the occurrence of
considerable limb activity after hatching the "excess" motoneuron
numbers were retained (Oppenheim, 1982b). Thus, after hatching
neuromuscular blockade no longer appears necessary for maintaining
the "excess" motoneurons. (However, it is not at present known
precisely when during development that the survival of "excess"
motoneurons is no longer dependent on neuromuscular blockade).
Beginning the neuromuscular blockade at any time prior to the
cessation of natural neuronal death (i.e. before E10) prevents the
degeneration of cells. The reduction of cell death can be induced
by either pre- or postsynaptic (both competitive and depolarizing)
blockade of neuromuscular transmission (Pittman and Oppenheim,
1979; Oppenheim and Maderdrut, 1981).

Neuromuscular blockade does not affect cell number in either DRG
or sympathetic ganglia but rather appears to affect only cholinergic
motoneurons in the spinal cord and brain-stem (e.g., Creazzo and
Sohal, 1979). Furthermore increased muscular activity induced by
chronic electrical stimulation of the chick hindlimb in ovo between
E6 and E8 selectively increases the number of dying motoneurons in
the LMC, without any apparent effect on DRG or sympathetic ganglion
cells (Oppenheim and Nunez, 1982). Chronic treatment during the cell

death period with pharmacological agents that in the adult are known
to act as acetylcholine receptor (AChR) agonists (e.g., carbachol) or
which increase ACh at the synapse (eserine) also increase the loss of
motoneurons (Oppenheim and Maderdrut, 1981); however, two other
AChR agonists used in these experiments (nicotine and choline) did
not alter motoneuron numbers even at concentrations sufficient to
induce a paralysis equal to that caused by curare. Although the
reason for this result is not known, the ability to dissociate neuromuscular blockade (paralysis) from reduced cell death may provide an
important control for future experiments. Collectively, these
results are consistent with our contention that the survival of
embryonic motoneurons is related to neuronal and/or muscular
activity.

Neuromuscular blockade appears to induce an increased arborization of peripheral motoneuron axons as well as the sprouting of
axonal terminals within the muscle (Oppenheim and Chu-Wang, 1982).
Individual muscle fibers are multiply innervated and each NMJ is
contacted by a greater-than-normal number of axon terminals. Muscle
mass is greatly reduced following neuromuscular blockade. Since more
motoneurons are maintained despite the reduced muscle mass, it seems
plausible that reduced neuromuscular activity is associated with an
increased supply of trophic agent.

The observation that chronic neuromuscular blockade results in
the prevention of natural motoneuron death was an unexpected result;
its underlying cellular mechanisms are still not well understood. We
have previously suggested (e.g., Pittman and Oppenheim, 1979) that
the level and/or distribution of AChR in the muscle membrane is
critically involved; muscular inactivity would alter muscle membrane
properties (e.g., induce more AChR's) so that a single muscle fiber
is able to support a greater number of axonal terminals than normal, thereby increasing the likelihood of neuronal survival. Recent
evidence (Bursztajn and Oppenheim, in preparation) indicates that
following the prevention of cell death by neuromuscular blockade
the total number of AChR's and the number of AChR clusters in a
number of fast and slow muscles are increased two-three fold.
Although it is conceivable that the AChR is the trophic agent for
motoneurons it seems more likely that the AChR merely defines the
site at which the putative agent is released or taken up. Whatever
the result of future analysis will be, I wish to emphasize that
the inhibition of neuromuscular function per se is probably not the
primary cause of neuronal survival. Rather, normal synaptic and/or
muscular activity, although of obvious importance, is merely a link
in the chain of events regulating the availability of a target-
derived trophic agent.

3. Target Development and Neuronal Death

Because motoneurons innervate their targets at a stage when
muscle cells are still in the myoblast or myotube stage, there very
likely are crucial reciprocal interactions between embryonic motoneurons and muscle which are involved in the differentiation and
survival of both cell types. For instance, embryonic motoneurons may
regulate some property or properties of muscle for which they compete
and which is essential for their own survival. Therefore, it seems
important to characterize embryonic muscle properties during the time
span in which motoneurons are dying both in the normal situation and
following treatments which alter neuron survival (e.g. curare
treatment).

In contrast to the situation in amphibians, where many properties of striated muscle cells can develop and survive relatively
normally in the absence of innervation (e.g., Harrison, 1904), the
muscles of birds and mammals require innervation in the embryonic
and fetal stages to differentiate beyond the myotube stage
(Goldspink, 1980; Holtzer, 1970). Moreover, once they have differentiated, avian and mammalian striated muscle requires the continued
presence of nerves for the maintenance of certain histological, biochemical and physiological properties.

Some aspects of avian and mammalian muscle which are either
wholly or partly dependent on normal innervation for their development and/or maintenance include the following: myofibrillar adenosine
tripsophatase (ATPase) activity, the activation of myosin-specific
proteins that are characteristic of different muscle or fiber types
(slow, fast); the synthesis and distribution of membrane AChRs; the
synthesis and distribution of the collagen-tailed (16-20S), synapse-
specific, form of acetylcholinesterase (AChE); levels of cyclic nuc-
leotides, cGMP and cAMP and their associated enzymes; calcium levels;
and a number of electrophysiological properties (e.g., resting potentials, input resistance, ACh sensitivity, and sensitivity to tetrodotoxin (TTX) (see the following reviews: Fambrough, 1979; Edwards,
1979; Drachman, 1974; Massoulie and Bon, 1982; Schaub and Watterson,
1981; Dennis, 1981; Gauthier, et al., 1982; Vrbova et al., 1978).

One of the major issues in this field during the past 10-15 years
has been the extent to which the innervation-dependent properties of
muscle development, as well as the maintenance of adult muscle proper
ties, are associated with activity-related versus nonactivity related
cellular interactions. There is a substantial amount of evidence
showing that the blockade of neuromuscular transmission can mimic
many of the effects of surgical denervation on the development and
maintenance of muscle and that direct electrical stimulation of
denervated or inactive muscle can prevent or reverse many of these
effects (Lomo, 1980 for a review). However, there is also an
increasing amount of evidence showing that at least some of the

normal properties of muscle can develop and be maintained when
either denervated or aneural, and thus physiologically inactive,
cultured muscle cells are exposed to crude or partially purified
extracts of nerve tissue. Until these putative trophic factors are
better characterized and shown to influence muscle events in vivo,
however, it is not possible to fully assess their role in the normal
regulation of muscle properties.

In the chick embryo, motoneuron axons begin to invade trunk and
limb muscles at a time when the muscle cells have just begun to differentiate from primitive mesenchyme into myoblasts and myotubes.
For instance, growing nerves first enter the chick hindlimb on E4 and
24-36 hours later spontaneous neuromuscular limb activity begins
(Hamburger, 1975; Landmesser and Morris, 1975). It seems likely that
growing nerve terminals begin to release ACh almost immediately following contact with a muscle cell (Cohen, 1980; Blackshaw and
Warner, 1976). Specific limb muscles first begin to cleave or
separate out of the dorsal and ventral muscle masses about 12 days
after innervation (Romer, 1927; Sullivan, 1962). The earliest neuromuscular contacts are primarily on myotubes and only rarely on
myoblasts (Oppenheim and Chu-Wang, 1982). Despite the fact that
neuromuscular contacts are sparse at these early stages, muscular
activity is often vigorous; it is likely that this situation
results from widespread electrical coupling between embyronic myotubes (Dennis, 1981).

At the onset of innervation and for several days thereafter
embryonic muscle is composed of clusters of primary and secondary
myotubes all contained within a common basement membrane (Ontell,
1977; Ontell and Dunn, 1978; Ashmore, et al., 1972; Kikuchi and
Ashmore, 1976); with further development these clusters break up
into individual myotubes which later differentiate into myofibers.
The adult complement of muscle fibers within a given muscle is only
gradually attained over a period of several days following innervation, a process which overlaps temporally with the period of naturally-occurring death of motoneurons (Oppenheim and Chu-Wang, 1982;
McLennan, 1981). The prevention of motoneuron death by neuromuscular
blockade is associated with a significant reduction in the volume
of specific limb muscles owing primarily to the presence of fewer
myofibers in these preparations (Oppenheim and Chu-Wang, 1982).

In the chick embryo, accumulations of AChE and AChRs occur at
the site of the NMJ a few days after the onset of physiological
activity (Atsumi, 1981; Burden, 1977; Betz, et al., 1980); prior to
this time there are relatively high levels of AChE and AChR at both
junctional and extrajunctional regions of the muscle fiber.

Avian NMJs become polyneuronally innervated at a relatively
late stage of embryonic development (Bennett and Pettigrew, 1974;
Oppenheim and Chu-Wang, 1982; Pockett, 1981; Atsumi, 1977); there-

fore, the normal loss of polyneuronal innervation is not associated with the death of motoneurons (Oppenheim and Majors-Willard, 1978). It has been suggested, however, (Weeds, 1978; Gauthier, et al., 1982), that the complete expression of adultlike fast and slow muscle properties is causally associated with the loss of polyneuronal innervation.

Skeletal muscle fibers of birds and mammals can be generally classified into two types based on their function. Those which maintain posture are called slow because they contract relatively slowly with a sustained pattern of activity, whereas fast muscles contract or shorten more rapidly and are used for rapid bursts of vigorous activity. Many muscles in the chicken are composed of mixtures of these two fiber types. Some examples of relatively homogenous fasttype muscles are the biceps, the posterior latissimus dorsi (PLD, a wing muscle) and the breast muscle, pectoralis major. Examples of slow-type muscles are the anterior latissimus dorsi (ALD), and the lateral adductor and sartorius (leg muscles)(Hess, 1970; Stockdale et al., 1981; Gauthier et al., 1982; Ashmore et al., 1973, 1978). In adult birds, slow-type fibers are characterized by a multiply or distributed type of innervation, "en grappe" NMJs, by low levels of myosin ATPase which are stable following alkali incubation and labile in acid incubation, and by reacting exclusively with anti-bodies against slow-type myosin proteins. The slow-tonic ALD muscle of the adult chicken contains myofibers which histochemically do not strictly correspond to either mammalian fast or slow fibers (e.g., they stain intensely for myosin ATPase after both acid and alkali preincubation). Avian fast-type fibers have the opposite characteristics to those of slow fibers (i.e., focal innervation, "en plaque" NMJs, etc.).

Although controversy exists over the specific sequence of changes that characterize the differentiation of slow and fast muscles (Weeds, 1978), at present it appears that initially all embryonic muscle fibers (presumptive slow and fast) are slow contracting react histochemically for both slow and fast myosin ATPase properties and contain myosin or myofibrillar proteins characteristic of both slow and fast fibers (Carraro et al., 1981; Stockdale et al., 1982; Ashmore et al., 1972; MacNaughton, 1974; Butler and Cosmos, 1981). There also appear to be specific embryonic forms of myosin which are not present in the adult (e.g., Gauthier et al., 1982).

In the case of the avian wing muscles, ALD and PLD, these muscles can first be distinguished on the basis of their ATPase and myosin protein properties on E7 (Butler and Cosmos, 1981) which is during the period of naturally-occurring death of brachial motoneurons (Oppenheim and Majors-Williard, 1978). Adult chicken fast-twitch muscles (e.g., PLD and pectoralis) contain primarily the 16-20S form of AChE, whereas, the adult slow-tonic ALD muscle

lacks this form of AChE. Interestingly, the 16-20S form of AChE is
transiently present in embryonic ALD muscle but disappears after
hatching (Lyles and Barnard, 1980). In the fast-twitch pectoralis
and PLD muscles, the 16-20S form of AChE becomes predominant
between E14 and E18 (Lyles et al., 1979); prior to E14 both the
heavy and light AChE forms are present in about equal amounts in
these muscles.

As noted above, the differentiation and maintenance of many of
these properties that distinguish fast and slow muscle fiber types
are regulated by motor nerves, particularly by the pattern of electrical activity produced by the motoneurons (see Vrbova et al., 1978
for a review). Much of this evidence, however, is based on studies
performed during early postnatal or posthatching stages. It is not
clear to what extent innervation and especially neuromuscular transmission during embryonic and fetal stages is involved in the differentiation of slow and fast muscles. And more important for the
present discussion, it is not known whether the differentiation of
slow and fast muscle properties are associated with the survival of
motoneurons during the cell death period.

Despite our present lack of understanding of the specific
events in the development of striated muscle that are associated with
the survival of motoneurons, it seems likely that a muscle-derived
trophic agent (or agents) will be shown to be critically involved.

4.   Trophic Factors and Neuronal Death

Since the discovery and characterization of NGF as a neurotrophic agent involved in the growth, differentiation and survival
of specific neuronal crest derivatives (e.g., sympathetic and spinal
ganglion cells), it has been assumed that similar growth factors
must exist for other neuronal populations (see Varon and Bunge,
1978 for a review). However, lacking the fortunate set of circumstances that marked the NGF story (Levi-Montalcini, 1975), efforts
to discover other specific trophic factors have been hindered by a
number of technical difficulties.

Recently, there has been a resurgence of interest in discovering
other NGF-like factors in the vertebrate nervous system; largely
because of technical advances these efforts have met with initial
success. Recent investigations in this field have usually followed
the methodological precedent set by previous NGF work in using in
vitro preparations for isolating and characterizing putative neurotrophic factors. However, once a trophic factor has been purified (or
even partially purified) its effects in vivo must be characterized.
The development of antibodies against a purified neurotrophic agent
also provides a powerful technique for assessing its biological significance during normal development.

In addition to trophic factors thought to be involved in neuromuscular development (reviewed below), crude extracts or partially
purified factors have also been isolated from various target tissues
and shown to influence the in vitro growth and survival of ciliary
neurons (Nishi and Berg, 1981; Hendry and Hill, 1980), other parasympathetic neurons (Coughlin et al., 1981), trigeminal sensory
neurons (Chan and Haschke, 1981), and a population of non-NGF
sensitive sympathetic neurons (Edgar et al., 1981).

Muscle-derived trophic factors have been shown to influence
the survival, choline acetyltransferase (CAT) activity and neurite
out-growth of embryonic spinal motoneurons (or ventral spinal cord
neu-rons) in vitro (Bennett et al., 1980; Smith and Appel, 1981;
Pollack and Muhlach, 1981; Pollack, 1980; Driben & Barrett, 1980;
Godfrey et al., 1980). Muscle-derived proteins have also been
shown to be retrogradely transported to rat spinal cord in vivo
where they enhance CAT activity (Gilmer-Waymire and Appel, 1981);
it was also shown by these investigators that one week of chronic
treatment with α-bungarotoxin (α-BTX) caused a 2-fold increase in
both the amount of muscle proteins that were transported and their
ability to enhance spinal cord CAT activity. In at least one study,
the age of the donor of the muscle and spinal cord tissue significantly affected the in vitro activity of a putative muscle-derived
trophic factor (Pollack and Muhlach, 1981; Pollack, 1980). In
another study, chick spinal cord neurons from only a restricted
age range of donor embryos were able to form synapses with skeletal
muscle in vitro (Ruffolo et al., 1978). This temporal specificity
for synapse formation may be associated with changes in the amount
of a molecule located on the surface of embryonic muscle cells and
reported to mediate adhesions between nerve and muscle (Grumet et
al., 1982); antibodies against this factor prevent synapse formation in vitro. Specific antigens associated with the synaptic
basal lamina of muscle may be candidates for this molecule (Sanes
et al., 1978; Sanes and Hall, 1979; Burden et al., 1979).

In addition to muscle-derived or muscle associated factors which
can influence neuronal development, other putative trophic molecules
have been isolated from brain, spinal cord and peripheral nerve and
shown to influence the development of skeletal muscle. These enhance
the mitotic activity and differentiation of muscle (Popiela and Ellis,
1981), and significantly increase the synapse specific form (16-20S)
of AChE, and increase AChRs and the number of AChR clusters in cultured myotubes (Lentz et al., 1981; Bostwick and Appel, 1981;
Markelonis et al., 1982; Christian et al., 1978; Cohen and Weldon,
1980; Jessell et al., 1979). Denervation-induced changes in adult
muscle can also be prevented by treatment with peripheral nerve
extracts, both in vivo (Davis, 1981) and in vitro (Hasegawa and Kurmi,
1978). The in vivo results of Davis (1981) suggest that even crude
extracts of tissue which contains putative trophic molecules can
produce detectable changes in specific target organs in vivo.

In the final analysis, suspected trophic factors will have to be shown to possess biological activity when tested in vivo and to act in a fashion that mimics or closely approximates normal neuro-genetic events. Despite the pace of recent progress in this field, it seems likely that we are still several years away from being able to conclude that specific trophic agents are the primary means by which developing cells regulate the survival and maintenance of other cells. It needs to be remembered that only after a quarter of a century of investigation of the NGF has substantial evidence appear-ed (albeit indirect) to support the notion that this trophic molecule is critically involved in the survival of various neural crest deri-vatives in vivo (Gorin and Johnson, 1980a,b; Hamburger et al., 1981; Oppenheim et al., 1982a; Hendry, 1976; Thoenen et al., 1979).

5.   Neuronal Death and Error Correction

One of the intuitively most appealing suggestions for the adap-tive value of neuronal death is that it serves to remove errors in the pattern of connections between neurons and their targets. Although some developmental errors of this sort undoubtedly occur (see Jacobson, 1978; Landmesser, 1980; Lamb, 1981, for examples) present evidence indicates that their magnitude is not sufficiently great to account for the massive cell loss that occurs in many neural units.

In two of the best studied cases, the chick and frog hindlimb motoneurons, it has been shown that virtually all motoneurons, even those that will die, send axons to the limb and that the vast major-ity of these projections are correct with reference to the adult situation. That is, prior to cell death, each muscle is innervated by motoneuron pools that are located in the same position in the spinal cord as in the adult animal (Lamb, 1976; Landmesser, 1980; Hollyday, 1980). (For a somewhat different view on this issue see Pettigrew, et al., 1979). Furthermore, in the chick, experimental-ly-induced inappropriate connections between motoneurons and muscles are maintained throughout the normal cell death period even when they are in competition with the appropriate connections in the same muscle (Lance-Jones and Landmesser, 1981). Finally, the prevention of virtually all motoneuron death in the chick spinal cord by neuro-muscular blockade does not alter the position of motoneuron pools for specific fore- or hindlimb muscles (Oppenheim, 1981b). Conse-quently, in this case one must also conclude that the projection pattern of motoneuron pools was generally correct at the time that neuromuscular blockade was initiated on E5, that is, before the cell death period.

It has been suggested that neurons may not die because of a simple mismatch between the location of their soma and their target but rather because of a mismatch between their target and presynaptic inputs (e.g., Lewis, 1980). According to this view, if the inputs to a motoneuron are not appropriate for producing functionally adaptive contractions of its target muscle, then it will be at a competitive disadvantage and is more likely to die. An argument against this possibililty, however, is the observation that the near total removal of both intrinsic and extrinsic afferents to spinal motoneurons does not alter natural neuronal death (Wenger, 1950; Hamburger, et al., 1966; Okado and Oppenheim, 1981). It is also difficult to explain cell death in the ciliary ganglion in this way since the two populations of ciliary neurons, the ciliary and choroid, both receive highly specific and appropriate presynaptic inputs prior to cell death, yet 50% of the cells in each population subsequently die (Landmesser and Pilar, 1972).

Another way in which cell death might be involved as a means of error correction would be if neurons were somehow specified to form connections in specific regions within a grossly appropriate target. For instance, cells within a motoneuron pool might project topographically onto specific regions or fiber types of their target muscle (Burke et al., 1977; English and Ledbetter, 1982; Swett et al., 1970), or neurons within the central nervous system may project to specific cell types or neuronal regions, such as dendrites vs soma, within their normal target. Although this is an interesting notion, whether significant errors of this type occur, and if so, whether they are eliminated by cell death remains to be substantiated (but see Bennett and Lavidis, 1982).

A final case that needs to be discussed in this context is the isthmo-optic nucleus in the chick. The beautiful studies of Clarke and Cowan (1976) and Clarke et al., 1976 on the isthmo-optic nucleus are perhaps the most widely and often inappropriately, cited evidence in support of the significant role of cell death as an error correction mechanism. (We might add that the authors, themselves, are more cautious in their conclusions on this issue.) These studies have shown that 60% of the neurons within the normal confines of this nucleus die despite having projected axons to their normal target region, the contralateral retina. Prior to cell death, about 10-20% of all isthmo-optic neurons are located outside of, or ectopic to, the normal confines of the nucleus and another 1% or so send axons to the incorrect, ipsilateral, eye. Originally it was reported that virtually all of the ectopic and ipsilateral cells degenerated. However, by the use of more sensitive retrograde tracer techniques it has recently been shown that a substantial number of these cells survive the normal period of cell death and are even retained in the adult chicken (Hayes and Webster, 1981; O'Leary and Cowan, 1981). Thus, of the almost 14,500 ION neurons that undergo natural death, little if any of this loss can be directly attributed to error correction, at least errors of the type being considered here.

In conclusion, in those few systems that have been examined in some detail, error correction appears to be either non-existent or

only minimally associated with natural neuronal death. Many more
cases need to be examined, however, before any general conclusions
can be reached on this issue.

6.   Evolutionary Significance of Neuronal Overproduction

     This topic has been the major focus of an interesting article by
Katz and Lasek (1978). The authors point out that the nervous system
is organized in the form of sets of "matching populations"; that is,
a proportional relation exists between a given neuron population and
its target. If a single genetic change occurs only in one partner,
which disturbs the match, then ontogenetic buffer mechanisms must op-
erate to restore the match. Otherwise, the mutation is not adaptive.

     The overproduction of neurons, which can be viewed as such a
unilateral genetic change, has often been considered as a "safety
factor" to guarantee the appropriate numerical innervation of the
target. The authors go a step further and envisage in the overproduction a potential for evolutionary change. For instance, in the
case of the neuromuscular system, the excess motoneurons can be considered as a reservoir that would permit a considerable enlargement
of the musculature without the necessity of a concomittant genetic
change in the nervous system.

     From this point of view, Katz and Lasek suggest that embryo-
logical manipulations can be considered as experimental tests for
evolutionary speculations. For instance, the transplantation of a
supernumerary limb, resulting in the utilization of some of the excess motoneurons (Hollyday and Hamburger, 1976) would mimic, so to
speak, an evolutionary enlargement at the target; partial limb removal which results in an enhanced loss of motoneurons, would be
the other side of the coin. Another example that can illuminate
evolutionary considerations is an early experiment by Twitty (1932).
One eye primordium of a small salamander species, Ambystoma punc-
tatum was replaced by an eye primordium of the larger species,
A. tigrinum. In later larval stages, the population of cells in the
optic tectum had increased to match the larger retinal cell population. However, in this instance, it is not known whether altered
cell death is the mechanism by which the adjustment is achieved
(Kollros, 1982).

     In a more general vein, neuronal death may only be the most ex-
treme case of what is actually a continuum of regressive, neurogenetic events that have both ontogenetic and phylogenetic significance.
Cellular overproduction, exuberant growth of axonal and dendritic
processes and excessive synapse formation may reflect only the most
obvious cases in which regression acts to mold the final product
(for recent expressions of this view see Innocenti, 1982; Oppenheim,
1981c; Purves and Lichtman, 1980).

7. Naturally-Occurring Neuronal Death and Neuropathology

It follows from the preceding section that if ontogenetic buffer mechanisms are defective and therefore incapable of neutralizing certain genetic changes in one partner of a matched population, then maladaptive, but potentially viable pathological conditions might result. It has, in fact, been suggested that certain kinds of neuromuscular disorders might involve a primary alteration in motoneuron numbers. Preliminary data from the mutant mouse Wobbler (wr/wr), a model for infantile spinal muscular atrophy in the human, indicated that there is a reduced number of spinal motoneurons (50% of normal) on E18, which is near the end of the normal cell death period for mouse spinal motoneurons (Hanson and Strominger, 1980). Similarly, the mutant mouse Sprawling (Swl), in which there is a signficant numerical depletion of neurons in the DRG, has a marked increase in the number of pyknotic DRG cells during the normal period of cell death in this population, that is, between E11 and E20, implying that altered cell death is involved (Scaravilli and Duchen, 1980).

By contrast, the situation in the case of the avian model of forelimb muscular dystrophy is presently confusing in that one author reports fewer brachial motoneurons (Murphy, 1977), one reports more brachial motoneurons (Sushella et al., 1980), and our own studies have found no differences in the number of brachial motoneurons at any time from E6 to 3 weeks posthatching (Oppenheim et al., 1982b).

The human disorder familial dysautonomia is a genetic disease which primarily affects individuals of Ashkenazic Jewish descent. This disease is manifest at birth and primarily involves deficits in sensory and sympathetic ganglia (Breakfield, 1981). It is pertinent that the number of neurons in the sympathetic ganglia and the intermediolateral column (i.e., the sympathetic preganglionic neurons) is reduced in patients with this disorder (Pearson and Pytel, 1978). Because of the parallel between these findings and those from mice treated with the antiserum to β- Nerve Growth Factor (Levi-Montalcini 1972), it was suggested that Nerve Growth Factor might somehow be altered in these patients (Pearson et al., 1974). In fact, the protein from patients has only about 10% of the biological activity of the normal protein (Schwartz and Breakfield, 1980). Recent evidence implicating Nerve Growth Factor as a trophic agent directly involved in the survival of embryonic sensory (Hamburger et al., 1981; Gorin and Johnson, 1980a,b) and sympathetic preganglionic neurons (Oppenheim et al., 1982a) raises the possibility that altered cell death may be one of the effects of the abnormal NGF which characterize this disease.

Although the evidence is still scanty, the possibility that altered naturally-occurring cell death is a factor in various neuropathological disorders cannot be ignored. Genetic defects in the

cell death process could alter cell numbers either directly or transneuronally (e.g., Oppenheim et al, 1982a), or both, with the possibility of long term repercussions on neuronal function. Environmental
factors such as drugs given to pregnant females could also affect
neuronal numbers by altering the normal cell death process. Conceivably, even benign neurobehavioral differences between "normal"
individuals could, in some instances, be associated with differences
in neuron numbers resulting from subtle genetic or environmentally-
induced alterations in neuronal death.

8.   Concluding Remarks

      The phenomenon of neuronal death is an integral part of a
broader neuro-embryological problem for which one can use the term
"systems-matching" that has been coined by Gaze and Keating (1972)
in a similar context. What is required is a quantitative matching
of neuron populations with target areas: these can be synaptic sites
on muscles or on other neurons, or arborizations. This need not be
a one-to-one relation; however, it is assumed that a fixed
quantitative relationship of some sort between the two systems is
required for optimal functional activity.

      How is the systems-matching achieved? It has been demonstrated
in virtually all examples of neuronal death that there is an initial
overproduction in the neuronal populations supplying the targets,
followed by an elimination process. In other words, system-matching
is achieved in a 2-step procedure. Although the two aspects are in-
tricately interwoven in the attainment of the end result, nevertheless overproduction and elimination of neurons are regulated by two
entirely different and independent developmental mechanisms. This
point will be elaborated in the hope that it may lead to a better
understanding of the curious indirect method by which systems-
matching is accomplished.

      I turn first to the question: how does the overproduction come
about? In confronting this question, one should realize a crucial
difficulty inherent in systems-matching, that is, that as a rule the
two systems which have to be matched develop topographically as separate entities, usually at some distance from each other; and they
undergo critical initial steps of development, including proliferation, independently of each other. The important point is that,
whatever the factors are which regulate proliferation of neuronal
units, the target area is not involved. This has been demonstrated
in several instances and it may be a general rule. A clear example
is the way in which the lateral motor columns in the spinal cord of
chick embryos are assembled. These neurons are derived from the
ventral neuroepithelium (basal plate) in the brachial and lumbar
segments of the neural tube. They are produced during a restricted
period by a precisely controlled number of mitotic cycles. This we
conclude from the fact that there is relatively little individual

variation in the maximal (pre-elimination) population size
(Hamburger, 1975). The proliferation process is independent of the
target area, i.e., the limbs, since the full numerical complement of
the lateral motor column can be formed in the absence of the limb
buds (Hamburger, 1958; Oppenheim et al., 1978).

The same independence can be demonstrated for the proliferation
process in the optic tectum of the chick embryo, which is unaffected
by the early removal of the optic vesicle (Cowan et al., 1968); and
it probably holds for other systems. The few claims that the target
actually does influence the mitotic activity in neuronal units need
to be re-examined. In the case of a decrease of mitotic figures in
chick spinal ganglia following wing extirpation, and increase following the addition of a transplanted wing (Hamburger and Levi-
Montalcini, 1949), it is not possible to distinguish between proli-
ferating neuronal and glial precursors. Kollros (1953) has found
that mitotic activity in the optic tectum of frog embryos is
reduced following extirpation of its major source of afferents from
the optic vesicle. But Currie and Cowan (1974) who repeated the
experiment, presented evidence that it is the production of glia
not neurons that is affected by the absence of optic fibers. More
recent experiments by Kollros (1982), however, provide additional
support for his original contention that <u>neuronal</u> number in the
frog optic tectum is at least partially under the control of the
ganglionic afferents from the eye via the regulation of precursor
proliferation.

Most available data, however, indicate that the factors which
regulate neuron proliferation reside in the neuroepithelium. In the
case of sensory and autonomic ganglia, proliferation also seems to be
regulated by intrinsic factors, although there is no direct proof
for this contention (Bibb, 1978). This implies that an understanding of the mechanisms that regulate initial cell numbers will
most likely be based on information concerning these intrinsic
regulatory factors. In addition, such information must account for
the very high rate of overproduction. It is not immediately obvious
why there should be a redundancy of 50%, if it were primarily a
matter of providing a safety factor to guarantee adequate nerve
supply to the target.

Let me pursue this thought more explicitly, using again the
formation of the lateral motor column as an example. Several
factors determine the final maximum (pre-elimination) population
size of the lateral motor column: the initial number of (hypothetical) founder or progenitor cells located in a segment of the ventral
neural epithelium (basal plate), and the number of mitotic cycles
which they undergo. The latter could be programmed within the
founder cells; or else it is determined by a factor in their
immediate environment which turns off the cycling. The production
process is regulated very precisely, since, as we have seen, the

maximum population numbers show a remarkable constancy with little individual variation. The rigorous control of the production process must have evolved independently of, and without concern for, the actual later demand at the target. Let us assume for the sake of argument that at a given period there are 10,000 precursor cells each with the capacity for another mitotic cycle and that the requirement eventually will be for 13,000 motor neurons. If proliferation stops at 10,000, then the target would be undersupplied, and natural selection would eliminate such individuals with malfunctioning muscles. If, on the other hand, entering another cycle were an all-or-none proposition for all 10,000 cells, then the overproduction would be inevitable, and, indeed, the closest approach to fulfilling the actual demand. I am aware that this model is unrealistic since the assumption of a synchronized simultaneous mitotic cycle of all 10,000 cells is improbable. The purpose of this model is to demonstrate that there is a way of understanding the high overproduction rate of 50% strictly in terms of developmental mechanisms intrinsic to the neural epithelium, without reference to the possible adaptive value of the redundancy. (The same explanation of the high rate of overproduction has been proposed independently by M. Katz and U. Grenander: personal communication). Of course, once the excess numbers are produced, they are available for adaptive use, such as systems matching and error elimination.

In summary, systems matching between neuronal populations and their targets is achieved in 2 steps: overproduction; and elimination of unsuccessful neurons. I have argued that the first step is independent of the second, and will show next that the reverse is also true. The elimination process is predicated on 2 related premises. The first is that embryonic neurons can sustain themselves only for a limited period. Sooner or later, they become dependent on trophic factors which are provided by the targets. The second premise is that the trophic factors are available only in limited supply, and its corollary, that neurons are in competition for the agent. This notion is supported by strong indirect evidence, which may be summarized briefly again: the parallelism in the spatial-temporal pattern of normally-occurring and experimentally induced death; the rescue of neurons which would have died, by experimental-enlargement of the target; and the finding that normally occurring death in the dorsal root and sympathetic ganglia can be alleviated or completely prevented by supplementing the available trophic agent with exogenously introduced Nerve Growth Factor (Hamburger et al., 1981; Oppenheim et al., 1982a; Hendry and Campbell, 1977).

The above form of competition hypothesis has been challenged by Lamb (1979, 1980, 1981). In a recent experiment, he has reported that if in a frog embryo one limb bud is extirpated and its nerve supply is manipulated so as to grow into the contralateral intact limb, the total number of motor neurons in both lateral motor columns

is significantly greater than the normally surviving number on one
side. However, as Purves (1980) has pointed out, a simple linear
one-to-one relation is not expected if neurons regulate the target
property which they compete for (i.e., the production or release of
the trophic factor). And, as mentioned previously, the prevention of
motoneuron cell death by neuromuscular blockade in which a greatly
reduced muscle mass is able to maintain many more neurons than normally, shows that experimental findings which at first sight seem
to contradict the competition hypothesis, can be easily accommodated
in it.

     Another challenge to the quantitative matching form of the com-
petition hypothesis, namely, that neuronal death serves to eliminate
heterospecific, that is, grossly inappropriate, connections has
also been repudiated. At best, cell death may only remove small-
scale projection errors and although these probably cannot account
for the massive elimination which is the rule, this remains an open
question.

     Finally, one can ask: competition for what? One finds in the
literature occasional references to "competition for synaptic sites
or for a trophic agent." The apparent need for alternatives is
probably motivated, in part, by the fact that dorsal root ganglia
which are also subject to neuronal death have no preipheral synaptic
contacts, although they do have terminal contacts with receptor
cells, in addition to free nerve endings. We can readily avoid the
notion of alternatives by assuming that wherever we are dealing with
synaptic or terminals contacts, they are the sites at which trophic
agents are internalized. In other words, competition is not for
synaptic sites but for trophic substances released and taken up at
synaptic or terminals sites. Justification for this assumption comes
from well-known experiments on sympathetic neurons in which it was
shown that the Nerve Growth Factor is actually internalized at
adrenergic terminals and transported retrogradely (Hendry et al.,
1974; review in Thoenen and Barde, 1980).

     In summary, we arrive at the unifying hypothesis that competi-
tion for a trophic agent is the overriding factor in explaining natural neuronal death. Our experience with the Nerve Growth Factor has
taught us that an agent can reach an embryonic neuron by retrograde
axonal transport or by diffusion. Of well known examples of neuronal death, the motoneurons, the ciliary ganglion and the retino-tectal
system belong to the first category, and the early differentiating
ventrolateral cells of chick dorsal root ganglia seem to take up the
growth factor along both routes. Other cases must exist in which
agents delivered by orthograde axonal transport via afferents are
important in regulating cell survival (e.g., Parks, 1979), or in
which a balance of some sort between both retrogradely and ortho-
gradely supplied trophic agents is involved (Cunningham, 1982).

Despite the overriding focus here on trophic agents as the key to understanding cellular interactions in general and naturally-occurring neuronal death in particular, I would like to close this chapter on a note of caution on this issue. There almost certainly are going to be a number of ways in which neurons interact with one another to control neurogenesis. To devote all or even most of our efforts to isolating, purifying and developing antibodies against putative trophic agents may be counterproductive. As promising as this approach is, other approaches must also be encouraged. Over 50 years ago Ross Harrison (1933) in a general discussion of the embryological concept of determination had these wise words of counsel which seem to apply equally well to the present situation:

> "A score of different factors may be involved and their
> effects most intricately interwoven...Success will be
> measured by the simplicity, precision and completeness
> of our descriptions rather than by a specious facility
> in ascribing causes to particular events. There is
> always room for fallacy, even when the logical pro-
> cedure may seem unimpeachable, and no conclusion in
> embryology is safe if based upon but a single
> proof" (p. 319).

References

Ashmore, C.R., Addies, P.B., Doerr, L. and Stokes, M., 1973, Development of muscle fibers in the complexus muscle of normal and dystrophic chicks, J. Histochem. Cytochem. 21:266-278.

Ashmore, C.R., Kikuchi, T. and Doerr, L., 1978, Some observations on the innervation pattern of different fiber types of chick muscles, Exp. Neurol. 58:272-284.

Ashmore, C.R., Robinson, D.W., Rattray, P. and Doerr, L., 1972, Biphasic development of muscle fibers in the fetal lamb, Exp. Neurol. 37:241-255.

Atsumi, S., 1977, Development of neuromuscular junctions of fast and slow muscles in the chick embryo: a light and electron microscopic study, J. Neurocytol. 6:691-709.

Atsumi, S., 1981, Localization of surface and internal acetylcholine receptors in developing fast and slow muscles of the chick embryo, Dev. Biol. 86:122-135.

Bennett, M.R., Lai, K. and Nurcombe, V., 1980, Identification of embryonic motoneurons in vitro: their survival is dependent on skeletal muscle, Brain Res. 190:537-542.

Bennett, M.R. and Pettigrew, A., 1974, The formation of synapses in striated muscle during development, J. Physiol. 241:515-545.

Bennett, M.R. and Lavidis, N.A., 1982, Development of the topographical projection of motor neurons to amphibian muscles accompanies motor neuron death, Dev. Brain Res. 2:448-452.

Betz, H., Bourgeois, J.P. and Changeux, J.P., 1980, Evolution of cholinergic proteins in developing slow and fast muscles in chick embryos, J. Physiol. 302:197-218.

Bibb, H.D., 1978, Neuronal death in the development of normal and hyperplastic spinal ganglia, J. Exp. Zool., 206:65-72.

Blackshaw, S.E. and Warner, A., 1976, Onset of acetylcholine sensitivity and endplate activity in developing myotome muscles of Xenopus, Nature 262:217-218.

Bostwick, J.R. and Appel, S.J., 1981, Effects of brain extracts on the number of acetylcholine receptors in primary cultures of rat myotubes, Soc. Neurosci. Abstract 7:553.

Breakfield, X.O., Altered nerve growth factor in familial dysautonomia: discovering the molecular basis of an inherited neurologic disease, Neurosci. Comm. 1:28-32.

Burden, S.J., 1977, Development of the neuromuscular junction in the chick embryo: the number, distribution and stability of acetylcholine receptors, Dev. Biol. 57:317-329.

Burden, S.J., Sargent, P.B. and McMahan, U.J., 1979, Acetylcholine receptors in regenerating muscle accumulate at original synaptic sites in the absence of the nerve, J. Cell Biol. 82:412-425.

Burke, R.E., Strick, P.L., Kanda, C. and Walmsley, B., 1977, Anatomy of medial gastrocnemius and soleus motor nuclei in cat spinal cord, J. Neurophysiol. 40:667-680.

Butler, J. and Cosmos, E., 1981, Differentiation of the avian latissimus dorsi primordium: analysis of fiber type expression using the myosin ATPase histochemical reaction, J. Exp. Zool. 218:219-232.

Carraro, U., Libera, L.D. and Catani, C., 1981, Myosin light chains of avian and mammalian slow muscles: evidence of intraspecific polymorphism, J. Muscle Res. Cell Motility 2:335-342.

Chan, K.Y. and Haschke, R.H., 1981, Action of a trophic factor(s) from rabbit corneal epithelial culture on dissociated trigeminal neurons, J. Neurosci. 1:1155-1162.

Christian, C.N., Daniels, M.P., Sugiyama, H., Vogel, Z., Jaques, J. and Nelson, P.G., 1978, A factor from neurons increases the number of acetylcholine receptor aggregates on cultured muscle cells, Proc. Natl. Acad. Sci. USA. 75:4011-4015.

Chu-Wang, I.-W. and Oppenheim, R.W., 1978a, Cell death of motoneurons in the chick embryo spinal cord. I. A light and electron microscopic study of naturally-occurring and induced cell loss during development, J. Comp. Neurol. 177:33-58.

Chu-Wang, I.-W. and Oppenheim, R.W., 1978b, Cell death of motoneurons in the chick embryo spinal cord. II. A quantitative and qualitative analysis of degeneration in the ventral root, including evidence for axon outgrowth and limb innervation prior to cell death, J. Comp. Neurol. 177:59-86.

Clarke, P.G.H. and Cowan, W.M., 1976, The development of the isthmo-
    optic tract in the chick, with special reference to the occur-
    rence and correction of developmental errors in the location
    and connection of isthmo-optic neurons, J. Comp. Neurol.
    167:143-163.
Clarke, P.G.H., Rogers, L.A. and Cowan, W.M., 1976, The time of
    origin and the pattern of survival of neurons in the isthmo-
    optic nucleus of the chick, J. Comp. Neurol. 167:125-141.
Cohen, S.A., 1980, Early nerve-muscle synapses in vitro release
    transmitter over postsynaptic membrane having low acetylcholine
    sensitivity, Proc. Natl. Acad. Sci., USA 77:644-648.
Cohen, M.W. and Weldon, P.R., 1980, Localization of acetylcholine
    receptors and synaptic ultrastructure at nerve-muscle contacts
    in culture: dependence on nerve type, J. Cell. Biol. 86:388-401.
Coughlin, M.D., Bloom, E.M. and Black, I.B., 1981, Characterization
    of a neuronal growth factor from mouse heart-cell-conditioned
    medium, Dev. Biol. 82:56-68.
Cowan, W.M., 1973, Neuronal death as a regulative mechanism in the
    control of cell number in the nervous system. in: Development
    and Aging in the Nervous System, (M. Rockstein, ed.), New York,
    Academic Press, pp. 19-41.
Cowan, W.M., Martin, A.H. and Wenger, E.L., 1968, Mitotic patterns
    in the optic tectum of the chick during normal development and
    after early removal of the optic vesicle, J. Exp. Zool.
    169:71-92.
Creazzo, T.L. and Sohal, G.S., 1979, Effects of chronic injections of
    β-bungarotoxin on embryonic cell death, Exp. Neurol. 66:135-145.
Cunningham, T.J., 1982, Naturally-occurring neuron death and its
    regulation by developing neural pathways, in: International
    Review of Cytology, (G.H. Bourne and J.F. Danielli, eds.),
    New York, Academic Press, pp. 163-186.
Currie, J. and Cowan, W.M., 1974, Some observations on the early
    development of the optic tectum in the frog (Rana pipiens), with
    special reference to the effects of early eye removal on mitotic
    activity in the larval tectum, J. Comp. Neurol. 156:123-142.
Davis, H.L., 1981, Effect of nerve extract on atrophy of denervated
    or immobilized muscles, Soc. Neurosci. Abstract 7:946.
Dennis, M., 1981, Development of the neuromuscular junction:
    inductive interactions between cells, Ann. Rev. Neurosci.
    4:43-68.
Detwiler, S.R., 1936, Neuroembryology, Macmillan, New York.
Drachman, D.B. (ed.), 1974, Trophic Functions of the Neuron, New York
    Academy of Sciences, New York.
Dribin, L.B. and Barrett, J.N., 1980, Conditioned medium enhanced
    neurite outgrowth from rat spinal cord explants, Dev. Biol.
    74:184-195.
Edgar, D., Barde, Y.-A. and Thoenen, H., 1981, Subpopulations of
    cultured chick sympathetic neurons differ in their requirements
    for survival factors, Nature 289:294-295.

Edwards, C., 1979, The effects of innervation on the properties of acetylcholine receptors in muscle, Neurosci. 4:565-584.

English, A.W. and Ledbetter, W.D., 1982, Anatomy and innervation patterns of cat lateral gastrocnemius and plantaris muscles, Amer. J. Anat. 164:67-77.

Fambrough, D.M., 1979, Control of acetylcholine receptors in skeletal muscle, Physiol. Rev. 59:165-227.

Fox, G.Q. and Richardson, G.P., 1981, Cell death and proliferation in the electric lobes of Torpedo mamorata, Soc. Neurosci. Abstract 7:293.

Gauthier, G.F., Lowey, S., Benfield, P.A. and Hobbs, A.W., 1982, Distribution and properties of myosin isozymes in developing avian and mammalian skeletal muscle fibers, J. Cell. Biol. 92:471-484.

Gaze, R.M. and Keating, M.J., 1972, The visual system and "neuronal specificity", Nature 237:375-378.

Gilmer-Waymire, K. and Appel, S.H., 1981, The appearance of muscle derived proteins in nerve and their enhancement with α -BTX in vivo, Soc. Neurosci. Abstract 7:767.

Glucksmann, A., 1951, Cell deaths in normal vertebrate ontogeny, Biol. Rev. 26:59-86.

Godfrey, E.W., Schrier, B.K. and Nelson, P.G., 1980, Source and target cell specificities of a conditioned medium factor that increases choline acetyltransferase activity in cultured spinal cord, Dev. Biol. 77:403-418.

Goldspink, D.F. (ed.), 1980, Development and Specialization of Skeletal Muscle, Cambridge, England, Cambridge University Press.

Gorin, P.D. and Johnson, E.M., 1980a, Effects of exposure to nerve growth factor antibodies on the developing nervous system of the rat: an experimental approach, Dev. Biol. 80:313-323.

Gorin, P.D. and Johnson. E.M., 1980b, Effects of long-term nerve growth factor deprivation on the nervous system of the adult rat: an experimental autoimmune approach, Brain Res. 198:27-42.

Gould, S.J., 1977, Ontogeny and Phylogeny, Cambridge, MA., Belknap.

Grumet, M., Rutishauser, U. and Edelman, G.M., 1982, Neural cell adhesion molecule is on embryonic muscle cells and mediates adhesion to nerve cells in vitro, Nature, 295:693-695.

Hamburger, V., 1958, Regression versus peripheral control of differentiation in motor hypoplasia, Amer. J. Anat. 102:365-410.

Hamburger, V., 1975, Cell death in the development of the lateral motor column of the chick embryo, J. Comp. Neurol. 160:535-546.

Hamburger, V., Brunso-Bechtold, J.K. and Yip, J., 1981, Neuronal death in the spinal ganglia of the chick embryo and its reduction by nerve growth factor, J. Neurosci. 1:60-71.

Hamburger, V. and Levi-Montalcini, R., 1949, Proliferation, differentiation and degeneration in the spinal ganglia of the chick embryo under normal and experimental conditions, J. Exp. Zool. 111: 457-502.

Hamburger, V. and Oppenheim, R.W., 1982, Naturally-occurring neuronal death in vertebrates. Neurosci. Comment 1. 2:39-55.

Hamburger, V., Wenger, E. and Oppenheim, R.W., 1966, Motility in the chick embryo in the absence of sensory input, J. Exp. Zool. 165:133-160.

Hanson, P.A. and Strominger, N.L., 1980, Intrauterine motor neuron death in normal mouse and in the Wobbler mutant, Soc. Neurosci. Abstract 6:669.

Harris-Flanagan, A., 1969, Differentiation and degeneration in the motor horn of foetal mouse, J. Morph. 129:281-305.

Harrison, R.G., An experimental study of the relation of the nervous system to the developing musculature in the embryo of the frog, Amer. J. Anat. 3:197-220.

Harrison, R.G., 1933, Some difficulties of the determination problem, Amer. Nat. 67:306-321.

Hasegawa, S. and Kuromi, H., 1978, Ventral part of spinal cord contains the neurotrophic factor for the action potential of cultured muscle, Brain Res. 157:153-156.

Hayes, B.P. and Webster, E.E., 1981, Neurons situated outside the isthmo-optic nucleus and projecting to the eye in adult birds, Neurosci. Lett. 26:107-112.

Hendry, I.A., 1976, Control in the development of the vertebrate sympathetic nervous system, Rev. Neurosci. 2:149-193.

Hendry, I.A. and Campbell, J., 1976, Morphometric analysis of rat superior cervical ganglion after axotomy and nerve growth factor treatment, J. Neurocytol. 5:351-360.

Hendry, I.A. and Hill, C.E., 1980, Retrograde axonal transport of target tissue-derived macromolecules, Nature 287:647-649.

Hendry, I.A., Stockel, K., Thoenen, H. and Iverson, L.L., 1974, The retrograde axonal transport of nerve growth factor, Brain Res. 68:103-131.

Hess, A., 1970, Vertebrate slow muscle fibers, Physiol. Rev. 68:103-131.

His, W., 1884, Unsere Korperform und das Physiologische Problem ihrer Entstehung, Leipzig, Vogel.

Hollyday, M., 1980, Motoneuron histogenesis and the development of limb innervation. in: Current Topics in Developmental Biology, Neural Development, vol. 15, (R.K. Hunt, ed.), New York, Academic Press, pp. 181-215.

Hollyday, M. and Hamburger, V., 1976, Reduction of the naturally occurring motor neuron loss by enlargement of the periphery, J. Comp. Neurol. 170:311-320.

Hollyday, M. and Hamburger, V., 1977, An autoradiographic study of the formation of the lateral motor column in the chick embryo, Brain Res. 132:197-208.

Holtzer, H., 1970, Myogenesis, in: O.A. Schjkeide and J. DeVellis (eds.) Cell Differentiation, New York, Van Nostrand Reinhold.

Hughes, A.F., 1968, Aspects of Neural Development, London, Logos.

Innocenti, G., 1982, Transitory structures as a substrate for developmental plasticity of the brain. in: Recovery from Brain Damage, (M.W. Van Hof and J. Mohn, eds.), Amsterdam, Elsevier (in press).

Jacobson, M., 1978, Developmental Neurobiology, New York: Plenum.

Jessel, T.M., Siegel, R.E. and Fischbach, G.D., 1979, Induction of acetylcholine receptors on cultured skeletal muscle by a factor extracted from brain and spinal cord, Proc. Natl. Acad. Sci. USA. 76:5397-5401.

Katz, M.J. and Lasek, R.J., 1978, Evolution of the nervous system: role of ontogenetic buffer mechanisms in the evolution of matching populations, Proc. Natl. Acad. Sci. USA. 75:1349-1352.

Kelly, J.P. and Cowan, W.M., 1972, Studies on the development of the chick optic tectum. III. Effects of early eye removal. Brain Res. 42:263-288.

Kikuchi, T. and Ashmore, C.R., 1976, Developmental aspects of the innervation of skeletal muscle fibers in the chick embryo, Cell Tiss. Res. 171:233-251.

Kollros, J.J., 1953, The development of the optic lobes in the frog. I. The effects of unilateral enucleation in embryonic stages, J. Exp. Zool. 123:153-187.

Kollros, J.J., 1982, Peripheral control of midbrain mitotic activity in the frog, J. Comp. Neurol. 205:171-178.

Laing, N. and Prestige, M., 1978, Prevention of spontaneous motoneurone death in chick embryos, J. Physiol. 282:33-34P.

Lamb, A.H., 1976, The projection patterns of the ventral horn in the hindlimb during development, Dev. Biol. 52:82-99.

Lamb, A.H., 1979, Ventral horn cell counts in Xenopus with naturally occurring supernumerary hindlimbs, J. Embryol. Exp. Morph. 49:13-16.

Lamb, A.H., 1980, Motoneurone counts in Xenopus frogs reared with one bilaterally-innervated hindlimb, Nature 284:347-350.

Lamb, A.H., 1981, Target dependency of developing motoneurons in Xenopus laevis, Comp. Neurol. 203:157-171.

Lance-Jones, C. and Landmesser, L., 1981, Pathway selection by embryonic chick motoneurons in an experimentally altered environment, Proc. Roy. Soc. Lond. B, 214:19-52.

Lance-Jones, C., 1982, Motoneuron cell death in the developing lumbar spinal cord of the mouse, Dev. Brain Res. (in press).

Landmesser, L., 1980, The generation of neuromuscular specificity, Ann. Rev. Neurosci. 3:279-302.

Landmesser, L. and Morris, D.G., 1975, The development of functional innervation in the hind limb of the chick embryo, J. Physiol. 249:301-326.

Landmesser, L. and Pilar, G., 1972, The onset and development of transmission in the chick ciliary ganglion, J. Physiol. 222:691-713.

Landmesser, L. and Pilar, G., 1974, Synapse formation during embryogenesis on ganglion cells lacking a periphery, J. Physiol. 241:714-736.

Landmesser, L. and Pilar, G., 1978, Interactions between neurons and
    their targets during in vivo synaptogenesis, Fed. Proceed.
    37:2016-2022.
Lentz, T.L., Addis, J.S. and Chester, J., 1981, Partial purification
    and characterization of a nerve trophic factor regulating muscle
    acetylcholinesterase activity, Exp. Neurol. 73:542-557.
Levi-Montalcini, R., 1972, The morphological effects of immunosym-
    pathectomy. in: Immunosympathectomy, (G. Steiner and
    E. Schonbaum, eds.) New York, Elsevier, pp. 55-78.
Levi-Montalcini, R., 1974, NGF: an uncharted route in: The Neuro-
    sciences: Paths of Discovery, (F.G. Worden, J.P. Swazey and
    G. Adelman, eds.), Cambridge, MIT Press pp. 245-265.
Levi-Montalcini, R. and Levi, G., 1942, Les conséquences de la des-
    truction d'un territoire d'innervation périphérique sur le
    développment des centres nerveux correspondants dans l'embryon
    de poulet, Arch. Biol. 53:537-545.
Levi-Montalcini, R. and Levi, G., 1944, Correlazioni nello sviluppo
    tra varie parti del sistema nervoso. I. Consequenze della demo-
    lizione dell'abbozoo di um arto sui centri nervosi cell'embrione
    di pollo, Comment. Pontif. Acad. Sci. 8:527-578.
Lewis, J., 1980, Death and the neurone, Nature 284:305-306.
Lomo, T., 1980, What controls the development of neuromuscular
    junctions? Trends Neurosci. 3:126-219.
Lyles, J.M. and Barnard, E.A., 1980, Disappearance of the endplate
    form of acetylcholinesterase from a slow tonic muscle, FEBS
    Lett. 109:9-12.
Lyles, J.M., Silman, I. and Barnard, E.A., 1979, Developmental
    changes in levels and forms of cholinesterases in muscles of
    normal and dystrophic chickens, J. Neurochem. 33:727-738.
MacNaughton, J.V., 1974, An ultrastructural and histochemical study
    of fibre types in the pectoralis thoracica and iliotibialis
    muscles of the fowl, J. Anat. 118:171-186.
McLennan, I.S., 1981, Size of motoneuron pool is related to number of
    myotubes in developing muscle, Soc. Neurosci. Abstract, 7:291.
Maderdrut, J.L., and Oppenheim, R.W., 1982, Reduction of naturally-
    occurring cell death in the thoraco-lumber and sacral pregan-
    glionic cell column of the chick embryo following blockade of
    ganglionic transmission, Soc. Neurosci. Abstract 8:1638.
Markelonis, G.J., Oh, T.H., Elderfrawi, M.E. and Guth, L., 1982,
    Sciatin: A myotrophic protein increases the number of acetyl-
    choline receptors and receptor clusters in cultured skeletal
    muscle, Dev. Biol. 89:383-361.
Massoulie, J. and Bon, S., 1982, The molecular forms of cholinester-
    ase and acetylcholinesterase in vertebrates, Ann. Rev. Neurosci.
    5:57-106.
Murphy, B.J., 1977, An analysis of myogenic and neurogenic influences
    on the development of muscular dystrophy in the chick embryo,
    Dissertation, Louisiana State University Medical Center.

Nishi, R. and Berg, D., 1981, Two components from eye tissue that differentially stimulate the growth and development of ciliary ganglion neurons in culture, J. Neurosci. 1:505-513.

Nurcombe, V., McGrath, P.A. and Bennett, M.R., 1981, Postnatal death of motor neurons during the development of the brachial spinal cord of the rat, Neurosci. Lett. 27:249-254.

Okada, N. and Oppenheim, R.W., 1981, Developmental changes in the lateral motor column of the chick embryo following either spinal transection or neural crest removal, Soc. Neurosci. Abstract. 7:291.

O'Leary, D.D.M. and Cowan, W.M., 1981, Further observations on the development of the nucleus of origin of centrifugal fibers in the avian retina, Soc. Neurosci. Abstract 7:293.

Ontell, M., 1977, Neonatal muscle: an electron microscopic study, Anat. Rec. 189:669-690.

Ontell, M. and Dunn, R.F., 1978, Neonatal muscle growth: a quantitative study, Amer. J. Anat. 152:539-556.

Oppenheim, R.W., 1975, The role of supraspinal input in embryonic motility: a re-examination in the chick, J. Comp. Neurol. 160:37-50.

Oppenheim, R.W., 1981a, Neuronal cell death and some related regressive phenomena during neurogenesis: a selective historical review and progress report. In: Studies in Developmental Neurobiology, Essays in Honor of Viktor Hamburger, (W.M. Cowan, ed.), New York, Oxford University Press, pp. 74-133.

Oppenheim, R.W., 1981b, Cell death of motoneurons in the chick embryo spinal cord. V. Evidence on the role of cell death and neuromuscular function in the formation of specific peripheral connections, J. Neurosci. 1:141-151.

Oppenheim, R.W., 1981c, Ontogenetic adaptations and retrogressive processes in the development of the nervous system and behavior. A neuroembryological perspective, in Maturation and Development: Biological and Psychological Perspectives, (K. Connolly and H. Prechtl, eds.), Philadelphia, J.P. Lippincott, pp. 73-109.

Oppenheim, R.W., 1982, Preformation and epigenesis in the origins of the nervous system and behavior: Issues, concepts and their history. In: Perspectives in Ethology, vol. 5 . (P. Bateson and P. Klopfer, eds.), New York, Plenum, (in press).

Oppenheim, R.W., 1982, Reduction of neuronal death by embryonic neuromuscular blockade persists after hatching, Soc. Neurosci. Abstract 8:708.

Oppenheim, R.W., and Chu-Wang, I.-W., 1977, Spontaneous cell death of spinal motoneurons following peripheral innervation in the chick embryo, Brain Res. 125:154-160.

Oppenheim, R.W. and Chu-Wang, I.-W., 1982, Aspects of naturally-occurring cell death in the chick spinal cord: somatic motoneurons. In: Somatic and Autonomic Nerve-Muscle Interactions, (G. Burnstock, G. Vrbova and R. O'Brien, eds.), Elsevier/North-Holland, Amsterdam (in press).

Oppenheim, R.W. and Maderdrut, J.L., 1981, Pharmacological modulation of neuromuscular transmission and cell death in the lateral motor column of the chick embryo, Soc. Neurosci. Abstract 7:291.

Oppenheim, R.W., Maderdrut, J.L. and Wells, D., 1982, Cell death of motoneurons in the chick embryo spinal cord VI. Reduction of naturally-occurring cell death in the thoraco-lumbar column of Terni by nerve growth factor, J. Comp. Neurol. (in press).

Oppenheim, R.W. and Majors-Willard, C., 1978, Neuronal cell death in the brachial spinal cord of the chick is unrelated to the loss of polyneuronal innervation in wing muscle, Brain Res. 154:148-152.

Oppenheim, R.W. and Nunez, R., 1982, Electrical stimulation of hindlimb increases neuronal cell death in chick embryo, Nature 295:57-59.

Oppenheim, R.W., Rose, L.L. and Stokes, B., 1982, Cell death of motoneurons in the chick embyro spinal cord. VII. The survival of brachial motoneurons in dystrophic chickens, Exp. Neurol. (in press).

Oppenheimer, J., 1967, Essays in the History of Embryology and Biology, Cambridge, MIT Press.

Parks, T.N., 1979, Afferent influences on the development of the brain stem auditory nuclei of the chicken; otocyst ablation, J. Comp. Neurol. 183:665-678.

Pearson, J., Axelrod, F. and Dancis, J., 1974, Current concepts of dysautonomia: neuropathological defects, Neurol. 21:486-493.

Pearson, J. and Pytel, B.A., 1978, Quantitative studies of sympathetic ganglia and spinal cord intermedio-lateral gray columns in familial dysautonomia, J. Neurol. Sci. 39:47-59.

Pettigrew, A.G., Lindeman, R. and Bennett, M.R., 1979, Development of the segmental innervation of the chick forelimb, J. Embryol. Exp. Morph. 49:115-137.

Pittman, R. and Oppenheim, R.W., 1979, Cell death of motoneurons in the chick embryo spinal cord, IV. Evidence that a functional neuromuscular interaction is involved in the regulation of naturally occurring cell death and stabilization of synapses, J. Comp. Neurol. 187:425-446.

Pockett, S., 1981, Elimination of polyneuronal innervation in proximal and distal leg muscles of chick embryos, Dev. Brain Res. 1:299-302.

Pollack, E.D., 1980, Target-dependent survival of tadpole spinal cord neurites in tissue culture, Neurosci. Lett. 16:269-274.

Pollack, E.D. and Muhlach, W.L., 1981, Stage dependency in eliciting target-dependent enhanced neurite outgrowth from spinal cord explants in vitro, Dev. Biol. 86:259-263.

Popiela, H. and Ellis, S., 1981, Neurotrophic factor: characterization and partial purification, Dev. Biol. 83:266-277.

Prestige, M., 1967, The control of cell number in the lumbar ventral horn during the development of Xenopus laevis tadpoles, J. Embryol. Exp. Morph. 18:359-387.

Purves, D., 1980, Neuronal competition, Nature 287:585–586.

Purves, D. and Lichtman, J.W., 1980, Elimination of synapses in the developing nervous system, Science 210:153–157.

Romer, A. 1927, The development of the thigh musculature of the chick, J. Morph and Physiol. 43:347–385.

Roux, W., 1894, The problems, methods, and scope of developmental mechanics (transl. by W.M. Wheeler) in Woods Hole Biological Lectures, Marine Biological Station, Woods Hole, 8th Lecture: 149–189.

Ruffolo, R.R., Eisenbarth, G.S., Thompson, J.M. and Nirenberg, M., 1978, Synapse turnover: a mechanism for acquiring synaptic specificity, Proc. Natl. Acad. Sci. USA. 75: 2281–2285.

Sanes, J.R. and Hall, Z.W., 1979, Antibodies that bind specifically to synaptic sites on muscle fiber basal lamina, J. Cell Biol. 83:357–370.

Sanes, J.R., Marshall, L.M. and McMahan, U.J., 1978, Reinnervation of muscle fiber basal lamina after removal of myofibers, J. Cell Biol. 78:176–198.

Scaravilli, F. and Duchen, L.W., 1980, Electron microscopic and quantitative studies of cell necrosis in developing sensory ganglia in normal and Sprawling mutant mice, J. Neurocytol.9:373–380.

Schaub, M.C. and Watterson, J.G., 1981, Control of the contractile process in muscle, Trends Pharmacol. Sci. 2:279–282.

Schwartz, J.P and Breakfield, X.O., 1980, Altered nerve growth factor in fibroblasts from patients with familial dysautonomia, Proc. Natl. Acad. Sci. USA 77:1154–1158.

Silver, J., 1978, Cell death during development of the nervous system, in: Handbook of Sensory Physiology, vol. 9 (M. Jacobson, ed.), Berlin, Springer, pp. 419–436.

Singer, M., 1959, The influence of nerves on regeneration, in: Regeneration in Vertebrates, (C.S. Thornton, ed.), Chicago, University of Chicago, pp. 59–80.

Smith, R.G. and Appel, S.H., 1981, Evidence for a skeletal muscle protein that enhances neuron survival, neurite extension and acetylcholine (ACh) synthesis, Soc. Neurosci Abstract 7:144.

Stockdale, F.E., Raman, N. and Baden, H., 1981, Myosin light chains and the developmental origin of fast muscle, Proc. Natl. Acad. Sci. USA. 78:931–935.

Sullivan, G.E., 1962, Anatomy and embryology of the wing musculature of the domestic fowl, Austral. J. Zool. 10:458–518.

Susheela, A.K. Seraydarian, M. and Abbott, B.C., 1980, Increase of alpha motor neurons in chicken afflicted with muscular dystrophy, Exp. Neurol. 67:453–458.

Swett, J., Eldred, E. and Buchwald, J.A., 1970, Somatotopic cord-to-muscle relations in efferent innervation of cat gastrocnemius, Amer. J. Physiol. 40:762–766.

Thoenen, H. and Barde, Y.-A., 1980, Physiology of nerve growth factor, Physiol. Rev. 60:1284–1335.

Thoenen H., Otten, U., and Schwab, M., 1979, Orthograde and retro-
    grade signals for the regulation of neuronal gene expression:
    the peripheral sympathetic nervous system as a model. In: The
    Neurosciences, Fourth Study Program, (F.O. Schmitt and F.G.
    Worden eds.), Cambridge, Massachusetts, MIT Press, pp. 911-928.
Twitty, V., 1932, Influence of the eye on the growth of its associ-
    ated structures, studied by means of heteroplastic transplant-
    ation, J. Exp. Zool. 61:333-374.
Varon, S.S. and Bunge, R.P., 1978, Trophic mechanisms in the periph-
    eral nervous system, Ann. Rev. Neurosci. 1:327-361.
Vrbova, G., Gordon, T. and Jones, R., 1978, Nerve-Muscle Inter-
    actions. London, Chapman and Hall.
Weeds, A., 1978, Myosin: polymorphism and promiscuity, Nature
    274:417-418.
Wenger, E.L., 1950, An experimental analysis of relations between
    parts of the brachial spinal cord of the embryonic chick,
    J. Exp. Zool. 114:51-85.

THE SPROUTING AND DISTRIBUTION OF SENSORY NERVE ENDINGS

Jack Diamond

Department of Neurosciences
McMaster University
Hamilton, Ontario, Canada

INTRODUCTION

The innervation of skin provides an instructive system for revealing some of the mechanisms that regulate the sprouting and distribution of axonal endings at target tissues.

The Stimulus for Nerves to Sprout

The sprouting of cutaneous sensory nerves appears to result from the action of sprouting agents manufactured in the skin itself. Ramon y Cajal (1919) noted that during primary development axons destined to innervate epithelial tissues begin extensive sprouting only when they arrive at their target tissues, and was the first to suggest that such tissues must be the source of sprouting agents. In preliminary experiments with Xenopus tissues (Mearow et al., 1981), in which explants of whole skin or of separated epidermis were co-cultured with explants of sensory ganglia, we observed that neurite outgrowth was not only more profuse from the side of the ganglion explant nearer to the skin but the neurites that appeared to survive for more than 1-2 weeks were those that actually invaded the explant; neurites that originally grew out into the medium away from the skin fragment soon tended to regress. Additional evidence for the ability of skin to promote sprouting of cutaneous nerves comes from the observation that an increase in skin thickness in vivo, produced by a variety of means, is associated with an extensive invasion of neurites into the "extra" cutaneous tissue (Fitzgerald et al., 1975). Experimentally the most convenient way of evoking sprouting (in this instance of mature nerves that already

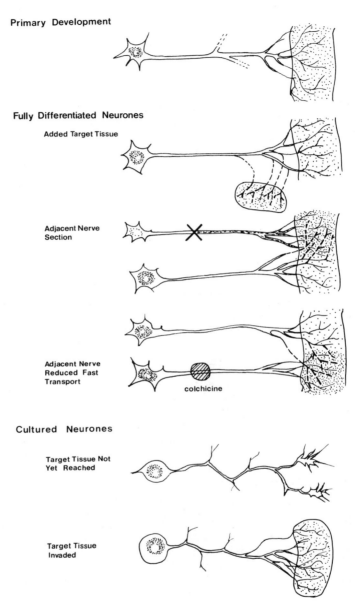

Figure 1. Diagrammatic representation of various conditions in which neurons sprout because of influences exerted by their target tissues; the tissues are shown on the right. The dashed lines in the examples of the sprouting of differentiated neurons represent new collaterals.

have made their functional contacts with their target tissue) is
the partial denervation of the tissue; both in the salamander and
in the mammal (Diamond et al., 1976), such deprived skin eventually
becomes functionally invaded by collateral growth from the remaining, spared, axons. Dorsal root ganglion (DRG) neurons are known
to be sensitive to nerve growth factor (NGF) only during embryonic
life (Johnson et al., 1980; Gorin and Johnson, 1980), so the presumed factors in skin that evoke the sprouting of cutaneous sensory
nerves in the adult are not identical with NGF. This hypothesis
has not yet been tested, however, by evoking sprouting into denervated skin in animals treated with anti-NGF serum (Levi-Montalcini
and Angeletti, 1968).

The Biological Function of Sprouting

     Sprouting is a mechanism that provides the target tissue with
an adequate number of endings. That the sprouting is largely confined to the target tissue itself, however, needs further comment.
Evolutionary pressures seem to have forced a minimum size on peripheral target tissues (muscles and skin). If all the possible
target sites within tissues were to be innervated by individual
neurons, or shared to only a minor degree among the arriving axons,
then the peripheral nerves, and the various fiber tracts and pathways within the central nervous system (CNS), would need to be dis-
proportionately large relative to the sizes of organisms that have
evolved. Of course the space problem could have been resolved if
all axons had very small diameters. Clearly the disadvantage of
the very slow conduction velocities associated with fine fibers has
made this an unviable solution, and the much more favorable one of
having at least a population of larger axons traversing the major
part of nerve pathways has evolved. Thus a single axon can convey
high velocity impulses to the vicinity of the target tissue and
then, through the provision of a multitude of fine (slowly con-
ducting) collaterals, accommodate a relatively unimportant incre-
ment of time to cover the short distance that remains to the final
target sites. Along with this solution go the additional advantages of having a target tissue supplied by a number of neurons
that differ in the extent of their individual control of that
tissue, largely through differences in the number of functional
collaterals they make. This means of ensuring that a given number
of axons provides enough endings for a much larger number of target
sites is found to be associated with another apparently advantageous feature, namely the ability of the target tissue itself to
provide the necessary stimulus for axons to sprout. Thus the gross
size of the target tissue is likely to be an important factor in
evoking an appropriate amount of sprouting. What seems to have
evolved is a means of producing a local excess of sprouting, with
the development of ancillary mechanisms for the regulation of competition among endings for target sites, the subsequent synaptogenesis and the elimination of excess endings.

How Could Endings Become Appropriately Distributed in the
Absence of Recognizable Targets?

    The two basic questions considered here are what determines
the number of sprouts that will survive, and where these will end
within a target tissue in which there are no specific target cells
or target sites. An hypothesis can be suggested to explain the ap-
propriateness of the distribution of endings, particularly those
within skin, based upon the local provision of sprouting factors
from the target tissue itself. If the elongation of individual
sprouts were also dependent on these sprouting factors, then any
mechanism that could reduce the effective concentration of these
factors, or offset their activity in some way, could help regulate
both the number of sprouts being produced and the extent of their
elongation. The problem was noted by Ramon y Cajal (1919) who
reasoned that the likeliest entity that could effectively regulate
the provision of the hypothesized local growth factor would be
the nerves themselves. We ourselves, starting from a somewhat different consideration than did Cajal, arrived at a similar conclusion;
we were dealing not with primary development as did Cajal, but with
the axonal sprouting that occurs within tissues that have been partially denervated (Aguilar et al., 1973). We hypothesized that the
explanation of such sprouting could be (a) that nerves are normally
involved in a continual suppression either of the provision, or the
effectiveness, of sprouting agents produced locally by the skin,
and (b) that the maintenance of this neural function could well
depend upon the continual provision of some appropriate agents supplied to the terminals by (fast) axoplasmic transport. When nerves
are cut the supply of these agents is eventually eliminated, leading
to a reduction in the periphery of the neural "neutralizing" influence, and a consequent increase in the effectiveness of the local
sprouting factors. Spared axons would then be stimulated to produce more sprouts until their suppressive influence was able to
restore an equilibrium. Such a mechanism could explain the sprouting (and its eventual cessation) that occurs both during primary
development and also that evoked by partial denervation. We tested
the hypothesis by using colchicine to reduce the fast transport in
selected nerves in the salamander (Aguilar et al., 1973); the
result was that untreated neighboring nerves sprouted to hyperinner-
vate the skin (and indeed the muscles) already innervated by the
colchicine-treated nerves. Although the latter retained their
normal sensory functions (Cooper et al., 1977), the untreated
nerves sprouted just as though the colchicine-treated ones had been
cut. These findings were consistent with our hypothesis, although
we cannot deduce from them whether the effect of the nerves is to
release an agent that interferes with the production or the action
of the proposed sprouting factors produced by the skin, or whether
nerve sprouts reduce the local level of these factors by active uptake into the terminals (Diamond, 1982a). What our results did
suggest is that some agent(s) carried continually in axoplasmic

transport are required for the regulatory action of the nerves to
be expressed. The hypothesis could, of course, be applicable to
the nervous system generally. Figure 1 summarizes various conditions that have in common the promotion of sprouting by target
tissues in which presumed sprouting agents are effective either
because of an absent or reduced innervation, or because of a reduced axoplasmic transport in some of the nerves. Of great relevance to the hypothesized role of nerves in the regulation of
sprouting agents are the findings that the level of NGF in rat iris
is high when the tissue is denervated, and low when innervated
(Ebendal et al., 1980).

     In skin, the consequence of such mechanisms operating at nerve
endings is that individual terminals would eventually be surrounded
by a local territory within which the effective sprouting stimulus
would be too low to evoke either the further sprouting, or the continued elongation, of the particular ending within that territory
(Fig. 2A). A further likely consequence would be a roughly uniform
distribution of endings, and this is what presumably occurs. Many
nerve endings in skin induce the differentiation of specific end
organs [e.g., the Pacinian corpuscle (Zelena, 1980), and Grandry
corpuscles (Saxod, 1978)] and we may suppose that the inductive influence can only become effective when the growth of the ending has
ceased. The possibility certainly exists that sprouting agents may
not be produced uniformly across the skin, and therefore that non-
uniform populations of specific types of endings, with or without
associated end organs, will occur.

The Role of Specific Target Cells: The Merkel Cells

     The provision of specific target cells that arriving sensory
axons could recognize (and possibly be attracted to) would mean that
the distribution of the endings is determined by the distribution of
the targets.   We have provided evidence that in the epidermis of
lower vertebrates the scattered Merkel cells do indeed act as specific targets for low-threshold mechanosensory axons (Scott et al.,
1981a). Moreover, both in lower vertebrates (Tweedle, 1978) and in
the mammal (Lyne and Hollis, 1971; Hashimoto, 1972; Call and Bell,
1979) epidermal Merkel cells can be distinguished in the electron
microscope before their innervation is detectable, thus it seems
likely that in the mammal too Merkel cells differentiate as targets
for the arriving nerves. We cannot be certain though whether in
the mammal this differentiation of Merkel cells would occur if the
nerves were prevented totally from having access to the skin during
development; in recent experiments we are finding that there is a
nerve dependency of a population (about half) of the Merkel cells
within the touch domes of adult rat skin (Nurse et al., 1982).   In
the salamander however, all the Merkel cells seem to survive denervation, and act as targets for nerves; moreover in newly regenerated skin, even that which can develop on a limb that is totally

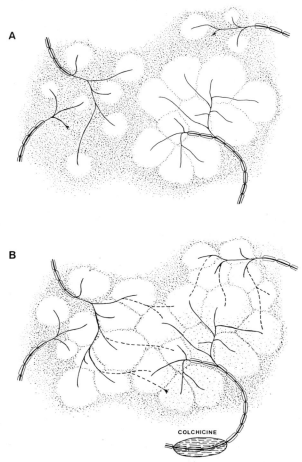

Figure 2. Diagrammatic representations of situations predicted by
the sprouting hypothesis: A. Nerve endings eventually become
associated with individual local territories within the target
tissue. B. When fast transport is reduced in one axon, its terminal
territories are invaded by collaterals (shown dashed) from neighboring normal axons. In both diagrams the density of the stippling
indicates the effective level of presumed sprouting factor in the
target tissue.

denervated, new Merkel cells differentiate, and these too act as targets for nerves that are allowed to regenerate back into that region (Scott et al., 1981a).

The hypothesis described above (Section 3) to account for the distribution of "free" nerve endings is compatible with the existence of specific target cells, such as Merkel cells, which may be the source of appropriate sprouting factors, and may also be able to instruct the neurites that contact them to cease their growth. We have suggestive evidence in the salamander that the sprouting of intact untreated nerves which results from the reduction of axoplasmic transport in neighboring nerves may result in the hyperinnervation of "touch spots" supplied by the treated nerves (Cooper et al., 1977; see Fig. 2B); a touch spot probably includes a single Merkel cell, and in normal skin this is innervated by endings of a single axon [although one axon may innervate many Merkel cells (Cooper and Diamond, 1977)]. We can infer therefore that the target character of the Merkel cell is itself regulated by the nerve, and that this regulation too is dependent upon some agent carried in the fast axoplasmic transport.

The provision by Merkel cells of a specific sprouting factor for a specific group of sensory axons would not be surprising. In the leech (Blackshaw et al., 1982) when a cell of one cutaneous sensory modality is eliminated, only axons of that modality sprout in response, suggesting the possibility that there are specific sprouting factors for axons subserving different sensory modalities. However, all such findings (including ours described above) are also consistent with the existence of a single sprouting factor produced by skin, coupled with an ability of different nerves to recognize their appropriate target sites, and only then to develop their characteristic sensory functions.

Thus another role for target cells could be the triggering of the differentiation of the nerve endings into functional sensory receptors; this differentiation might occur automatically when elongation of the neurite ceased and, as was suggested above, one function of the target cell could be to cause the neurite to stop growing. While it is true that the ends of regenerating sensory axons may be more susceptible than usual to non-characteristic stimuli [for example regenerating pain nerves are readily excited by mechanical stimulation, hence Tinel's sign in humans (Henderson, 1948)], it seems that specific sensory functions only develop when the endings are within the skin, and have presumably ceased or drastically reduced their elongation, perhaps because they have arrived at characteristic end-sites within that tissue.

Finally, the type of physiological function that the sensory nerve ending will develop could itself be determined by a target cell, i.e. the latter could be instructive, and not merely permis-

sive, in this regard. A recent report has suggested the possibility
that carotid body glomus cells transplanted to skeletal muscle sites
could become contacted by mechanosensory axons which then develop
chemosensitivity while maintaining mechanosensitive properties
(Monti-Bloche et al., 1981). It has yet to be shown however, that
among the axons in muscle available to innervate such transplanted
glomus tissue, there were not some already chemically sensitive
ones which were therefore being "selected" as appropriate to innervate the chemosensory cells; there is evidence that skeletal muscle
is normally supplied by large diameter, but mechanically relatively
insensitive, axons which are excited by the kind of ischemic conditions that are appropriate for producing carotid body chemosensory
discharges (Hink and Payne, 1965). The exact role of glomus cells
in the chemosensory transduction process is still unclear (McDonald,
1981), as is that of Merkel cells in mechanosensory function.

Competition Among Nerve Endings for Targets

     The evoking of collateral sprouting by factors made in target
tissues was suggested above as very likely to result in an initial
excess of terminals, even though the axons themselves could be
responsible for eventually eliminating the effectiveness of the
sprouting stimulus at their endings. It would not be surprising
though if, during the attainment of the final equilibrium situation,
more endings were produced than a population of targets or target
sites could accommodate. There would then be a potential, or real,
competition among the endings for these sites. Such competition
could in theory occur at any stage, e.g. after endings had made
contact with targets [i.e. after an initial hyperinnervation of
targets had occurred (see Diamond, 1979)], or earlier, when growing
terminals had not yet reached their targets. Eventually the excess
endings (the losers in the competition) would probably need to be
eliminated, although the continued existence of non-functioning terminals is a possibility, and could even confer advantages on the
organism possesssing them (e.g. Cass et al., 1973); it should be
pointed out however that in vivo there is no direct evidence for the
occurrence of maintained non-functional terminals.

     Many conditions have been identified in skin which suggest how
the outcome of competition among nerves can be influenced, and these
have been discussed in detail elsewhere (Diamond, 1982a, b). Some
observations of special relevance to the present discussion will be
mentioned. From what has been said earlier, it appears that fast
axoplasmic transport is involved in the regulation by nerves not
only of the sprouting factors, but of the target character of target
cells. In the salamander this axonal influence is very potent, and
except in one experimental circumstance Merkel cells seem never to
become innervated (at least functionally) by the endings of more
than one axon (Scott et al., 1981a, b); the exception is the situation described above in which reduced transport in some of the

nerves supplying skin was followed by an apparent hyperinnervation
of touch spots, and thus probably of single Merkel cells (Cooper et
al., 1977). Since the evidence was physiological the latter probability can only be inferred. Our salamander studies suggest that
in the competition, the first ending to arrive at a nerve-free
Merkel cell captured it, and caused its target character to disappear
(Diamond, 1979). This latter effect depends on a maintained transport in the axons; when this was reduced not only did other axons
sprout (due to the increased effectiveness of the local supply of
sprouting factor) but those sprouts were now able to recognize
Merkel cells still innervated by endings of the treated axon, and
to make functional associations with them. In the salamander then,
the most important item (other things being equal) in a potential
competition among nerve endings would seem to be the timing; the
first to arrive wins. Nevertheless this simple strategy could, in
theory, be upset by variations among competing axons in the fast
transport in them of the agent(s) involved in this target regulation.

In mammalian skin a comparable competitive situation can be produced, but here timing is not the most important consideration,
since later-arriving nerves can displace those already resident and
functioning in the target tissue. In these experiments the skin of
rats was denervated, and subsequently became invaded by collateral
sprouts from intact, spared, nerves in neighboring skin; later the
originally cut nerves regenerated, and both the high-treshold noci-
ceptive fibers (Devor et al., 1979; Diamond, 1981) and the low-
threshold mechanosensory ones (Jackson and Diamond, 1981) invaded
the regions occupied by the sprouted nerves, which functionally
seemed to disappear from this territory. We are particularly interested in the competition specifically for the mechanosensory structures in the skin known as touch domes, each of which contains
scores of Merkel cells (Nurse et al., 1981; Nurse et al., in
press). At the height of the struggle between the two classes of
nerves the mechanical stimulation of identified domes evokes impulses
in both the sprouted and the regenerated nerve. Our preliminary
results (Diamond et al., in press) indicate that this competition
for touch domes occurs at the level of the individual Merkel cells,
since endings of both the sprouted and the regenerated nerve were
revealed on a single cell. Eventually however the sprouted ones
disappear. Could it be that the axoplasmic transport of presumed
agents to the sprouted endings is insufficient to permit an adequate
structural association to be formed? This might be the consequence
of the terminal fields of the neurons having become too large to be
adequately "nourished" from the soma (see e.g. Wigston, 1980).
There are other possible explanations (see Diamond, 1982a).

Recently we have obtained indications that during development
there is a true hyperinnervation of single Merkel cells within rat
touch domes, the excess endings disappearing over the first few
weeks of life to reach the normal adult situation of a single ending

per innervated Merkel cell (Diamond et al., in press). When this
hyperinnervation involves two axons (as in our investigated situations) we can invoke similar explanations involving differences in
axoplasmic transport.

Finally, the known characteristics of membranes that are likely
to be involved in adhesion between cells (e.g. Gottleib and Glasser,
1980) can be used to construct hypotheses to explain how, at the
molecular level, one ending could displace another from target cells
(Diamond, 1982a); the proposed mechanisms can be made readily compatible with a role for specific axoplasmically transported agents.
We can anticipate that eventual molecular descriptions of the phenomenon of competition will tie in closely with those of the action
and regulation of sprouting factors.

Acknowledgements

The investigations mentioned in this article were supported by a
grant from the Medical Research Council of Canada, and by U.S. Public
Health Services Research Grant (NS 15992).

References

Aguilar, C.E., Bisby, M.A., Cooper, E. and Diamond, J., 1973,
      Evidence that axoplasmic transport of trophic factors is
      involved in the regulation of peripheral nerve fields in
      salamanders, J. Physiol., 234:449-464.
Blackshaw, S.E., Nicholls, J.G., and Parnas, I., 1982, Expanded
      receptive fields of cutaneous mechanoreceptor cells after
      single neurone deletion in leech central nervous system,
      J. Physiol. (Lond), 326:261-268.
Call, T.W. and Bell, M., 1979, Ultrastructural features of Merkel
      cells during murine ontogenetic differentiation, Anat. Rec.,
      193:495.
Cass, D.T., Sutton, T.J. and Mark, R.F., 1973, Competition between
      nerves for functional connexions with Axolotl muscle, Nature,
      243:201-203.
Cooper, E., and Diamond, J., 1977, A quantitative study of the
      mechanosensory innervation of salamander skin, J. Physiol.,
      264:695-723.
Cooper, E., Diamond, J., and Turner, C., 1977, The effects of nerve
      section and of colchicine treatment on the density of mechano-
      sensory nerve endings in salamander skin, J. Physiol. (Lond.),
      264:725-759.
Devor, M., Schonfield, D., Seltzer, Z., and Wall, P.D., 1979, Two
      modes of cutaneous reinnervation following peripheral nerve
      injury, J. Comp. Neurol., 185:211-220.

Diamond, J., 1979, The regulation of nerve sprouting by extrinsic influences, in: The Neurosciences Fourth Study Program, (F.O. Schmitt and F.G. Worden, editors-in-chief), M.I.T. Press, Cambridge, Mass., pp. 937-955.

Diamond, J., 1981, The recovery of sensory function in skin after peripheral nerve lesions, in: Post-Traumatic Peripheral Nerve Regeneration: Experimental Basis and Clinical Implications, (A. Gorio et al., eds.), Raven Press, N.Y., pp. 533-548.

Diamond, J., 1982a, Modelling and competition in the nervous system: clues from the sensory innervation of skin, Curr. Top. Dev. Biol., 17:147-205.

Diamond, J., 1982b, The patterning of neuronal connections, Amer. Zool., 22:153-172.

Diamond, J., Cooper, E., Turner, C. and Macintyre, L., 1976, Trophic regulation of nerve sprouting, Science, 193:371-377.

Diamond, J., Macintyre, L., Nurse, C.A., and Visheau, B., in press, Modelling and remodelling within a cutaneous mechanosensory structure in rats, J. Physiol., (abstr.).

Ebendal, T., Olson, L., Seiger, A., and Hedlund, O., 1980, Nerve growth factors in the rat iris, Nature, 286:25-28.

Fitzgerald, M.J.T., Folan, J.C., and O'Brien, T.M., 1975, The innervation of hyperplastic epidermis in the mouse: a light microscopic study, J. Invest. Dermatol., 64:169-174.

Gottleib, D.I., and Glasser, L., 1980, Cellular recognition during neural development, Ann. Rev. Neurosci., 3:303-318.

Gorin, P.D. and Johnson, E.M., 1980, Effects of long-term nerve growth factor deprivation on the nervous system of the adult rat: an experimental autoimmune approach, Brain Res., 198:27-42.

Hashimoto, K., 1972, The ultrastructure of the skin in human embryos, J. Anat., 111:99-120.

Henderson, W.R., 1948, Clinical assessment of peripheral nerve injury. Tinel's test, Lancet, 2:801.

Hnik, P., and Payne, R., 1965, Spontaneous activity in nonproprioceptive sensory fibres from de-efferented muscles, J. Physiol., 180:25-26P.

Jackson, P.C., and Diamond, J., 1981, Regenerating axons reclaim sensory targets from collateral nerve sprouts, Science, 214:926-928.

Johnson, E.M., Gorin, P.D., Brandeis, L.D., and Pearson, J., 1980, Dorsal root ganglion neurons are destroyed by exposure in utero to maternal antibody to nerve growth factor, Science, 210:916-918.

Levi-Montalcini, jR., and Angeletti, P.A., 1968, Nerve growth factor, Physiol. Rev., 48:534-569.

Lyne, A.G., and Hollis, D.E., 1971, Merkel cells in sheep during fetal development, J. Ultrastruc. Res., 34:464-472.

Macintyre, L., and Diamond, J., 1981, Domains and mechanosensory nerve fields in salamander skin, Proc. Roy. Soc. Lond. B., 211:471-499.

McDonald, D.M., 1981, Peripheral chemoreceptors: structure-function relationships of the carotid body, in: Regulation of Breathing. Part I, (Hornbein, T.F., Ed.) Marcel Deker, Inc., N.Y., pp. 105-317.

Mearow, K.M., Nurse, C.A., Visheau, B., and Diamond, J., 1981, Interactions between co-cultured amphibian sensory neurons and mechanosensory target tissues, Soc. for Neurosci. Abstr., 7:547.

Monti-Bloch, L., Stensaas, L.J., and Ezyaguirre, C., 1981, Induction of chemosensitivity in a muscle nerve after grafting the carotid body into the muscle, Soc. for Neurosci. Abstr., 7:469.

Nurse, C.A., Mearow, K.M., Vishea, B., Holmes, M., and Diamond, J., 1981, Comparison of the distribution of mechanosensory target (Merkel) cells in mammalian and amphibian epidermis using quinacrine fluorescence as a marker, Soc. for Neurosci. Abstr. 7:417.

Nurse, C.A., Macintyre, L., and Diamond, J., 1982, Effect of sensory denervation on the postnatal development of Merkel cells within the rat touch dome, Soc. for Neurosci. Abstr., 8:756.

Nurse, C.A., Mearow, K.M., Holmes, M., Visheau, B., and Diamond, J., (in press), Merkel cell distribution in various tissues using quinacrine fluorescence as a marker, Cell and Tiss. Res.

Ramon y Cajal, S., 1919, Studies on Vertebrate Neurogenesis, L. Guth trans., Charles C. Thomas (1960), Springfield, Ill.

Saxod, R., 1978, Avian mechanoreceptive corpuscles, in: Handbook of Sensory Physiology, Vol. 9, (M. Jacobson, Ed.), Springer-Verlag, N.Y., pp. 337-417.

Scott, S.A., Cooper, E., and Diamond, J., 1981a, Merkel cells as targets of the mechanosensory nerves in salamander skin, Proc. Roy. Soc. Lond. B., 211:455-470.

Scott, S.A., Macintyre, L.A., and Diamond, J., 1981b, Competitive reinnervation of salamander skin by regenerating and intact mechanosensory nerves, Proc. Roy. Soc. Lond. B., 211:501-511.

Tweedle, C.D., 1978, Ultrastructure of Merkel cell development in aneurogenic and control Amphibian larvae (Ambystoma), Neuroscience, 3:481-486.

Wigston, D.J., 1980, Suppression of sprouted synapses in axolotl muscle by transplanted foreign nerves, J. Physiol., 307:355-366.

Zelena, J., 1980, Rapid degeneration and regeneration of receptor organs, Brain Res., 187:97-111.

NERVE GROWTH-PROMOTING ACTIVITIES IN EMBRYONIC AND ADULT TISSUES

Ted Ebendal

Department of Zoology
Uppsala University
Uppsala, Sweden

ABSTRACT

Methods to establish the presence in tissues of nerve growth factor (NGF) and other promoters of nerve fiber growth are described. Evidence for a NGF-like activity in the rat iris and sciatic nerve obtained by bioassay is reviewed. Data are presented to indicate that the iris of the adult chick can also produce a NGF-like factor in culture. It is described that many tissues from the rat and embryonic chick contain additional substances eliciting fiber outgrowth in ciliary neurons not susceptible to the actions of NGF.

INTRODUCTION

How is nerve fiber growth regulated during the organization of an embryo? A concept generally accepted among developmental neurobiologists is that target areas provide messages to support the ingrowth of nerves and survival of innervating neurons. To reveal the nature of such target influences is a challenging task. As early as 1910, Harrison saw the possibility of studying nerves growing in culture in order to detect "attracting" influences from target tissues. Indeed, from the discovery of the protein NGF and its drastic stimulation of nerve fiber growth and neuron survival in vitro as well as in vivo it became clear that specific molecules can serve as target-to-neuron signals (Cohen et al., 1954; Levi-Montalcini, 1966; Thoenen and Barde, 1980).

Tissue explants were also found to stimulate neurite outgrowth in co-cultured ganglia (Ebendal and Jacobson, 1977). Such observa-

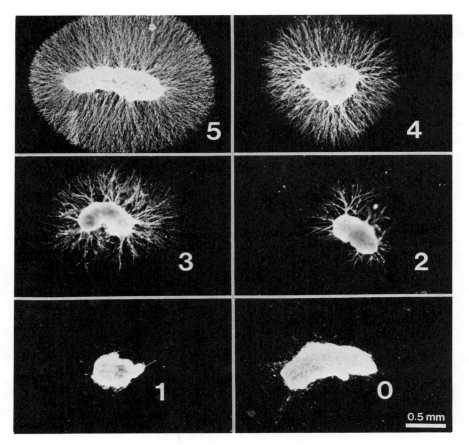

Fig. 1.   Graded fiber outgrowth responses to mouse NGF. Chick
sympathetic ganglia explanted to a collagen gel are shown. Scores
for ranking outgrowth densities are indicated. Note that the
ganglion scored zero shows total absence of nerve fibers although
some fibroblast-like cells show up around the explant. Dark-
field micrographs of living cultures, two days after initiation.

tions have prompted analysis of the substances evoking nerve fiber
outgrowth (by Varon and Adler, 1980). The present paper describes
work to establish the presence of NGF and other factors promoting
nerve growth in tissues of embryos and adults.

BIOASSAY OF NERVE GROWTH FACTOR

NGF bioassay is carried out in the author's laboratory with ganglia explanted to collagen gels. These gels are satisfactory for their resemblance to connective tissue matrices, their transparency (Elsdale and Bard, 1972) and their lack of endogenous factors evoking fiber growth. We routinely use sympathetic ganglia rather than the commonly used spinal ganglia from the chick embryo. In our experience the sympathetic neurons depend totally on added growth factors for neurite production. They also show minimum outgrowth of fibroblast-like cells.

In the first section it will be demonstrated how the cultures react to NGF from the mouse submandibular gland. By ranking the intensity of the neurite outgrowth as shown in Fig. 1 it is possible to determine the local levels of NGF sensed by the neurons (Campenot, 1977). Fig. 2 thus shows the relation between the concentration of NGF added to the gel and the resulting fiber ougrowth score obtained in blind tests. The classical 1 BU (biological unit) response is based on the maximum fiber outgrowth observed at the plateau of the dose-response curve (thus score 5 in Fig. 1). Increasing the level of NGF further results in successively thinner and more fasciculated fibers, until no fibers at all are seen projecting from the ganglion. The minimum amount of NGF that can be reliably detected in this bioassay is about 0.5-1 ng/ml (Fig. 2). Most useful for the identification of NGF in the bioassay is its specific antiserum. Fig. 3 shows the outcome of a titration of rabbit anti-NGF antiserum against a constant amount of mouse NGF. It is evident from the graph that anti-NGF blocks the fiber outgrowth response effectively, in this case up to 8,000-fold dilutions, whereas normal rabbit serum, even when present at 10% by volume, does not interfere with the detection of NGF. A limitation in the use of anti-NGF to identify NGFs from other species is the lowered cross-reactivity with increasing phylogenetic distance (Bailey et al., 1976; Harper and Thoenen, 1980b).

NGF DETECTION IN TISSUES

The NGF molecule purified from mouse salivary glands and from some other very rich sources (Chapman et al., 1979; Harper and Thoenen, 1980a, b) has been held as the model for target-supplied trophic factors likely to act in the growth of the nervous system (Varon and Adler, 1980). A role for NGF outside the salivary glands and the other localized sources is implied by the destructive effects on sympathetic neurons by injected anti-NGF antiserum (Levi-Montalcini, 1966) suggested to neutralize endogenous supplies of NGF (Ennis et al., 1979).

It is a paradox, however, as pointed out in extensive reviews by Thoenen and collaborators (Harper and Thoenen, 1980a, b; Thoenen and Barde, 1980), that critical attempts to directly demonstrate the

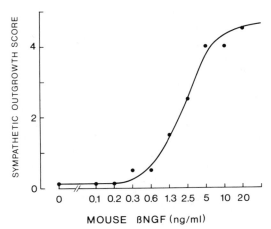

Fig. 2.   Does response of fiber outgrowth evoked by NGF. Sympathetic ganglia were scored as shown in Fig. 1 after two days of
incubation.   Scores were determined blind with the culture dishes
in random order.   The result shown is the outcome from one actual
experiment, but repeated experiments gave similar results.   The
NGF was prepared according to the method of Mobley et al. (1976)
and the protein content determined by the absorbance at 280 nm.

presence of NGF in tissues receiving sympathetic and sensory innervation have had little success.   One of the problems to measure NGF by
bioassay is that many living tissues put into culture (in order to
test conditioned media or to confront ganglia with tissue explants)
raise their apparent levels of NGF (Harper et al., 1980).   Also the
competition radioimmunoassays often used may give incorrect values
of NGF in homogenates due to interference from NGF-binding components (e.g. present in serum; see Suda et al., 1978; Harper and
Thoenen, 1980b).

The section below will describe work from our laboratory aimed
at establishing the presence of NGF in peripheral tissues.   In all
cases sympathetic ganglia from the chick embryo were used in the
collagen gels to probe NGF-like activity in the immediate environment of tissue explants.

NGF in the Adult Rat Iris

Studies of the rat iris were carried out in collaboration with
Drs. Lars Olson and Ake Seiger, Department of Histology at the
Karolinska Institute in Stockholm, Sweden.

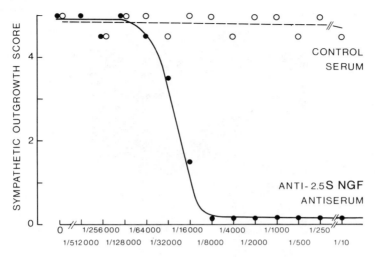

Fig. 3. Titration of anti-NGF antiserum. Nerve fiber outgrowths were determined as described in legends to Figs. 1 and 2. A constant amount of 20 ng/ml of NGF was present in the collagen gels also receiving serial dilutions of rabbit anti-2.5S NGF anti-serum (obtained commercially from Laref, Switzerland) or normal rabbit serum (serving as control). The normal serum from the rabbit did not interefere with neurite growth whereas the antiserum totally inhibited the fiber outgrowth at dilutions of 1:8,000 and lower (final dilution in the culture medium). The graph shows the actual result from one experiment but identical results were obtained in several tests.

Living explants of the iris released easily detectable amounts of NGF possible to block with antiserum to mouse NGF (Ebendal at al., 1980). An example of the response in a sympathetic ganglion to a co-cultured living rat iris is shown in Fig. 4.

In order to measure the level of NGF present initially, rather than after a day in culture, we used a protocol by which the iris was killed immediately after dissection by freezing and thawing. The killed tissue was then explanted to the collagen gel (Ebendal et al., 1980). This treatment did not harm the NGF-like activity accumulated in cultured irides. However, in normal irides little or no NGF was detected in general accordance with the findings by Harper et al. (1980).

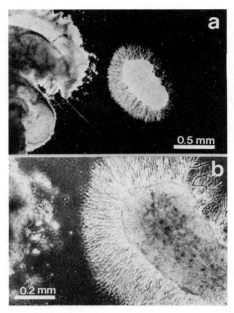

Fig. 4.   NGF-like activity released from a normal living rat iris
indicated by a heavy fibre outgrowth in a nearby sympathetic ganglion
(right). a, dark-field micrograph. b, close up of the interexplant
zone, phase contrast. The two tissues had been co-cultured for 22
hours when the photographs were taken. As described by Ebendal et
al. (1980) the response can be blocked with antiserum to mouse NGF.

        The method allowed us to study whether the low levels of de-
tectable NGF was linked through some mechanism to the full innervation of the iris.

        Such a relation did indeed exist. Killed explants prepared
little over one week after sensory denervation of the iris, showed
increased amounts of NGF (Ebendal et al., 1980). Sympathetic denervation had a similar but less dramatic effect on the amount of
NGF-like activity. These findings suggest that the presence of
nerve endings depress the NGF level, possibly by draining off NGF
or by inhibiting its synthesis. The extent to which nerves, other
than sensory and sympathetic, participate in the regulation of the
NGF level would be interesting to study.

NGF in the Rat Sciatic Nerve

An intriguing aspect is whether the NGF content of other tissues in the rat is also under similar nerve control. To examine this in neural pathways, possibly stimulating axonal regrowth after injury, the prsent bioassay was used to study the sciatic nerve of the rat as a source for NGF (in collaboration with Dr. Peter M. Richardson, Division of Neurosurgery, Montreal General Hospital, Canada). Once again we found only low levels of NGF-like activity in the sciatic nerve when killed by freezing and thawing immediately after removal from the leg (Richardson and Ebendal, 1982). As living explants, the sciatic nerve released NGF in considerable amounts. The same was true for sciatic nerves as autografts. A most interesting finding was that degenerating nerves distal to a cut contained increased levels of NGF two days after the operation, whereas after two weeks virtually no NGF-like activity was found (Richardson and Ebendal, 1982). Obviously, manipulating the nerve altered the amounts of detectable NGF. It is, however, not known whether the mechanism is the same as for the iris.

NGF in the Chick Iris

To demonstrate NGF in birds has been more difficult than in mammals. Firstly, no rich sources for an avian NGF are known. Secondly, antibodies to mouse NGF injected into chicks do not cause immunosympathectomy (e.g. unpublished results by I.A. Barde cited by Harper and Thoenen, 1981). The mere fact that avian neurons respond to NGF and can transport it retrogradely (Brunso-Bechtold and Hamburger, 1979) may be the best indications for a physiological role for an avian NGF. If so, the failure of antiserum to mouse NGF to effectively block endogenous avian NGF might be ascribed to the phylogenetical distance as mentioned above.

Nevertheless, there are claims in the literature that chick fibroblasts and ganglionic glial cells in culture release a molecular species cross-reacting with anti-(mouse) NGF (Varon et al., 1974; Young et al., 1975; Riopelle and Cameron, 1981). However, little support was found for the presence of NGF-like activity in homogenates of embryonic chick tissues (Riopelle and Cameron, 1981; Ebendal et al.; 1982).

To further study this paradox, the iris from one-year-old chicks was studied in a manner similar to that employed for the rat iris. The chick iris killed immediately evoked no obvious NGF-like response (Fig. 5) nor did anti-NGF significantly interfere with the few nerve fibers present (Table 1). In contrast, sympathetic ganglia co-cultured with a living chick iris, or confronted with a killed iris previously cultured for a day or two (Fig. 5), showed fairly dense fiber halos by the addition of anti-NGF (Fig. 5 and Table 1) indicating at least partial recognition between the growth-

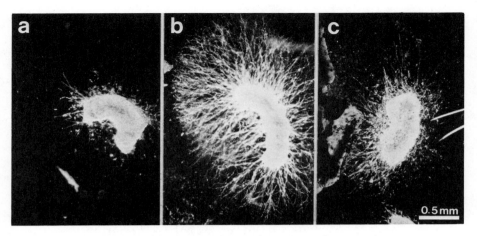

Fig. 5.   Cultures indicating the existence of an avian NGF cross-
reacting with anti-(mouse)NGF antiserum. a, sympathetic ganglion
co-explanted with an iris (to the left) taken from a one-year-old
chick and immediately killed by freezing-thawing. Only a weak
fiber outgrowth was evoked by this normal iris. b, a corresponding
iris cultured for two days before being frozen and thawed and explanted in a second culture gel with a sympathetic ganglion. A
fairly dense fiber halo is seen under these conditions. c, similar
to b but with antiserum to mouse 2.5S NGF (Laref) included in
the gel (final dilution 1:500). The inclusion of anti-NGF
distinctly lowered the fiber outgrowth response. Dark-field micrographs of cultures incubated for two days.

stimulating substance and anti-bodies to mouse NGF. This finding of
a source for an avian NGF-like activity is parallel to the results
from the rat iris and encourage the view that there are basic
similarities between birds and mammals concerning neuronal growth
factors and their regulation.

NON-NGF FACTORS PROMOTING NERVE GROWTH

Rat Tissues

     It is clear from what has been said that the nerve growth-
promoting activity detectable in tissues fits with the definition
of NGF-like actions in the bioassay (Fig. 6, top frame). In addition, however, there seem to be other factors present that enhance
nerve growth and show another spectrum of affected neurons. Thus we
found (Ebendal et al., 1980) that the rat iris stimulated neuron

Table 1. Sympathetic outgrowth scores obtained with frozen and thawed explants of iris from one-year-old chicks

	Normal iris	Cultured iris
Control medium	0.7±0.18(15)	4.2±0.08(18)[b]
Anti-NGF medium	1.3±0.34(12)[a]	2.1±0.28(18)[c]

Values given are the mean ± S.E.M.

Number of observations is given within parenthesis.

a

  Not significantly different from control medium (t-test)

b

  Significantly elevated outgrowth score compared with the normal, non-cultured iris (P<0.001)

c

  Significant depression by anti-2.5S-NGF antiserum from rabbit added at 0.2% to the culture medium (P<0.001).

survival and neurite outgrowth in the chick ciliary ganglion through a NGF-independent mechanism only weakly affecting the sympathetic ganglia (Fig. 6, bottom frame). This non-NGF activity did not change in any apparent way as a result of manipulating the iris.

A similar, possibly identical, active substance (or substances) was found also in the rat sciatic nerve (Richarson and Ebendal, 1982). Also mouse peripheral nerve has been demonstrated to be rich in factors, only some corresponding NGF, that support neuron development in culture (Riopelle et al., 1981).

In addition to the iris and sciatic nerve, many other organs in the rat carry a similar activity when tested as explants or homogenates in the ciliary bioassay. Macromolecules with the ability to support the survival of ciliary neurons in culture were also described by McLennan and Hendry (1978), Bonyhady et al. (1980), Bennett and Nurcombe (1970), Nurcombe et al. (1981), Coughlin et al.

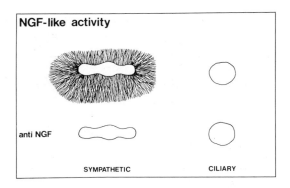

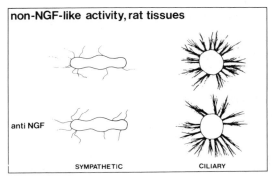

Fig. 6.   Top frame shows the definition of NGF-like activity in
the present culture system. Sympathetic ganglia respond by a dense
fiber outgrowth fully suppressible by antiserum to NGF whereas the
ciliary ganglion from the chick orbit is left unaffected by both
NGF and its antiserum. The bottom frame shows an additional kind
of nerve growth-promoting activity seen in a number of tissues from
the rat. The main characteristic is stimulation of outgrowth of
neurite fascicles from the ciliary ganglion and a mild effect on
fiber formation in the sympathetic ganglia, none of which are
suppressed by anti-NGF antiserum.

(1981). The interrelationship between these factors is at present
unknown.

Embryonic Chick Tissues

     It was shown in this laboratory that various embryonic chick
tissues stimulated nerve fiber extension from nearby ganglia

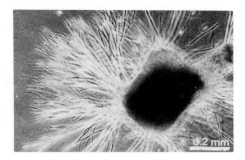

Fig. 7.   Fiber outgrowth in a ciliary ganglion in response to an extract of the 18-day-old chick embryo. The extract was passed over a CM-Sepharose bed at neutral pH (under which conditions the active factor is rejected; Ebendal and Belew, 1980) before being dialyzed and added to the culture dish. Phase contrast of a two-day culture.

(Ebendal and Jacobson, 1977). Based on the failure of antiserum to NGF to block the fiber outgrowth and on the fact that the ciliary ganglion was stimulated also by these tissues (Ebendal, 1979), it was concluded that NGF is not the growth-inducing signal in this case.

The active material from the chick tissues stimulates ciliary, sympathetic and sensory ganglia equally well in a dose-dependent fashion (Ebendal et al., 1982). The effects on the ciliary ganglion are shown in Fig. 7. The extracts are effective in promoting both survival and fiber development also in dissociated neurons from these three ganglia seeded in the collagen gels. It was demonstrated that the growth-promoting activity is widely distributed in the chick embryo and that the activity increases 400-fold in the carcass from the first to the third week of development (Ebendal et al., 1982). Similar findings regarding age-related increases and lack of regional specificity in chick embryo extracts were reported also by Hill et al. (1981).

The properties of the active substance indicate a protein with isoelectric point around pH 5 and molecular weight of about 40,000 daltons (Ebendal et al., 1979; Ebendal and Belew, 1980). A scheme for the purification of this factor, aiming at acceptable recovery, is currently worked out in collaboration with Drs. Jerker Porath and Makonnen Belew at the Biochemistry Department of Uppsala University. One approach taken to get the active substance in sufficient amount involves large-scale preparation of embryonic chick extract.

A trophic activity for dissociated ciliary neurons has also
been studied by Varon and Adler with collaborators, focusing their
attention on the choroid coat of the chick embryo (Adler et al.,
1979; Landa et al., 1980). The factor partially purified from the
eye shows actions and chromatographic properties (Manthorpe et al.,
1980; Barbin et al., 1981) similar to those we find for the activity in the total chick embryo extract. Possibly the factors are
identical. The relation between these substances and the non-NGF
factor in rat tissue stimulating the ciliary ganglion (Fig. 6) is
not clear, but strict identity is not suggested from our bioassay.

The connection between the factors operating on peripheral
neurons and materials supporting growth of CNS neurites (e.g. in
retinal cultures, see Carri and Ebendal, 1982) is worth further
attention.

CONCLUSIONS AND GENERAL OUTLOOK

When screening tissues for factors stimulating nerve growth,
one finds, under some circumstances, an activity similar to that of
NGF from the mouse salivary gland. The chemistry of the NGF produced in small amounts in tissues like the iris is not known in any
detail. In addition, one is faced with a number of other less well
characterized factors provoking responses in the bioassay.

A primary step in any attempt to sort out the diversity is the
establishment of a bioassay that will discriminate between various
groups of factors. The use of sympathetic versus ciliary neurons to
identify NGF is an example of this approach. Another important
tool is specific antibodies to the growth factor under study. So
far, only antibodies to NGF are available for use in the bioassay.
An immunological approach to study the various factors involved in
nerve growth can also allow the preparation of immunosorbents.
Furthermore, antibodies injected in developing embryos may help to
reveal the roles during development for NGF and other not yet fully
characterized nerve growth factors.

Supported by grants from the Swedish Natural Science Research
Council (B 2021-100, S-FP 4024-101).

REFERENCES

Adler, R., Varon, S., 1980, Cholinergic neuronotrophic factors: V.
    Segregation of survival- and neurite-promoting activities in
    heart-conditioned media, Brain Res., 188:437-448.
Adler, R., Landa, K.B., Manthorpe, M., Varon, S., 1979, Cholinergic
    neuronotrophic factors: Intraocular distribution of trophic
    activity for ciliary neurons, Science, 204:1434-1436.

Bailey, G.S, Banks, B.E.C., Carstairs,J.R., Edwards, D.C., Pearce, F.L., Vernon, C.A., 1976, Immunological properties of nerve growth factors, Biochim. Biophys. Acta, 437:259-263.

Barbin, G., Manthorpe, M., Varon, S., 1981, Molecular behaviors of the ciliary neuronotrophic factor(s), Soc. Neurosci. Abstr. 7:554.

Bennett, M.R., Nurcombe, V., 1979, The survival and development of cholinergic neurons in skeletal muscle conditioned media, Brain Res., 173:543-548.

Bonyhady, R.D., Hendry, I.A., Hill, C.E., McLennan, I.S., 1980, Characterization of a cardiac muscle factor required for the survival of cultured parasympathetic neurones, Neurosci. Lett., 18:197-201.

Brunso-Bechtold, J.K. and Hamburger, V., 1979, Retrograde transport of nerve growth factor in chicken embryo, Proc. Natl. Acad. Sci. USA, 76:1494-1496.

Campenot, R.B., 1977, Local control of neurite development by nerve growth factor, Proc. Natl. Acad. Sci. USA, 74:4516-4519.

Carri, N.G. and Ebendal, T., 1982, Organotypic cultures of neural retina: Neurite outgrowth stimulated by brain extracts, Develop. Brain Res., (in press).

Chapman, C.A., Banks, B.E.C., Carstairs, J.R., Pearce, F.L., Vernon, C.A., 1979, The preparation of nerve growth factor from the prostate of the guinea-pig and isolation of immunogenically pure material from the mouse submandibular gland, FEBS Lett. 105: 341-344.

Cohen, S., Levi-Montalcini, R., Hamburger, V. 1954, A nerve growth-stimulating factor isolated from sarcomas 37 and 180, Proc. Natl. Acad Sci. USA, 40:1014-1018.

Coughlin, M.D., Bloom, E.M., Black, I.B., 1981, Characterization of a neuronal growth factor from mouse heart-cell-conditioned medium, Develop. Biol., 82:56-68.

Ebendal, T., 19769, Stage-dependent stimulation of neurite outgrowth exerted by nerve growth factor and chick heart in cultured embryonic ganglia, Develop. Biol., 72:276-290.

Ebendal, T. and Jacobson, C.-O., 1977, Tissue explants affecting extension and orientation of axons in cultured chick embryo ganglia, Exp. Cell Res., 105:379-387.

Ebendal, T. and Belew, M., 1980, Chick heart factor controlling neurite extension, Eur. J. Cell Biol., 22:409.

Ebendal, T., Belew, M., Jacobson, C.-O., Porath, J., 1979, Neurite outgrowth elicited by embryonic chick heart: Partial purification of the active factor, Neurosci. Lett., 14:91-95.

Ebendal, T., Olson, L., Seiger, A., Hedlund, K.-O., 1980, Nerve growth factors in the rat iris, Nature, 286:25-28.

Ebendal, T. Norrgren, T., Hedlund, K.-O., 1982, Nerve-growth promoting activity in the chick embryo, in manuscript.

Elsdale, T., Bard, J., 1972, Collagen substrata for studies on cell behavior, J. Cell Biol., 54:626-637.

Ennis, M., Pearce, F.L., Vernon, C.A., 1979, Some studies on the
    mechanism of action of antibodies to nerve growth factor,
    Neuroscience, 4:1391-1398.
Harper, G.P. and Thoenen, H., 1980a, Nerve growth factor: Biological
    significance, measurement, and distribution, J. Neurochem.,
    34:5-16.
Harper, G.P. and Thoenen, H., 1980b, The distribution of nerve growt
    factor in the male sex organs of mammals, J. Neurochem., 34:
    893-903.
Harper, G.P. and H. Thoenen, 1981, Target cells, biological effects,
    and mechanism of action of nerve growth factor and its anti-
    bodies, Ann. Rev. Pharmacol. Toxicol., 21:205-229.
Harper, G.P., Pearce, F.L., Vernon, C.A., 1980, The production and
    storage of nerve growth factor in vivo by tissues of the mouse,
    rat, guinea pig, hamster, and gerbil, Develop. Biol.,
    77:391-402.
Harrison, R.G., 1910, The outgrowth of the nerve fiber as a mode
    of protoplasmic movement, J. Exp. Zool., 9:787-846.
Hill, C.E., Hendry, I.A., Bonyhady, R.E., 1981, Avian parasympathe-
    tic neurotrophic factors: Age-related increases and lack of
    regional specificity, Develop. Biol., 85:258-261.
Landa, K.B., Adler, R., Manthorpe, M., Varon, S., 1980, Cholinergic
    neuronotrophic factors. III. Developmental increase of trophic
    activity for chick embryo ciliary ganglion neurons in their
    intraocular target tissues, Develop. Biol., 74:401-408.
Levi-Montalcini, R., 1966, The nerve growth factor: Its mode of
    action on sensory and sympathetic nerve cells, Harvey Lect.,
    60:217-259.
Manthorpe, M., Skaper, S., Adler, R., Landa, K., Varon, S., 1980,
    Cholinergic neuronotrophic factors: Fractionation properties of
    an extract from selected chick embryonic eye tissues,
    J. Neurochem., 34:69-75.
McLennan, I.S., Hendry, I.A., 1978, Parasympathetic neuronal surviva
    induced by factors from muscle, Neurosci. Lett., 10:269-273.
Mobley, W.C., Schenker,A., Shooter, E.M., 1976, Characterization and
    isolation of proteolytically modified nerve growth factor,
    Biochemistry, 15:5543-5552.
Nurcombe, V., Penman, E.A., Hill, M.A., Catanzaro, D., Bennett, M.R.
    1981, Partial purification of an extract from skeletal muscle
    required for the survival of embryonic cholinergic neurons,
    Proc. Austr. Physiol. Pharmacol. Soc., 12:120 P.
Richardson, P.M. Ebendal, T., 1982, Nerve growth activities in rat
    peripheral nerve, Brain Res., in press.
Riopelle, R.J., Cameron, D.A., 1981, Neurite growth promoting factor
    of embryonic chick - ontogeny, regional distribution, and
    characteristics, J. Neurobiol., 12:175-186.
Riopelle, R.J., Boegman, R.J., Cameron, D.A., 1981, Peripheral nerve
    contains heterogeneous growth factors that support sensory
    neurons in vitro, Neurosci. Lett., 25:311-316.

Suda, K., Barde, Y.A., Thoenen, H., 1978, Nerve growth factor in mouse and rat serum: Correlation between bioassay and radio-immunoassay determinations, Proc. Natl. Acad. Sci. USA, 75:4042-4046.

Thoenen, H., Barde, Y.-A., 1980, Physiology of nerve growth factor, Physiol. Rev., 60:1284-1335.

Varon, S., Adler, R., 1980, Nerve growth factors and control of nerve growth, Curr. Top. Develop. Biol., 16 (2):207-252.

Varon, S., Raiborn, C., Burnham, P.A., 1974, Implication of a nerve growth factor-like antigen in the support derived by ganglionic neurons from their homologous glia in dissociated cultures, Neurobiology, 4:317-327.

Young, M., Oger, J., Blanchard, M.H., Asdourian, H., Amos, H., Arnason, B.G.W., 1975, Secretion of a nerve growth factor by primary chick fibroblast cultures, Science, 187:361-362.

MACROMOLECULAR FACTORS INVOLVED IN THE REGULATION OF THE SURVIVAL

AND DIFFERENTIATION OF NEURONS DURING DEVELOPMENT

Hans Thoenen

Max-Planck-Institute for Psychiatry
Department of Neurochemistry
Federal Republic of Germany

INTRODUCTION

It is a well-established, almost universal phenomenon that, during the ontogenesis of the peripheral and central nervous systems of vertebrates, neurons are initially produced in excess and that the subsequent selective neuronal death occurs as a normal event (Cowan, 1973; Jacobson, 1978). The topographically selective regulation of survival is an important mechanism for the formation of the final structure and function of integrated neuronal systems. The possible mechanism(s) involved in the regulation of neuronal survival have mainly been investigated in the peripheral nervous system, which is relatively simply organized, both structurally and functionally, and which is therefore better suited for detailed analysis than the more complex central nervous system.

Ablation and transplantation experiments dating back to the beginning of this century showed that the size of the field of innervation determines the degree of survival of the corresponding sensory and motor neurons (cf. Hamburger, 1977). Similar observations were also made for the autonomic nervous system (cf. Landmesser and Pilar, 1976; Dibner and Black, 1976). Although these experiments firmly established the importance of the target tissues for the survival of the innervating neurons, they did not provide any information on the possible underlying mechanism(s). The extension of these transplantation experiments in chick embryos, using sarcoma tissue rather than wing or leg buds (Bueker, 1948; Levi-Montalcini et al., 1954) led to the detection of Nerve Growth Factor (NGF)(cf. Levi-Montalcini and Angeletti, 1968; Thoenen and Barde, 1980). The eluci-

idation of the physiological function of this protein provided one
possible mechanism by which peripheral target cells have a trophic
influence on innervating neurons (cf. Thoenen and Barde, 1980;
Schwab and Thoenen, 1983). It has been demonstrated that NGF acts
as a retrograde messenger between target tissues and innervating
sympathetic and spinal sensory neurons. NGF is taken up by the corresponding nerve terminals by a highly specific, saturable mechanism. The rate-limiting step in this uptake process is the number of
available NGF-receptors at the nerve terminals. The specific binding of NGF is followed by internalization and transfer to the perikaryon in membrane-confined compartments by rapid retro-grade axonal
transport at a rate of 5-10 mm/hr. In the perikaryon, the NGF molecules effect their characteristic biochemical actions, namely the
selective induction of enzymes (tyrosine hydroxylase (TH) and
dopamine-β-hydroxylase (DBH)) involved in the synthesis of the
adrenergic transmitter norepinephrine (cf. Schwab and Thoenen, 1983).
More recently an enhanced formation of specific peptides such as
substance P (Kessler and Black, 1980; Otten et al., 1980) and somastatin (Kessler and Black, 1981) have been demonstrated. Moreover,
retrogradely transported NGF has a general growth-promoting action on
the target neurons (Hendry, 1977), which is more pronounced in early
stages of ontogenesis than in adult, fully differentiated neurons
(cf. Levi-Montalcini and Angeletti, 1968; Thoenen and Barde, 1980).
The physiological significance of this retrograde transport of NGF is
reflected by the fact that its interruption by axotomy (Hendry, 1975,
or by the blockade of axonal transport with drugs causing depolymeri-
zation of microtubules (Menesini et al., 1977; Johnson, 1978) or the
destruction of nerve terminals (Levi-Montalcini et al., 1975), leads
in early stages of embryonic development, to the degeneration of the
corresponding neurons and, in differentiated neurons, to an impairment of their specific functions as reflected, for instance, in
adrenergic neurons by a reduction of TH and DBH (cf. Thoenen and
Barde, 1980; Schwab and Thoenen, 1983). That the impaired functions
resulting from the blockade of axonal transport are caused by the
accompanying impairment of the transfer of NGF form the periphery
to the perikaryon is indicated by the fact that the same impairment
of functions (in adults) or neuronal death (in earlier neurogenesis)
of endogenous NGF by the administration of specific antibodies to NGF
(cf. Thoenen and Barde, 1980; Harper and Theonen, 1981). Furthermore, the deleterious effects of the blockade of axonal transport
can be prevented by the simultaneous administration of NGF.

The physiological role of NGF, demonstrated by the effect of
NGF-antibodies in vivo, also becomes apparent in vitro under
appropriate experimental conditions. The survival of cultured sensory and sympathetic neurons depends on the addition of NGF to the
culture medium, and the induction of neurotransmitter-synthesizing
enzymes and of neurite outgrowth by NGF can be shown in vitro as
well as in vivo (cf. Thoenen and Barde, 1980). The in vitro
approach has the advantage that it allows the mechanisms involved in

trophic factor-neuron interactions to be analyzed under precisely
defined conditions.

In the following we will give a survey of the strategies used to
characterize new survival factors in comparison to NGF, using tissue
culture procedures as a tool to answer questions such as: which populations of neurons depend on which survival factors at which stages
of their development? Do neurons depend on more than one survival
factor at a given stage of their development, or can they survive
with alternative factors?

Although the final goal is to obtain information on the situation in vivo, this has to be accomplished by detailed analyses in
vitro under very stringent criteria.

Culture Systems used for the characterization and purification of neuronal trophic factors

Neuronal explants

In the course of the analysis and purification of NGF, explants
of sensory and sympathetic ganglia played a very important role (cf.
Levi-Montalcini and Angeletti, 1968). Moreover, explants proved to
be a very useful system for experiments aimed at an understanding
whether the outgrowth of neuronal fibers is preferentially promoted
by, and directed to, explants of physiological target tissues (cf.
Burnstock, 1974; Ebendal and Jacobson, 1977).

However, in the analysis of survival factors from conditioned
media and tissue extracts, explant cultures also have their clear
limitations: the observed effects are difficult to interpret with
regard to neuronal survival, since enhanced fiber outgrowth can,
indeed, result from a survival effect on the neurons, but it can also
result from a promotion of fiber outgrowth from neurons whose survival does not depend on the added factor(s). In order to obtain
information on a possible survival effect under these circumstances
time-consuming neuronal cell counts have to be performed in histological serial sections. Even if a survival effect becomes apparent
in this manner, it cannot be decided whether it results from a direct
action on the neurons or from an indirect effect via surrounding non-
neuronal cells.

Cultures of isolated neurons

The drawbacks and limitations of tissue explants can be overcome
by the use of cultures of isolated neurons. However, with this
approach also, a series of conditions have to be fulfilled in order
to obtain unambiguous results:

1)   A dissociation procedure has to be used that gives a high yield
of neurons from the ganglia investigated, in order to avoid the possibility that the dissociation procedure selects specific subpopulations of neurons, whose properties are not necessarily typical of all
the neurons originally present.

In chick sensory and sympathetic ganglia it is possible to
obtain a virtually 100% yield of the neurons investigated. In other
species, for example rats, such a high yield of neurons has not been
obtained, in spite of the intensive efforts of many laboratories (see
for instance Chun and Patterson, 1977; Hefti et al., 1983).

2)   The non-neuronal cells must be eliminated from the cultures, in
order to demonstrate that the added trophic factors act directly on
neurons rather than via non-neuronal cells. Moreover, non-neuronal
cells may themselves produce survival factors (cf. Varon and Adler,
1981; Barde et al., 1982b, 1983).

3)   Culture conditions have to be chosen (either with or without
serum) under which no neurons survive unless the adequate survival
factors originating from conditioned media or tissue extracts are
added to the culture medium (Barde et al., 1980; Wakade et al.,
1982).

4)   The concentrations of the added trophic factors have always to
be "saturating", i.e. the addition of more factor should not increase
the number of surviving neurons. The use of such "saturating" concentrations precludes ambiguities in the interpretation of the
results which could occur, e.g., if added tissue extracts change not
only the concentration of survival factor(s) in the medium, but also
the substrate of the culture dish. The latter phenomenon could lead
to an augmented binding of survival factor(s) to the substrate,
which could, thus, result in a locally higher concentration of these
factor(s) in the immediate surroundings of the neurons and hence, to
an apparent potentiating effect.

5)   The criteria of survival have to be long-term, i.e. the survival
should be judged after an observation period of at least 48 hr and
it should be established that no major changes occur during the
subsequent days of culture.

Age-dependent changes in the requirements of sensory and
sympathetic neurons for different survival factors in vitro

Age-dependent requirements for NGF in vivo are also reflected
in vitro by the survival of differing proportions of neurons under
experimental conditions in which no neurons survive without the addition of specific macromolecular factors (Barde et al., 1980; 1982b).
As shown in Fig. 1, the survival with NGF alone for both sensory and
sympathetic neurons is low in cultures originating from E8 chick

Table I. Survival of cultured chick sensory neurons of different embryonic ages

Embryonic age (days)	% neuronal survival in response to				
	NGF	GCM	Brain Extract	NGF + GCM	NGF + Brain Extract
8	27 ± 3	13 ± 1	17 ± 2	80 ± 7	76 ± 6
10	42 ± 2	21 ± 1	32 ± 1	92 ± 8	68 ± 6
12	44 ± 0.5	52 ± 2	50 ± 3	76 ± 6	98 ± 6
14	25 ± 0.2	64 ± 6	47 ± 5	85 ± 5	98 ± 9
16	6 ± 0.5	74 ± 7	73 ± 4	76 ± 3	76 ± 1

Neurons were grown with NGF (5 ng/ml), conditioned medium by C6 glial tumor cells (GCM), brain extract and the combination of NGF with GCM or brain extract. Neurons were counted after 48 hr. Results are expressed as percentages of initially plated neurons ± SD. Without addition of NGF, GCM or brain extract less than 5% of neurons survived after 48 hr.

Table II. Survival of cultured chick sympathetic neurons of different embryonic ages

Embryonic age (days)	% neuronal survival in response to		
	NGF	HCM	HCM + NGF
8	5 ± 2	16 ± 3	65 ± 7
10	25 ± 2	36 ± 6	84 ± 9
12	37 ± 6	45 ± 3	88 ± 11
14	30 ± 4	56 ± 9	92 ± 8
16	18 ± 3	55 ± 11	84 ± 9

Neurons were grown with NGF (5 ng/ml), heart-conditioned medium (HCM) plus 500 ng/ml of anti-NGF antibodies or NGF plus HCM. Neurons were counted after 48 hr. Results are expressed as percentage of initially plated neurons ± SD. Without adding NGF or HCM less than 5% of neurons survived after 48 hr.

embryos. The proportion of surviving neurons then increases to a maximum between E10 and E12, and then declines again to low levels at E16 and E18.

After the initial observations that culture media conditioned by rat-glioma or chick heart cells have a survival effect on chick sensory, sympathetic and parasympathetic neurons (Helfand et al., 1976; Barde et al., 1978; Collins, 1978) in the presence of antibodies against NGF the analysis of the survival effects was further pursued with respect to the proportion of neurons surviving by the individual factors or by a combination of these factors with NGF during different stages of development (Barde et al., 1980; Edgar et al., 1981).

In the following, we will confine ourselves to the analysis of the sensory and sympathetic systems. In Table I, the proportions of sensory neurons surviving with NGF, conditioned media from C6 glioma cells, and rat brain extract are presented. Both brain extract and C6 glial-conditioned medium (in the presence of antibodies against NGF) maintain a steadily increasing proportion of neurons from E8 to E16, by which stage NGF alone can maintain virtually no neurons.

It is noteworthy that similar results were obtained with medium conditioned by rat brain astrocytes (Lindsay, 1979). This, together with the fact that the specific survival activity in rat brain extracts increases in parallel with the postnatal development of glial cells (Barde et al., 1980), is compatible with the assumption that the survival activity present in brain extract may originate from glial cells.

The combination of NGF with either glial-conditioned medium or brain extract results in the survival of 80-90% of the neurons plated over the whole observation period from E8 to E16 (Table I). From these results it can be concluded that, in particular in early stages of development, the survival activity of NGF and of glial-conditioned medium or brain extract are more than additive, suggesting that in these stages of the development a considerable population of neurons need more than one factor for survival.

In cultures of sympathetic neurons the situation is very similar, i.e. by the combination of NGF and heart-conditioned medium the majority of the neurons survive, in vitro (Table II) and also in this case there are neurons which need for survival more than one factor. Thus, in early stages of development the survival with either NGF or heart-conditioned medium alone is very low (5 and 16%, respectively) whereas the number of surviving neurons by the combination of NGF and heart-conditioned medium is much higher than expected from the addition of the two effects (Table II).

Changes in the "efficacy" and "potency" of survival factors by
macromolecules bound to the culture dish substrate

In recent experiments, it has been demonstrated that the extent
of the NGF-mediated survival of sympathetic neurons could be greatly
increased by changing the substrate of the culture dishes by the
addition of a protease-sensitive macromolecule(s), which alone had
no survival activity (Edgar and Thoenen, 1982b). The substrate
attached material changed the response of the sympathetic neurons to
such an extent that essentially all the neurons survived with NGF as
the only survival factor (85-90% for neurons from E8 to E16). The
mechanism by which this modulating factor(s) act is not known. Although the "dose-survival" curve for NGF is shifted to the left by
this modulating molecule(s) it produces not only an enhanced potency
of NGF but also a marked increase in "efficacy". It increases the
survival activity of supramaximal concentrations of NGF of 5% at E8
(minimal effect) and 37% at E12 (maximal effect) to 85-90% from E8
to E16. It is worth noting that the circumstances of the production
of this factor and the manner of its interaction with the polyornithine substrate of the tissue culture dishes is indistinguishable
from that of a neurite-promoting factor (Collins, 1978; Adler and
Varon, 1980; Adler et al., 1981; Lander et al., 1981). The neurite-
promoting factor is not only produced by chicken heart cells but also
by a large number of other cells and cell lines (Adler et al., 1981).
A particularly rich source is the medium conditioned by schwannoma
RN-22 cells, which is also a rich source for the substrate-mediated
enchancement of NGF survival in chick sympathetic neurons (Edgar,
unpublished observation). Both the neurite-promoting and NGF-
enhancing activity can be removed completely from the conditioned
media by adsorption to polyornithine substrate. It remains to be
established whether the molecule(s), which are responsible for the
potentiation of the survival effect of NGF and for the neurite-
promoting activity are identical and, if this should be the case,
whether the same domain of the molecule is responsible for the two
actions. It is to be expected that monoclonal antibodies produced
against the molecules bound to polyornithine will play an important
role in the elucidation of this problem.

In recent experiments it has been demonstrated that the potentiating effect of the polyornithine bound molecule(s) is not
restricted to the NGF survival effect on chick sympathetic neurons,
but also exists in sensory neurons. In this case, however, the
potentiation of NGF seems to be relatively small, but is quite
impressive for a newly-purified survival factor from pig brain
(Barde, in preparation).

The unexpected detection of this modulating macromolecule(s) in
tissue culture could be of great importance to the future elucidation
of the physiological role of new survival molecules, since such modulating factors may allow neurons to survive with alternative factors.

The administration of antibodies inhibiting the biological action of a given new survival factor may only become apparent if at the same time the action of possible modulating factor(s) is also blocked.

Survival of selective populations of neurons by different survival factors

The changing proportion of neurons surviving in response to different survival factors during development raises the question as to whether these populations of neurons can be distinguished from from each other by other criteria. We first investigated whether the changing survival activity of NGF during development is reflected by the presence or absence of NGF-receptors. In previous experiments, Herrup and Shooter (1975) demonstrated that in chick dorsal root ganglionic neurons of increasing embryonic age, there was a reduction in the number of NGF-receptors in parallel with the decreasing response (fiber outgrowth from explants) to NGF. However, these experiments did not distinguish between a general decrease in the number of receptors in all the neurons versus the disappearance of the receptors in a limited subpopulation of sensory neurons. An autoradiographic method developed by Rohrer and Barde (1982) permits this distinction to be made. Studies using this method indicated the existence of two sharply distinct populations of neurons, with labeled and unlabeled neurons being segregated in an astonishingly "black and white" manner. The cells were classified as unlabled when the pattern of neurites could not be displayed by the accumulation of silver grains above background. That this classification is valid can be deduced from the fact that by increasing the exposure time of the preparations no change in the proportion of labeled and non-labeled neurons occurred. This excludes the possibility that there was a significant population of faintly labeled neurons of an intermediate classification becoming apparent only after a longer exposure time.

As expected, the sensory neurons surviving with NGF alone were all labeled with ^{125}I-NGF. Nevertheless, at E10 80% of the neurons which did not survive with NGF but only with rat brain extract exhibited NGF receptors (Rohrer and Barde, 1982). With increasing age the proportion of NGF-receptor-positive neurons dropped to 30% at E16. But even then the proportion of labeled neurons was distinctly larger than the proportion of neurons surviving with NGF alone (compare Fig. 1, Table I). Thus, in cultures of sensory ganglia, the proportion of neurons with NGF-receptors is definitely higher than the proportion of neurons which survive with NGF alone. The difference between the proportion of neurons having NGF receptors and the proportion of neurons surviving with NGF alone is even more impressive in cultures of chick sympathetic neurons, in which from E8 to E16 virtually all the neurons (more than 95%) are labeled with ^{125}I-NGF (Edgar et al., 1982a), whereas the proportion of neurons surviving with NGF alone reaches a maximum of 37% at E14 (Table II). However, the presence of NGF-receptors on vitually all the sympathetic neurons

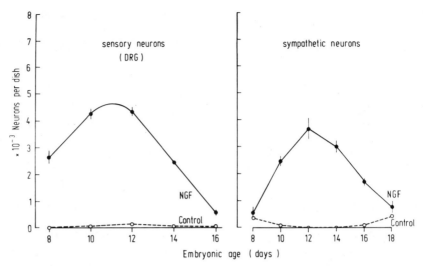

Figure 1.   Effect of NGF on the survival of sensory and sympathetic
neurons of different embryonic ages.   Dissociated neurons from dorsal
root and sympathetic ganglia of chick embryos of different embryo-
genic ages (E8 to E18) were grown with   5 ng/ml of 2.5S mouse NGF
and without addition (control).   10,000 cells were plated per 35 mm
culture dish.   Neurons were counted after 48 h in culture.   Results
are expressed as the mean of triplicate determinations ± SD.   Where
not shown SD is smaller than the symbols.   For experimental details
see Barde et al. (1980) and Edgar et al. (1981).

is a prerequisite for the modulating ability of the substrate-bound
macromolecule(s), which enhances the survival activity of NGF alone
so as to maintain 85-90% of the neurons plated (Edgar and Thoenen,
1982b).

     The characterization of the subpopulations of neurons surviving
with different survival factors with respect to specific biochemical
and functional properties has so far mainly been pursued in chick
sympathetic neurons.   Edgar et al. (1981) demonstrated that neurons
surviving at E12 with heart-conditioned medium alone showed a much
lower specific activity of TH than neurons surviving with NGF alone
(Table III).   The difference between these two populations of neurons
was even more impressive with respect to the specific activities of
choline acetyltransferase (CAT), which is about 8 times higher in
neurons surviving with heart-conditioned medium than in neurons
maintained by NGF alone.   The combination of the two factors results
in an average of the enzyme specific activities.   This, together with

Table III.   Enzyme pattern of chick sympathetic neurons maintained by NGF, heart-conditioned medium (HCM) or their combinations

	Choline acetyltransferase pmol ACH/min/mg protein	Tyrosine hydroxylase pmol Dopa/min/mg protein
After 48 h culture with		
NGF	102 ± 44	281 ± 75
HCM	842 ± 77	137 ± 31
NGF + HCM	855 ± 45	310 ± 40
After 48 h with NGF followed by 48 h with NGF + HCM	85 ± 30	210 ± 40

Cultures were set up with 50,000 – 80,000 sympathetic neurons from 12 day old chick embryos. After the culture periods shown, the neurons were rinsed twice with warm phosphate buffered saline and collected in 300 ul 50 mM tris-acetate buffer, pH 7.4 containing 0.1% (vol/vol) triton X-100, and stored at -70° until assayed. Biochemical assays were performed as described by Edgar et al. (1981).

the fact that neurons initially exposed to NGF alone (and thus selected for survival under these conditions) and then exposed to a
combination of heart-conditioned medium and NGF, did not change
their enzyme pattern, speaks in favor of a selection of a specific
population of neurons by the survival effects of NGF and heart-
conditioned medium, rather than for an induction of the corresponding enzymes by the two agents (Edgar et al., 1981).

Although specific antibodies to CAT are avilable (Eckenstein and
Thoenen, 1982) the quantity of enzyme present in the single neurons
in culture in early stages of the development is too small to be
visualized by immunohistochemical methods. However, in recent preliminary experiments (Edgar, unpublished observations) it could be
demonstrated that virtually all the neurons surviving with NG gave a
positive reaction with antibodies to TH and also exhibited a high
affinity uptake for norepinephrine (as visualized by autoradiographic
procedures) which could be blocked by desmethylimipramine. In
contrast, far fewer neurons surviving with heart-conditioned medium
gave a TH-positive reaction and showed a high-affinity norepinephrine
uptake. Interestingly, of the neurons surviving with NGF, only about
5-10% gave a positive reaction with antibodies to vasoactive intestinal peptide (VIP), whereas many more neurons maintained by heart-
conditioned medium were VIP-positive. It seems that the proportion
of VIP-positive neurons roughly parallels the level of CAT activity,
and the percentage of TH and VIP-positive neurons adds up to roughly
100%. It remains to be established by double labeling experiments
whether there is a small proportion of neurons which contain both TH
and VIP.

Importance of the purification of new trophic factors

The history of the research on NGF has impressively demonstrated
how essential it is to purify the molecules which are responsible for
the trophic effects of conditioned media or tissue extracts (cf.
Levi-Montalcini and Angeletti, 1968; Thoenen and Barde, 1980). Purified material is a prerequisite for the production of antibodies
against the molecules in question, and the administration of antibodies is the most crucial approach for obtaining information on the
physiological importance of these molecules, i.e. which populations
of neurons are dependent on which factors at which time of their
development.

The purification of NGF was made possible by the very fortunate
detection of rich sources of NGF, firstly snake venoms, then the male
mouse submandibular gland (cf. Levi-Montalcini and Angeletti, 1968)
and more recently also the prostate glands of guinea pig and bull
(cf. Harper and Thoenen, 1981). These rich sources have no significance for the physiological action of NGF on the peripheral sympathetic and sensory nervous system (cf. Thoenen and Barde, 1980; Harper
and Thoenen, 1981). So far, no convincing function for NGF has been

found in the saliva (including venom) and the seminal fluid, and the unimportance of these rich sources for the development and mainte- nance of function of the target neurons is indicated by the absence of any relationship between the presence or absence of these rich sources in a given species and the trophic action of NGF on the peri- pheral sympathetic and sensory nervous system in that animal (cf. Thoenen and Barde, 1980; Harper and Theonen, 1981). For example, there is no difference between the development of the sensory and sympathetic nervous system of male and female mice, although the amount of NGF in the salivary glands of the male is several thousand times higher than in females. Moreover, in other species, for ex- ample the rat, where no detectable quantities of NGF are present in the submandibular gland, the sympathetic and sensory nervous system depends on NGF to an equal extent as in mice (cf. Thoenen and Barde, 1980; Harper and Thoenen, 1981).

It is not to be expected that such rich sources of other trophic factors will be found, and their purification will therefore be more difficult. Indeed, within the last decade, a large number of trophic activities have been described in conditioned media and extracts of a great variety of tissues and cell lines (see Varon and Adler, 1981 and Barde et al., 1983 for reviews. For single examples of trophic factors present in conditioned media and tissue extracts see Adler and Varon, 1980; Adler et al., 1979; Barde et al., 1978; Bennett and Nurcombe, 1980; Bonyhady et al., 1980; Collins, 1978; Coughlin et al., 1981; Ebendal et al., 1979; Helfand et al., 1976; Lindsay 1979; Nishi and Berg, 1981) but so far NGF remains the only molecule with defined chemical properties (including amino-acid sequence) and established physiological functions evolving from the observations of the effects of anti-NGF antibodies on the sympathetic and sensory nervous system (cf. Thoenen and Barde, 1980).

Recently a new trophic factor has been purified from pig brain (Barde et al., 1982), which exhibits survival activity on peripheral sensory neurons and possibly also on some central neurons. The pro- tocol of the purification of this factor demonstrates the tremendous difficulties encountered in its purification as compared to NGF. In order to obtain a preparation of NGF with a purity of more than 95%, a purification factor of about 200 is necessary from the starting material of male mouse submandibular glands. In the case of the new trophic factor from pig brain, a purification factor of more than 1 million was necessary to obtain a preparation of comparable purity (Barde et al., 1982). This has implications for the future. As already mentioned, in order to evaluate the physiological function of a trophic factor, it is essential to produce specific antibodies. The method of the production of monoclonal antibodies in principle no longer requires the availability of highly purified antigens for immunization, as clones of hybridoma cells resulting from the fusion of myeloma tumor cells and antigen-activated spleen cells can be selected according to the specificity of the antibodies they produce (cf. Kohler and Milstein, 1976). However, this undoubtedly powerful method has also led to over-enthusiastic expectations, for example, that it could dispense with efforts to purify antigens altogether. However, unless the molecule of interest is an extremely potent antigen, it has to be borne in mind that the production of specific clones of hybridomas generally corresponds to the proportion of antigen used for the immunization. Thus, the chance of "hitting" the small number of activated B cells by fusion with the myeloma cells and of obtaining an active clone becomes extremely small for minor components in a mixture of injected antigens. This is especially emphasized if one considers the number of stable clones obtained from fusions following immunization with relatively pure fractions of macromolecules having good antigenic properties, as for example in the case of CAT (Eckenstein and Thoenen, 1982). Lucky shots that may occasionally happen should not lead to erroneous general expectations. In the case of the newly purified trophic factor from pig brain (Barde et al., 1982), available so far only in microgram quantities (quantities, however, which are sufficient to immunize a mouse against NGF), successful immunization has not yet been achieved, as judged by the absence of a positive titer in the serum of an immunized mouse. However, if one calculates the quantity of material to be injected after the first crude purification steps, without pursuing a further more rigorous purification, it would be necessary to inject a mouse with several grams of protein in order to administer the same quantity of antigen which, injected in pure form, was not able to elicit a positive titer. The delineation of this problem of quantity at this grotesque level only serves the purpose of stressing the problems to be encountered.

Not only the production of antibodies against neurotrophic agents is hampered by the small quantities of purified material available. It is also not possible to establish the "pharmacology" of such new factors in the intact animal in a manner comparable with that used for NGF unless one can find ways to produce these factors in larger quantities. The same is true for the determination of the binding kinetics of such factors to their target cells. Here the trivial basic information on the distinction between specific and non-specific binding-sites requires relatively large quantities of the ligand being studied. A possible approach for the future to resolve this problem is provided by new methods of gene technology which allow the insertion of the cDNA corresponding to the mRNA of the molecules in question in appropriate positions in plasmids or viral vectors, and then the production of these molecules in large quantities in bacteria or in eukaryotic cells (for review see Miozzari, 1981). However, although such an approach is possible in principle, the methodology for the isolation of the super-rare mRNAs and the production of the coresponding cDNA and their cloning remains to be established and will be a challenge for neurobiologically-oriented molecular geneticists. For a survey of these aspects, the reader is referred to a monograph edited by Schmitt et al.

(1982) in which the contemporary possibilities and problems of the
application of molecular genetics to neurobiology is discussed.

Concluding Remarks

During early stages of the ontogenesis of the vertebrate peripheral and central nervous system neurons are produced in excess. The
subsequent, topographically selective, regulation of neuronal survival represents an important mechanism for the formation of the final
structures and functions of the fully differentiated nervous system.

In chick sympathetic and sensory neurons, the regulation of
their survival in vivo is reflected in vitro by the fact that under
defined culture conditions in the absence of non-neuronal cells their
survival depends on the addition of specific macromolecular factors.
The requirement for the individual survival factors changes during
embryonic development. Some populations of neurons depend on more
than one survival factor, whereas others have the ability to survive
with alternative factors. Moreover, the survival effect of NGF and
of a newly purified factor from pig brain can be modulated by macro-
molecule(s) which strongly attach to the (polyornithine) substrate of
the culture dishes. This "substrate factor" has no survival activity
of its own, but markedly increases both the potency and efficacy of
the two survival factors. The populations of neurons selected by
individual survival factors can be distinguished from one another by
the levels of specific enzymes, neuronal peptides, plasma membrane
receptors or transport mechanisms for transmitters.

In order to evaluate the physiological significance of the macromolecules demonstrated to be important under analytical conditions
in vitro, it is necessary to purify them. This is the prerequisite
for establishing their "pharmacology" in vivo and, at least to some
extent, also for the production of antibodies, although the method
of monoclonal antibodies allows the production of selective clones
which recognize specific antigenic sites of individual molecules,
even if mixtures of antigens have been used for immunization. The
availability of antibodies allows one to determine in vivo which
neurons, at which stage of their development, depend on which survival factors, and whether these survival factors are also involved in
maintaining specific functions in differentiated neurons, as in the
case of NGF.

The history of the research on NGF strongly supports the necessity for purification of neurotrophic factors as the prerequisite for
establishing their physiological functions. It also demonstrates
that the relatively advanced information on NGF derives from the fact
that very rich sources of this protein were available. Astonishingly, none of these rich sources (submandibular gland of the male
mouse, the prostate glands of guinea pig and bull) have any import
importance for the regulation of the survival or maintenance of

specific functions of sympathetic and sensory neurons. The tremendous difficulties which arise if no such rich sources are available became apparent in the course of the isolation of the new trophic factor present in low concentrations in the mammalian brain. With a purification factor of more than one million (in comparison to several hundredfold for NGF) the microgram quantities of this molecule are too small to establish its "pharmacology" in vivo, and to perform complete binding kinetics. Even for the production of antibodies, the available quantities are barely sufficient. However, new methods of protein chemistry and recombinant DNA techniques might provide the keys to the resolution of these problems. Thus, it is to be expected that methods of molecular genetics will play a rapidly increasing role in developmental neurobiology, not only for analytical, but also for preparative purposes.

References

Adler, R. and Varon, S., 1980, Cholinergic neuronotrophic factors: V. Segregation of survival- and neurite-promoting activities in heart conditioned media, Br. Res., 188:437-448.

Adler, R., Landa, K.B., Manthrope, M., Varon, S., 1979, Cholinergic neuronotrophic factors: intraocular distribution of trophic activity for ciliary neurons, Science, 204:1434-1436.

Adler, R., Manthorpe, M., Skaper, S.D., and Varon, S., 1981, Poly-ornithine neurite-promoting factors, Br. Res., 206:129-144.

Barde, Y.-A., Edgar,D., and Thoenen, H., 1980, Sensory neurons in culture: changing requirements for survival factors during embryonic development, Proc. Natl. Acad. Sci. USA, 77:1199-1203.

Barde, Y.-A., Edgar, D., and Thoenen, H., 1982a, Purification of a new neurotrophic factor from mammalian brain, EMBO J., 1:549-553.

Barde, Y.-A., Edgar, D., and Thoenen, H., 1982b, Molecules involved in the regulation of neuron survival during development, in: Neuroscience Approached Through Cell Culture, Volume 1 (S. Pfeiffer, ed.) CRC Press, Boca Raton, in press.

Barde, Y.-A., Edgar, D., and Thoenen, H., 1983, New neurotrophic factors, Ann. Rev. Physiol., in press.

Barde, Y.-A., Lindsay, R.M., Monard, D., and Thoenen, H., 1978, New growth factor released by glioma cells supporting survival and growth of sensory neurones, Nature, 274:818.

Bennett, M.R. and Nurcombe, V., 1980, Identification of embryonic motoneurons in vitro: their survival is dependent on skeletal muscle, Br. Res., 190:537-542.

Bonyhady, R.E., Hendry, I.A., Hill, C.E., and McLennan, I.S., 1980, Characterization of a cardiac muscle factor required for the survival of cultured parasympathetic neurons, Neurosci. Lett., 18:197-201.

Bueker, E.D., 1948, Implantation of tumors in the hind limb of the embryonic chick and developmental response of the lumbosacral nervous system, Anat. Rec., 102:369-390.

Burnstock, G., 1974, Degeneration and orientation of growth of
    autonomic nerves in relation to smooth muscle in joint tissue
    cultures and anterior eye chamber transplants, in: Dynamics of
    Degeneration and Growth in Neurons (K. Fuxe, L. Olson, and Y.
    Zollerman, eds.), Pergamon Press, Oxford, 509-520.
Chun, L.L.Y. and Patterson, P.H., 1977, Role of nerve growth factor
    in the development of rat sympathetic neurons in vitro. I.
    Survival, growth, and differentiaton of catecholamine
    production, J. Cell Biol., 75:694-704.
Collins, F., 1978, Induction of neurite outgrowth by a conditioned-
    medium factor bound to the culture substratum, Proc. Natl.
    Acad. Sci. USA, 75:5210-5213.
Coughlin, M.D., Bloom, E.M., and Black, I.B., 1981, Characterization
    of a neuronal growth factor from mouse heart-cell-conditioned
    medium, Dev. Biol., 82:52-68.
Cowan, W.M., 1973, Neuronal death as a regulative mechanism in the
    control of cell number in the nervous system, in: Development
    and Aging in the Nervous System (Rockstein, ed.), Academic
    Press, New York, 19-41.
Dibner, M.D. and Black, I.B., 1976, The effect of target organ
    removal on the development of sympathetic neurons, Br. Res.,
    103:93-102.
Ebendal, T. and Jacobson, C.O., 1977, Tissue explants affecting ex-
    tension and orientation of axons in cultured chick embryo
    ganglia, Exp. Cell Res., 105-379-387.
Ebendal, T., Belew, M., Jacobson, C.-O. and Porath, J., 1979,
    Neurite outgrowth elicited by embryonic chick heart,
    Neurosci. Lett., 14:91-95.
Eckenstein, F. and Thoenen, H., 1982, Production of specific anti-
    sera and monoclonal antibodies to choline acetyltransferase:
    characterization and use for identification of cholinertic
    neurons, EMBO J., 1:363=368.
Edgar, D., Barde, Y.-A., and Thoenen, H., 1981, Subpopulations of
    cultured chick sympathetic neurones differ in their requirements
    for survival factors, Nature, 289:294-295.
Edgar, D. and Thoenen, H., 1982a, Modulation of NGF-induced neuronal
    survival by contact with factors attached to the culture
    substrate. Abstr. 3rd International Meeting International
    Society for Developmental Neurosciences, Patras, Greece.
Edgar, D. and Thoenen, H., 1982b, Modulation of NGF-induced survival
    of chick sympathetic neurons by contact with a conditioned
    medium factor bound to the culture substrate, Dev. Brain Res.,
    in press.
Hamburger, V., 1977, The developmental history of the motor neuron,
    Neurosci. Res. Program Bull., 15 (Suppl).:iii-37.
Harper, G.P. and Thoenen, H., 1981, Target cells, biological effects
    and mechanism of action of Nerve Growth Factor and its
    antibodies, Ann. Rev. Pharm. & Toxicol., 21:20-229.

Hefti, F., Gnahn, H., Schwab, M.E., and Thoenen, H., 1982, Induction of tyrosine hydroxylase by Nerve Growth Factor and by elevated K+ concentrations in cultures of dissociated sympathetic neurons, J. Neurosci., in press.

Helfand, S.L., Smith, G.A., and Wessells, N.K., 1976, Survival and development in culture of dissociated parasympathetic neurons from ciliary ganglia, Dev. Biol., 50:541-547.

Hendry, I.A., 1975, The effects of axotomy on the development of the rat superior cervical ganglion, Brain Res., 90:235-244.

Hendry, I.A., 1977, The effect of the retrograde axonal transport of nerve growth factor on the morphology of adrenergic neurons, Brain Res., 134:213-223.

Herrup, K., and Shooter, E.M., 1975, Properties of the β-NGF receptor in development, J. Cell Biol., 67:118-125.

Jacobson, M., 1978, Developmental Neurobiology (2nd ed.) Plenum Press, London, New York.

Johnson, Jr., E.M., 1978, Destruction of the sympathetic nervous system in neonatal rats and hamsters by vinblastine: prevention by concomitant administrtion of nerve growth factor, Brain Res., 141:105-118.

Kessler, J.A. and Black, I.B., 1980, Nerve growth factor stimulates the development of substance P in sensory ganglia, Proc. Natl. Acad. Sci. USA, 77:649-653.

Kessler, J.A. and Black, I.B., 1981, Similarities in development of substance P and somatostatin in peripheral sensory neurons: Effects of capsaicin and nerve growth factor, Soc. Natl. Acad. Sci. USA, 78:4644-4747.

Kohler, G., and Milstein, C., 1976, Derivation of specific antibody-producing tissue culture and tumor lines by cell fusion, Eur. J. Immunol., 6:511-519.

Lander, A.D., Fujii, D.K., Gospodarowicz, D., and Reichardt, L.F., 1981, A heparan sulfate glycoprotein indudes rapid-neurite outgrowth in vitro, Soc. Neurosci. Abstr., 7:348.

Landmesser, L. and Pilar, G., 1976, Fate of ganglionic synapses and and ganglion cell axons during normal and induced cell death, J. Cell Biol., 68:357-374.

Levi-Montalcini, R., and Angeletti, P.U., 1968, Nerve growth factor, Physiol. Rev., 48:534-569.

Levi-Montalcini, R., Meyer, H., and Hamburger, V., 1954, In vitro experiments as the effects of mouse sarcomas 180 and 37 on the spinal and sympathetic ganglia of the chick embryo, Cancer Res., 14:49-57.

Levi-Montalcini, R., Aloe, L., Mugnaini, E., Oesch, F., and Thoenen, H., 1975, Nerve growth factor induces volume increase and enhances tyrosine hydroxylase synethesis in chemically axotomized sympathetic ganglia of newborn rats, Proc. Natl. Acad. Sci. USA, 72:595-599.

Lindsay, R.M., 1979, Adult rat brain astrocytes support survival of both NGF-dependent and NGF-insensitive neurones, Nature, 282:80-82.

Menesini Chen, M.G., Chen, J.S., Calissano, P., and Levi-Montalcini, R., 1977, Nerve growth factor prevents vinblastine destructive effects on sympathetic ganglia in newborn mice, Proc. Natl. Acad. Sci. USA, 74:5559-5563.

Miozzari, G.F., 1981, Strategies for obtaining expression of peptide hormones in E. coli, in: Insulins, Growth Hormone, and Recombinant DNA Technology, (J.L. Gueriguian, ed.), Raven Press, New York, 13-31.

Nishi, R. and Berg, D.K., 1981, Two components from eye tissue that differentially stimulate the growth and development of ciliary ganglion neurons in cell culture, J. Neurosci., 1:505-513.

Otten, U., Goedert, M., Mayer, N., and Lambeck, F., 1980, Requirement of nerve growth factor for development of substance P-containing sensory neurones, Nature, 287:158-159.

Rohrer, H. and Barde, Y.-A., 1982, Presence and disappearance of nerve growth factor receptors on sensory neurons in culture, Dev. Biol., 89:309-315.

Rohrer, H., Barde, Y.A., Edgar, D., and Thoenen, H., 1982, Nerve growth factor receptor on sensory and sympathetic neurons in culture, in: Neuroreceptors (F. Hucho, ed.), Walter de Gruyter & Co., Berlin, New York, 65-75.

Schmitt, F.O., Bird, S.J., and Bloom, F.E., 1982, Molecular Genetic Neuroscience, Raven Press, New York.

Schwab, M.E. and Thoenen, H., 1983, Retrograde axonal transport, in: Handbook of Neurochemistry (A. Lajtha, ed.), Plenum Publishing Corporation, New York, in press.

Thoenen, H., and Barde, Y.-A., 1980, Physiology of nerve growth factor, Physiol. Rev., 60:1284-1335.

Varon, S. and Adler, R., 1981, Trophic and specifying factors directed to neuronal cells, in: Advances in Cellular Neurobiology Volume 2 (S. Fedoroff and L. Herz, eds.), Academic Press, New York, 115-163.

Wakade, A.R., Edgar, D., and Thoenen, H., 1982, Substrate requirement and media supplements necessary for the long-term survival of chick sympathetic and sensory neurons cultured without serum, Exp. Cell Res., in press.

A GENETIC ANALYSIS OF EARLY NEUROGENESIS IN DROSOPHILA

José A. Campos-Ortega, Ruth Lehmann,
Fernando Jiminez[+] and Ursula Dietrich

Institut für Biologie III
Freiburg, West Germany

Centro de Biologia Molecular[+]
Facultad de Ciencias
Universidad Autonoma
Canto Blanco-Madrid
Spain

INTRODUCTION

As in other animals, the central nervous system (CNS) of _Droso-phila_ consists of supracellular units called ganglia. Each ganglion contains a characteristic array of neurones integrated in a frequently complex spatial pattern, and is connected with other ganglia by means of appropriate fiber tracts. Nerve cells, neuronal assemblies and connections are three prominent features of nervous systems, which emphasize the differences between the CNS and other organs and tissues of the body. From this follows that any developmental study of the CNS should be aimed to answer particular questions related to the following three problems: 1) The origin of the neurones as opposed to other cell types; 2) the origin of structural and functional patterns of neuronal assemblies; 3) the origin of the pattern of connections between ganglia.

We are currently concerned with the first of these problems, the origin of the neurones, and have approached it from the viewpoint of genetics. Early during _Drosophila_ embryogenesis cells of the ectodermal germ layer become committed to either the central neural or the epidermal pathway of development. It is plausible to assume neu-

129

ral and epidermal cell determination to be mediated by differential
gene activity. It is our working hypothesis that distinct patterns
of genetic activity do specify CNS and epidermal cell precursors,
and we intend to experimentally test this hypothesis. Our goal is
to understand how the genome of Drosophila contributes to control
the origin of the neurones as opposed to epidermal cells. Here we
present results from this work.

     This paper is divided into three main sections. The first one
summarizes what is known about normal neurogenesis in the embryo of
Drosophila.   In the second part we describe the phenotype of mutations in seven different loci which are apparently involved in this
process, and discuss some of the properties of genes with neurogenic
effects. The third part deals with functional relationships of
those genes with each other and with other genes of the Drosophila
genome, that are relevant for CNS development.

EARLY NEUROGENESIS IN DROSOPHILA

     The CNS of Drosophila develops from precursor cells, neuro-
blasts, which segregate from the ectodermal germ layer early in
embryogenesis and move into the embryo. Neuroblasts are supposed to
derive from a region of the ectoderm that is called neurogenic field.
Morphogenic maps (Poulson, 1950) indicate that the neurogenic field
occupies about 20% of the circumference on either side of the ventral
midline along the posterior two thirds of the embryo, and extends
dorsolaterally within the anterior one third. From the latter part
originates the cephalic supraesophageal ganglion, from the former the
subesophageal ganglia and the ventral cord. It is not clear whether
all neuroblasts arise from the neurogenic field as it has been defined above; it is possible that a few segregate from more laterally located ectoderm. Moreover, the cellular composition of the
neurogenic region is not well understood. For example, it is not
known whether the neurogenic field is a continuous stripe of ectoderm, all cells of which develop into neuroblasts. Alternatively
neural and epidermal cell precursors might be intermingled. Histology does not provide the necessary evidence because neuroblast
segregation is a fast process which seems to be accomplished within
some 30 minutes. In sections of the early germ band conspicuous
clusters of large cells become evident in paramedian position in the
neighborhood of the mesoectodermal cells. Most, or all, neuroblasts
of the ventral cord derive from these clusters. Not all neuroblasts
of a given neuromere leave the ectoderm at the same time. Single
cells drop from the ventromedial ectoderm into the space limited by
mesoderm and ectoderm initiating development as neural cell precursors so that no invagination of the whole neural anlage takes place
in Drosophila. Therefore early neurogenesis in this animal cannot
be compared to the invagination of the neural plate in vertebrates,
where the sequence of events leading to the neural tube can easily
be followed. The clusters of presumptive neuroblasts vanish within

a short time, less than 30 min, apparently because single cells are
continuously being pushed into the embryo by laterally dividing ectodermal cells. The whole of the germ layer consists thereafter of
cylindrical cells arranged in a rather homogeneous epithelium. Most
of these cells are the dermatoblasts, which will divide 1-2 times
each (Szabad et al., 1979) to give rise to the larval epidermis; a
few of them will invaginate to form the anlagen of the imaginal epidermis, i.e. imaginal discs and histoblasts; and the remaining cells
will contribute to form the tracheal stem. The neuroblast complement
of each thoracic and abdominal neuromere consists of some 18-20
cells, the total number of differentiated neurones is about 300 per
neuromere (Poulson, 1950). The exact pattern of neuroblast divisions
is unknown, but it is assumed that ventral cord neuroblasts divide
only asymmetrically producing at each division a small cell called
ganglion mother cell (Bauer, 1904) and another neuroblast. Whereas
the ganglion mother cells are each thought to divide only once,
neuroblasts undergo asymmetric mitosis repeatedly, at least 8-10
times (Poulson, 1950). The size of the neuroblasts decreases from
mitosis to mitosis, so that during the last divisions asymmetry is
less evident. The polarity of neuroblast division is constantly the
same, and therefore new cells accumulate towards the inner side of
the embryo forming a column-like arrangement of related cells, with
the progenitor neuroblast towards the outside. Neuroblasts within
the prospective head region behave in a different way than those in
the developing ventral cord. For example, they become evident slightly earlier than ventral cord neuroblasts and do not separate from
the ectodermal germ layer for a few hours; they divide both symme-
trically, to produce two equal size neuroblasts, and asymmetrically
to give rise to smaller ganglion mother cells. Eventually the developing brain lobes become displaced into the head by the ingrowing
epidermis. The cephalic CNS anlage which leaves the ectoderm last
is the anlage of the imaginal optic lobes. This is a well defined
group of invaginating cells which joins the developing protocerebrum
at the end of the first one-third of embryogenesis. In addition to
optic lobe neuroblasts, which will proliferate during larval stages
to give rise to the imaginal optic lobes, other embryonic neuroblasts
retain their abilities to divide and later contribute to the imaginal CNS. However, except for the optic lobes, there is no information available about the number of imaginal neuroblasts nor about
their location within the larval brain.

The first signs of neuronal differentiation are visible midway
in Drosophila embryogenesis. Dorsally in the ventral cord and in
centrally located portions of the brain lobes, fibers appear which
apparently have grown from the oldest neurones. The topology of
those fibers reflects the peculiar polarity of division of Drosophila
neuroblasts described above, and suggests a defined polarity of the
neurones themselves from which the fibers grow. The volume of the
neuropil increases as time passes, and its final organization becomes
evident immediately after germ band shortening. Condensation of the

CNS continues until the posterior tip of the ventral cord comes to
lie at some 40% egg length towards the end of embryogenesis.

NEUROGENIC MUTANTS

     In the following we shall discuss Drosophila mutants which
affect early neurogenesis. These mutants have been found in the
course of a fairly extensive analysis of mutations which was performed with the aim of localizing the genes involved in the segregation
of neuroblasts and dermatoblasts from the ectoderm. As a result of
this analysis we have identified several loci that are involved in a
variety of ways in CNS development. The phenotypes produced by mutations in those genes have been discussed in several papers to which
the interested reader is referred (see Jiminez and Campos-Ortega,
1979, 1981; Campos-Ortega and Jimenez, 1980; Lehmann et al., 1981,
1982). In this paper we shall deal with mutations at seven different
loci, whose phenotypes indicate a participation of the mutated genes
in the segregation of neural and epidermal cell precursors. The
genetic loci to be discussed are listed in Table 1. All these
mutations produce essentially the same phenotype. It consists of an
initial misrouting into the neural pathway of development of ectodermal cells which in the wildtype would have given rise to epidermal cells. Consequently, the CNS of the mutants initiates
development with a larger number of neuroblasts than the wildtype,
whereas the surface of the ectoderm committed to form epidermis,
i.e. the number of epidermal cell precursors, is smaller. This
defect leads after completion of embryogenesis to clear hypertrophy
of the CNS of the mutants and, concomitantly, to hypotrophy of the
epidermis, important parts of which are lacking. The remaining
organs of the mutants, e.g. endoderm and mesoderm derivatives, are
not directly affected by these mutations (but only in as much as
secondarily conditioned by the huge CNS and the lack of epidermis).
In spite of a relatively normal cytodifferentiation of affected
parts, such mutant embyros cannot hatch and are necessarily lethal.

     Among the seven loci that were identified in our mutational
analysis, three correspond to new genes, big brain (bib), master mind
(mam) and neuralized (neu)(Lehmann et al., 1981). They were found
among embryonic lethals collected by Nusslein-Volhard and Wieschaus
(unpublished, and 1980) on the basis of their epidermal defects and
kindly given to us. The other four turned out to correspond to
already known genes. One of these genes is Notch (N), one of the
most thoroughly studied loci in Drosophila (Welshons, 1965, 1974;
Welshons and Keppy, 1981). It was also known that N affects neurogenesis since Poulson (1937) discovered the morphogenic defects
associated with hemizygous N embryos, and described this phenotype
and its embryonic development in subsequent papers (Poulson, 1940,
1945, 1968). We have isolated several new alleles of N, our study
confirming Poulson's findings in their major aspects. The other
three already known genes are Delta (Dl), Enhancer of split (E(spl))

Table 1.

Locus	Map Position	Cytology	Alleles
Notch	1-3.	3C7	26
almondex (amx)	1-27.7	8D	1
big brain (bib)	2-34.7	27A-31	7
master mind (mam)	2-70.3	50-51	10
neuralized (neu)	3-50	86C1-2-86D8	6
Delta (Dl)	3-66.2	92A1-2	29
Enhancer of split (E(spl))	3-89.1	associated with break- point in 96E-F	3

and almondex (amx). It was, however, not known that these genes affect neurogenesis in a similar way as N.

Notwithstanding the similarity in phenotype, there are conspicuous differences between the mutations which we would like to discuss. Dl and E(spl), like N itself, are haploinsufficient loci. Thus, heterozygous N/+, Dl/+ and E(spl)^R/+ flies, though perfectly viable, show defects in both compound eyes and wings, whereas homozygous embryos develop the defects mentioned above and are lethal. amx, on the other hand, is a maternal effect mutation, whereby homozygous females and hemizygous males are viable but their progeny is embryonically lethal displaying the mutant syndrome. Thus the gene product of amx+ is an essential maternal contribution to the development of the wildtype . The remaining three loci, bib, mam and neu, have been identified by recessive lethal mutations.

Further differences to be considered refer to the extent of the morphogenic defect which is attained by mutations at each locus. In its zygotic or maternal expression, each locus is able to reach a characteristic degree of neuralization. This fact enables ordering of the seven loci in a series ranging from Dl, with the strongest, to mam with the weakest expression. The actual sequence is Dl> E(spl)^R>amx>neu>N>bib>mam. Nevertheless it must be emphasized that we are dealing with graded differences in the same process, namely neuralization of increasing amounts of ectodermal cells. Dl,

$E(spl)^R$ and amx embryos show the most severe forms of the phenotype.
These mutations cause neuralization of the entire ventral half of
the ectoderm up to the tracheal anlagen, and of most of the head.
However, dorsal epidermis, as well as fore- and hindgut derivatives
along with endoderm and mesoderm derivatives are able to develop
normally. This differential behavior of ectodermal cells towards
neuralization is a striking finding to which we shall come back
later on.

The morphogenic anomaly produced by these mutations suggests
that the seven loci are sharing the same function during the
development of the wildtype. Wright (1970) proposed that N+
suppresses neuroblast production in some ectodermal cells and makes
possible their epidermal commitment. The lack of N+ function would
therefore result in additional neuroblasts and the absence of the
corresponding dermatoblasts. This hypothesis can also be applied to
explain the phenotype of the remaining six mutations. Thus we propose
that the functional integrity of at least seven genes is necessary to
keep the neurogenic field within the limits of the wildtype.

Maternal effects

The postulated common function of neurogenic genes makes it
necessary to reconsider the phenotypic differences found between the
mutants. Referring exclusively to the neuralizing capabilities of
the genes, if these genes share one function, why do they produce
quantitatively different phenotypes? One possibility to explain
phenotypic differences would be that the genes are maternally expressed. We have found that this is indeed the case for N and mam
(Jimenez and Campos-Ortega, 1982).

All neurogenic genes except amx, which as already mentioned is a
maternal effect mutation, were identified as zygotic lethal mutations.
This means that the zygotic expression of those genes is necessary
for normal development. Since the mutations are embryonic lethal
they are normally kept in heterozygous condition, i.e. over one copy
of the wildtype gene. Matings between heterozygous flies give rise
to the homozygous embryos that we study. If the genes under discussion would be active during oogenesis, then gene products from the
wildtype copy would be laid down in the unfertilized egg cell and
thus prevent, or modify, the full expression of the mutant zygotic
phenotype. In order to test this hypothesis we removed maternal
wildtype genes in the germ line of heterozygous females, by inducing
early in gametogenesis homozygosis for neurogenic mutations via
mitotic recombination. Consequently, clones of egg cells developed
in the absence of the respective maternal wildtype gene. To make
possible the identification of oocytes derived from homozygous mutant
germ line cells we used additional mutations which cause sterility of
heterozygous females by blocking oogenesis (Wieschaus, 1980). The
sterility is cell autonomous and germ line dependent; in other words,

it depends on the genotype of the germ line cell itself. Given the appropriate genotypic constitution, recombination can make a germ line cell simultaneously homozygous for the neurogenic mutation and wildtype in regard to the sterility gene. Thus, the only eggs to develop normally in such females will be the progeny of homozygous germ line cells. When crossed with appropriate males, embryos were obtained lacking both maternal and zygotic components of gene expression.

This experiment could be performed only with N and mam, since appropriate dominant female sterile mutations were only available for the chromosome arms in which these two genes map. Removing maternal and zygotic products of N+ and mam+ results in two important consequences: first, the morphogenic defect is stronger under these conditions than in control embryos, i.e. where maternal products are available; second, the phenotypes of N and mam embryos become virtually identical. It is noteworthy that the increased phenotypic severity of N and mam embryos devoid of maternal and zygotic components of gene expression reaches the level of, or is only slightly stronger than that of Dl deletions. In the context of phenotypic differences between control N and mam embryos the present results are conclusive in showing those differences to be due to different maternal contributions from each gene. Two main conclusions follow from these results: 1) N+ and mam+ have dual, maternal and zygotic, expression; 2) maternal and zygotic expression show additivity of effects, the total genetic contribution of each gene to neurogenesis being the same. A further important result of this analysis is that the maternal expression of N+ is necessary for viability of the wildtype embryo. Jimenez and Campos-Ortega (1982) found that embryos derived from N homozygous germ line cells are lethal irrespective of their own genomic constitution. By contrast, the maternal expression of mam+ is not necessary for wildtype viability. In other words, the zygotic expression of mam+ is both necessary and sufficient in this regard.

It must be pointed out at this place that amx+ does actually show the same duality of gene expression, whereby zygotic expression of amx+, like the maternal expression of mam+, is dispensable for the viability of the zygote. amx was already known to be a zygotically rescuable, maternal effect mutation. When homozygous amx females are crossed with amx males the whole progeny displays the mutant phenotype. However, a few larvae develop normally and even reach adulthood when wildtype males are used in the crosses (Shannon, 1972, 1973). Furthermore, the number of adult progeny increases considerably when the males carry two copies of amx+ by means of a duplication of the gene (Dp(1;1)lz^{+2}, Lehmann et al., 1982). This shows the genetic products contributed to the zygote by the paternal genome to be actually utilized to compensate for the lack of maternal amx+ function. We have asked ourselves whether the remaining neurogenic loci are also maternally expressed. Unfortunately the lack of appropriate dominant sterile mutations precludes using the same approach that was used in the cases of N and mam. In the case of Dl, however, whose zygotic phenotype closely approaches the most extreme form of the neurogenic syndrome, there is one piece of evidence that indicates this gene to not be maternally expressed in any appreciable way. In crosses of two different, non-complementing Dl alleles, one being weak and the other strong, the resulting embryos show a phenotype intermediate between the weak and the strong one. This intermediate phenotype is apparently the same irrespective of the paternal or maternal provenance of the strong allele. By performing similar reciprocal crosses with weak and strong alleles of N or of mam, the resulting intermediate phenotype is invariably stronger when the strong allele was provided by the mother (Lehmann, 1981). This reflects the maternal expression of N and mam and suggests that Dl is exclusively expressed during the development of the zygote. It is highly desirable to assess possible maternal expression of bib, neu and E(spl), and experiments in this direction are in preparation.

FUNCTIONAL INTERRELATIONSHIPS

The similarity, or identity in some cases, of the phenotype caused by the mutations under discussion strongly suggests related functions of the affected genes. In order to test possible functional interrelationships of neurogenic genes at the cellular level we are currently following two different approaches. In the first one, to enable estimations of possible additive effects in the activity of the seven loci we are studying embryos carrying two different mutant genes. With the second approach we intend to assess the modifiability of the mutant phenotype produced by a given mutant, by increasing the amount of wildtype gene products from each of the other neurogenic genes. None of these experiments is, however, finished; either because of the still pending synthesis of a few double mutant combinations, or due to the lack of appropriate duplications of bib+, mam+, neu+ and E(spl)+. Despite the incompleteness of our study some preliminary results have been obtained which merit to be discussed.

When using lethal alleles the first interesting finding is that strong Dl alleles which do not complement $E(spl)^{Rl-3}$, i.e. are embryonic lethal in heterozygosis over each other, although weak alleles of Dl are viable over any of the three $E(spl)^R$. This indicates closely related functions of Dl+ and E(spl)+. All remaining heterozygous combinations of the other genes are viable and therefore allow the production of double homozygous mutant embryos. These embryos behave according to two different patterns which depend on which genes have been combined. Combinations between lethal alleles of N, bib, mam and neu with each other have shown additive effects, in that the phenotype of the double mutant is more severe than any of the phenotypes of the combined mutations (unpublished observations; Lehmann, 1981). However, the increased severity of the double mutant phenotype only reaches a similar level of neuralization than that of Dl deletions, suggesting this to be the maximal possible extent of the neuralizing process to be attained. This tentative conclusion receives support from the results of combining amx, Dl or E(spl)^R with any other of the remaining four genes. The phenotype of such combinations closely corresponds to that of the stronger of the two combined mutations.

These results indicate functional interrelationships between neurogenic genes. On purely operational terms one could postulate some overlapping in the territory of action of, at least, N, bib, mam, and neu, the removal of two of those genes manifesting the functional overlapping with the increased severity of the double mutant phenotype. The fact that combinations using amx, Dl and E(spl)^R do not produce the same effect, does not mean that the latter genes are not interrelated to the former four, since it seems that the ability of the Drosophila embryo to be neuralized is already almost exhausted by the lack of function of amx+, Dl+ or E(spl)+ alone. Thus, one should not expect any further neuralization to be effected on embryos carrying one of those strong mutations by removing additional genes of the system.

The results of combining bib, mam or neu alleles with increasing doses of N+ by using different duplications of the N+ locus, do point in the same direction. Several different duplications of N+ have been made available by Lefevre (1952) and by Welshons (1965), which segregate with the first, the second or the third chromosome. They enabled the synthesis of homozygous bib, mam, neu, Dl and E(spl)^R embryos carrying up to six copies of N+. The assumedly higher amounts of N+ gene product present in those embryos are apparently able to partially rescue the phenotype of the three first mutations towards the wildtype, by reducing the extent of the neuralization; but those N+ gene products do not seem to exert any influence on Dl or E(spl)^R. Similarly, amx+ and Dl- duplications in up to four doses leave the phenotype of mutations in any of the other five genes without important modifications.

Although preliminary, these results emphasize a key role for N. Lethal N alleles of N+ duplications modify the phenotype of bib, mam and neu embryos. Therefore two groups of loci arise from this analysis, the elements of each of which seem to be related: the haplo-insufficient loci Dl and E(spl) together with N, on the one hand, and the recessive lethals bib, mam and neu also together with N, on the other hand. As to amx, the only predominantly maternal effect mutation of the series, there are as yet no indications for any kind of genetic interactions with the remaining neurogenic genes.

Topological specificity of neurogenic genes

A further important result of the analysis of double mutants is
the apparent incapability of some ectodermal regions, e.g. the anlage
of the dorsal epidermis and some fore- and hindgut derivatives, to be
neuralized by the lack of function of neurogenic genes. Apparently,
neurogenic genes are completely suppressed within certain regions of
the ectoderm, and conditionally expressable within the remaining
ones. Following on those lines one would have to accept the wildtype ectoderm to be compartmentalized, in that one half is susceptible to neurogenesis and able to react to mutations in neurogenic
genes, whereas the other half is insensitive to those mutations.
We would like to report here on a few experiments which support
this hypothesis, by showing the neuralizing ability of neurogenic
genes to be dependent on certain characteristics of the ectodermal
substrate on which they act.

Two additional mutations of Drosophila which change the dorsoventral polarity of the wildtype embryo have been used for this
purpose. Both are maternal effect mutations. One is dorsal (dl),
as it was called by its discoverer Nüsslein-Volhard (1980), because
it effects the complete dorsalization of the embryo. Embryos derived
from homozygous dl mothers do not develop any of the pattern elements
of the ventral and lateral regions but consist of dorsal structures
in all regions. This defect is due to an initial programming of
embryonic cells to form dorsal pattern elements in the whole circumferential extent of the embryo, rather than to impairment of the development of ventral cell precursors (Nüsslein-Volhard, 1980).
Accordingly there is no CNS in dl embryos, but a small conglomerate
of neurones within the presumptive head region, most probably derived
from the procephalic lobes (dorsally located in the wildtype). The
second mutation was discovered by Wieschaus and Nüsslein-Volhard (unpublished) and has been provisionally called Toll (Tl). Tl is a
dominant female sterile mutation. The progeny of Tl/+ females lacks
dorsal pattern elements and shows instead derivaties of the ventral
wildtype anlagen within both dorsal and ventral regions of the
mutant. We have brought N, amx and Dl alleles into a dl or a Tl
background, in order to see whether and to what extent neuralization
occurs in this highly modified ectoderm.

All neurogenic mutants tested behave in the same way. When combined with dl they do not effect any neuralization except for the
head region, where they cause a clear increase in volume of differentiated neural tissue at the expense of the cephalic epidermis.
Combinations of N and dl had already been studied by E. Wieschaus
(personal communication) who obtained the same result. We have extended the experiment to the observation of N;dl embryos derived from
homozygous germ line cells. The result is essentially the same: even
after removing its entire genetic activity, N only expresses itself
in the head territory, being unable to bring about neuralization of

thoracic and abdominal segments of the d1 embryo.

The situation is completely opposite in combinations of neurogenic mutations with Tl. With the exception of pharynx, eosphagus
and hindgut, all ectodermal derivatives of N;Tl or Dl/Tl embryos are
neuralized. The whole epidermis is absent, being substituted by
neural cells. However, endoderm and mesoderm derivatives are
unaffected.

The main conclusion of these observations is that the developmental history of the ectodermal cells, rather than merely their
location in the embryo, decides about their sensitivity to react with
neuralization upon mutation in neurogenic genes. The genetic system
that in the wildtype determines the spatial coordinates of the
embryonic pattern (dl, Tl and perhaps other still unknown genes) is
therefore epistatic over neurogenic genes. The former system
determines the positional values of ectodermal cells; the latter becomes active afterwards and contributes to translate those positional
values into the actual pattern. The whole ectoderm of thoracic and
abdominal segments of dl embryos lacks the ability to enter the
neural developmental pathway, its only possible commitment being the
epidermal one. Contrarily, this ability to develop into neural cell
precursors is shared by all ectodermal cells of the same segments in
Tl embryos. When comparing these findings with the wildtype
situation, it seems plausible to conclude the expressiveness of
neurogenic genes in the ventral ectoderm and its derivatives, and
their suppression in the dorsal ectoderm. Embryological studies mentioned above demonstrated the tracheal placodes to mark the limit of
neurogenic activity. In relation with this observation we should
like to briefly refer to another set of experiments, in which N
embryos were derived from mothers carrying weak alleles of dl,
e.g. dl^2. This allele (also recovered by Nüsslein-Volhard, 1979)
effects incomplete dorsalization of the embryo such that some more
ventrally located structures of the wildtype, e.g. tracheal stem and
rudiments of the denticle belts, do develop normally in the mutant.
However, dorsalization of the dl^2 ectoderm is considerable, most of
the ventral derivatives being absent. The CNS of these mutants is
reduced to a thin stripe of neurones along the germ band and to the
remnant of the protocerebrum in the head region. In $N;dl^2$ embryos
neuralization occurs ventrally at both thoracic and abdominal levels,
as well as within the head region. But neuralization in thorax and
abdomen exclusively affects ectodermal cells situated ventral to the
tracheal placodes of the mutants. Neurogenetic gene activity, therefore, seems to depend on spatial cues controlled by coordinate genes.

CONCLUSIONS

We want to emphasize three main conclusions, drawn from the observations reported above, which define the lines of our future work.

The first conclusion is the apparent validity of our working hypothesis: Differential gene activity is responsible for a normal neurogenesis in Drosophila. The following two arguments support this conclusion: 1) A small number of genes have been found to be involved in the segregation of neuroblasts and dermoblasts. Mutation in those genes results in abnormal neurogenesis due to the wrong commitment of precursor cells. Whether or not these seven loci represent all genes of the Drosophila genome to be involved in this process remains open; however, some evidence indicates this to be the case. 2) There is a topological specifity in the expression of these seven genes. The experimental results indicate that in the wildtype the genes are suppressed within all derivaties of the endoderm and mesoderm and some derivatives of the ectoderm, and conditionally expressed in the remaining ectoderm. Therefore, a distinct pattern of genetic activity is necessary for normal development of some embryonic regions, whereas this genetic activity is dispensable in the remaining regions. Experiments described above demonstrate differential expression of neurogenic genes to be subordinate to the genetic system that establishes egg polarity. dl and Tl, two genes of this system, are epistatic over neurogenic genes in that they determine the fate of embryonic cells, without necessarily implying direct involvement of dl+ and Tl+ in the activation of the neurogenic genes. Nevertheless these findings are suggestive of a temporal sequence of genetic activity, its first step being the activation of polarity genes, followed by that of steps form part of this sequence is unknown.

The second conclusion concerns the genetic system that contributes to control neurogenesis. It presents some peculiarities that might well be relevant in the context of its possible function during development. The first of these peculiarities is the combination of maternal and zygotic components of gene expression so far demonstrated for three of the seven genes (N, amx and mam). Removal of both components of gene expression has led to virtually identical phenotypes of the mutations investigated, and at the same time to the uncovering of comparable morphogenic defects produced by the lack of function form any of five genes (N, amx, mam, Dl and E(spl)). The genetic contribution to neurogenesis of each of those genes is therefore equivalent. Mutations in Drosophila are customarily classified as either zygotic or maternal, depending on the effects being dependent of the zygotic or the maternal genome. A dual, maternal and zygotic, gene expression is an exceptional situation, only a few instances of which are known in Drosophila (Fausto-Sterling et al., 1977; Shearn et al., 1978). In the case of N and mam both components evidently add their effects in such a way that the morphogenic defect is considerably stronger when the maternal products are removed along with the zygotic ones. Paradoxically the lack of maternal information by itself does not seem to produce any morphological defect when the zygotic component is present, although genetically wildtype embryos are lethal when derived from N homozygous

germ line cells. Apparently the zygotic component can compensate
for the lack of maternal gene products, at least concerning their
role in neurogenesis. The lethality of embryos derived from N homozygous germ line cells would be explained if N+ participates during
oogenesis in other vital functions, probably independent of neurogenesis.

The last conclusion refers to the functional interrelationship
of genes with neurogenic effects, a further peculiarity of the
system, which has been shown at several instances. The synergistic
effects of lethal alleles of N, bib, mam and neu; the partial suppression of the phenotype of homozygous bib, mam and neu by increasing doses of N+, and thus by assumedly increasing amounts of its
gene product, all these are examples of functional community of
these genes, which let envisage highly complex regulatory mechanisms
still poorly understood. From the side of transmission genetics a
host of experiments and tests must still be performed from which we
hope to complete the very fragmentary and dispersed body of data on
which we dispose nowadays. A deeper understanding of functional
relationships between neurogenic genes is to be expected from any
biochemical approach which would provide insight into the nature of
the different gene products (ref. to Thörig et al., 1981a and b).

ACKNOWLEDGEMENTS

We gratefully acknowledge Sigrid Krien for excellent technical
assistance, Gerd Jürgens, Chr. Nüsslein-Volhard and Eric Wieschaus
for mutants and discussions and the Deutsche Forschungsgemeinschaft
(SFB 46) for financial support.

REFERENCES

Bauer, V., 1904, Zur inneren Metamorphose des Centralnervensystems
    der Insecten. Zool. Jahrb. Abt. Anat. Ontog. Tiere,
    20:123-150.
Campos-Ortega, J.A. and Jiménez, F., 1980, The effect of X-chromosome
    deficiencies on neurogenesis in Drosophila, in: Development and
    Neurobiology of Drosophila, (Siddiqi, O., Babu, P., Hall, L.M.
    and Hall, J.C. eds.), Plenum Press, New York, pp. 201-222.
Fausto-Sterling, A., Weiner, A.J. and Digan, M.E., 1977, Analysis of
    a newly isolated temperature sensitive, maternal effect mutation
    of Drosophila melangoster, J. Exp. Biol., 200:199-210.
Jiménez, F. and Campos-Ortega, J.A., 1979, A region of the Drosophila
    genome necessary for CNS development, Nature, 282:310-311.
Jiménez, F. and Campos-Ortega, J.A., 1981, A cell arrangement specif-
    ic to thoracic ganglia in the central nervous system of the
    Drosophila embryo: its behaviour in homeotic mutants, Roux's
    Arch. Dev. Biol., 190:370-373.

Jiménez, F. and Campos-Ortega, J.A., 1982, Maternal effects of
    zygotic mutants affecting early neurogenesis in Drosophila,
    Roux's Arch. Dev. Biol., in press.
Lefevre, G., 1952, Dp (1;2)w^{51b7}, D.I.S.., 26:66.
Lehmann, R., 1981, Untersuchungen an zwei Mutanten der frühen
    Neurogenese bei Drosophila melanogaster, Diplomathesis, Univer-
    sity of Freiburg.
Lehmann, R., Deitrich, U., Jiménez, F. and Campos-Ortega, F.A., 1981,
    Mutations of early neurogenesis in Drosophila, Roux's Arch. Dev.
    Biol., 190:226-229.
Lehmann, R., Jiménez, F., Campos-Ortega, J.A. and Dietrich, U., 1982,
    in preparation.
Nüsslein-Volhard, Chr., 1979, Pattern mutants in Drosophila embryo-
    genesis, in: Cell lineage stem cells and cell determination (Le
    Douarin, N., ed.), Sinserm Symp. N 10, Elsevier, pp. 69-82.
Nüsslein-Volhard, Chr., 1980, Maternal effect mutations that alter
    the spatial coordinates of the embryo of Drosophila
    melanogaster, in: Determinants of spatial organization
    (Subtelney, S., and Konigsberg, I.R., eds.), Acad. Press, New
    York, pp. 185-211.
Nüsslein-Volhard, Chr. and Wieschaus, E., 1980, Mutations affecting
    segment number and polarity in Drosophila, Nature 287:795-801.
Poulson, D.F., 1937, Chromosomal deficiencies and the embryonic
    development of Drosophila melanogaster, Proc. Nat. Acad. Sci.,
    23:133-137.
Poulson, D.F., 1940, The effect of certain chromosome deficiences on
    the embryonic development of Drosophila melanogaster, J. Exp.
    Zool., 83:271-325.
Poulson, D.F., 1945, Chromosomal control of embryogenesis in
    Drosophila, Am. Anat., 79:340-363.
Poulson, D.F., 1950, Histogenesis, organogenesis and differentiation
    in the embryo of Drosophila melanogaster Meigen, in: Biology of
    Drosophila, (Demerec, M., ed.), Wiley, New York, pp. 168-274.
Poulson, D.F., 1968, The embryogenetic function of the Notch locus in
    Drosophila melanogaster, Proc. 12th Int. Congr. Genetics Tokyo,
    1:143.
Shannon, M.P., 1972, Characterization of the female sterile mutant
    almondex of Drosophila melanogaster, Genetica, 43:244-256.
Shannon, M.P., 1973, The development of eggs produced by the female-
    sterile mutant almondex of Drosophila melanogaster, J. Exp.
    Zool., 183:383-400.
Shearn, A., Hersperger, G., Hersperger, E., 1978, Genetic analysis
    of two allelic temperature-sensitive mutants of Drosophila
    melanogaster both of which are zyotic and maternal effect
    lethals, Genetica, 89:341-353.
Szabad, J., Schüpbach, T. and Wieschaus, E., 1979, Cell lineage and
    development of the larval epidermis, Devel. Biol., 73:256-271.
Thörig, G.E.W., Heinstra, P.W.H. and Scharloo, W., 1981, The action
    of the Notch locus in Drosophila melanogaster, I. Effects of

the Notch[8] deficiency on mitochondrial enzymes, Molec. Gen. Genet., 182:31-38.

Thörig, G.E.W., Heinstra, P.W.H. and Scharloo, W., 1981, The action of the Notch locus in Drosophila melanogaster. II. Biochemical effects of recessive lethals on mitochondrial enzymes, Genetics, 99:65-74.

von Halle, E.S., 1965, Localization of E(spl), D.I.S., 40:60.

Welshons, W.J., 1956, D.I.S., 30:157-158.

Welshons, W.J., 1965, Analysis of a gene in Drosophila, Science, 150:1122-1129.

Welshons, W.J., 1974, The cytogenetic analysis of a fractured gene in Drosophila, Genetics, 76:775-794.

Welshons, W.J. and Keppy, D.O., 1975, Intragenic deletions and salivary band relationships in Drosophila, Genetics, 80:143-155.

Wieschaus, E., 1980, A combined genetic and mosaic approach to the study of oogenesis in Drosophila, in: Development and Neurobiology of Drosophila, (Siddiqi, O., Babu, P., Hall, L.M. and Hall, J.C., eds.), Plenum Press, New York, pp. 85-94.

Wright, T.R.F., 1970, The genetics of embryogenesis in Drosophila, Adv. Genet., 15:262-395.

SEMANTICS AND NEURAL DEVELOPMENT

Gunther S. Stent

Department of Molecular Biology
University of California
Berkeley, California 94720

GENETIC INFORMATION

The latter-day success of molecular biology in providing a physical account of the structure and function of the hereditary material
was in large part due to the focus of its founders on the concept
of "genetic information". As was spelled out thirty-five years ago
by Erwin Schrödinger (1945) in his seminal book What Is Life?, the
gene can be viewed as an information carrier whose physical structure
corresponds to an aperiodic succession of a small number of isomeric
elements of a hereditary codescript. Eventually, the gene was identified as a segment of a double helical DNA molecule residing in
the chromosomes of the cell nucleus. The isomeric elements of the
hereditary codescript turned out to be the four nucleotide bases
adenine, guanine, thymine, and cytosine, which embody the genetic
information by their aperiodic linear sequence along the DNA molecule. And as far as the meaning of the information contained in
an individual gene is concerned, it was first put forward as an
a priori dogmatic postulate and later established as an empirical
fact, that the linear sequence of DNA nucleotide bases stands for
the linear sequence of amino acids of a particular protein molecule. The two sequences are related to each other via a genetic
code, under which each nucleotide base triplet stands for one of
the twenty kinds of amino acids of which protein molecules are built.
However, the chromosomal DNA also contain some nucleotide base sequence segments which do not stand for protein molecules, and,
strictly speaking, do not constitute genes. Some of these segments

145

serve as templates for the assembly of nucleic acid components of the cellular apparatus for protein synthesis, such as transfer and ribosomal RNA molecules, and other segments serve as control sites at which the expression of the genes is regulated. Thus there exists at present a reasonably satisfactory state of understanding of the nature of the informational content and meaning of the structural elements of the genetic material.

GENOME AND PHENOME

However, the present state of understanding the overall meaning of the entire DNA complement of an organism, or its genome, is much less satisfactory. What does the genome, in fact, mean? A not uncommon answer to this question is that the genome is a one-dimensional representation of the organism. For instance, Carl Sagan once suggested at a Conference on Communication with Extraterrestrial Intelligence (Sagan, 1973) that to transmit via radio signals the DNA nucleotide sequence of a cat to a Distant Alien Civilization is equivalent to sending the Aliens the cat itself. This suggestion, though made partly in jest, allows us to recognize that the correct answer to the question about the meaning of the genome is not so obvious. Rather, what is obvious is that the Aliens, even if they possessed a table of the terrestrial genetic code, would not be able to reconstruct the cat from its DNA nucleotide base sequence. To make this reconstruction, the Aliens would have to know a great deal more about terrestrial life than the formal relations between the DNA nucleotide base sequences and protein amino acid sequences.

What they would have to know, above all, is that the actual cat, or the feline phenome, arises from a fertilized egg containing the feline DNA nucleotide sequences in the course of embryonic development. Moreover, the Aliens would have to understand the developmental relation between phenome and genome, an understanding which we unfortunately still lack. As I shall try to show here, the Aliens could not, regardless of their level of intelligence and technical sophistication, discover the feline phenome by semantic analysis of the feline DNA, for the reason that the developmental relations cannot be abstracted from the DNA. And what goes for the Aliens goes for us too.

THE EPIGENETIC LANDSCAPE

As C.H. Waddington (1957) set forth long before the informational theories of molecular biology had even received their experimental validation, the information embodied in the genome does not represent an organism but merely some functional components of an epigenetic landscape. What Waddington meant by this poetic term is a plot of multivariant functional relations in multidimensional space. In this space, developmental time is the independent variable and the properties that describe both the organism and its environment are the

dependent variables. The functional relations from which this landscape is constructed are the chemical and physical processes which
relate the changes in these properties with the flow of developmental
pathways along which the embryo moves from fertilized egg to adult.
Waddington's main reason for using the landscape metaphor was to
point out that in this space the developmental pathways are bound to
form a system of interconnected valleys that slope "downward" from
the summit of the egg with developmental time towards the "sea level"
of the adult organism. This feature would assure that the pathways
are relatively resistant to perturbations of the functional relations
fluctuations in the dependent variables, and thus guarantee a reasonably invariant relation between genome and phenome. The role of the
genes in shaping this landscape derives from their control of critical
chemical processes in the developmental sequences, or (as we now
know) from their governance of the production of protein molecules
capable of catalyzing specific chemical reactions.

     The idea of the epigenetic landscape certainly brings us closer
to an understanding of the relation between the genetic information
and the organism to which it gives rise. And it can fairly be said
that the discovery of the functional relations of that landscape, or
as Francois Jacob (1973) has called them, "the algorithms of the
living world", is one of the main goals, if not the main goal, of
contemporary genetic biology. But I give it as my opinion that, thus
far at least, this goal has not generally been brought into sufficiently sharp conceptual focus, because of semantic difficulties
inherent in the notion of "phenome", on the one hand, and in the
notion of "meaning", as applied to the genetic information, on the
other hand.

OSTENSION AND CONNOTATION

     It is not without irony that the problem of meaning is no less
troublesome in the domain of human communication, for which the scientific concept of information was developed in the first place,
than in the study of the genome-phenome relation to which semantic
notions have been extended by molecular geneticists. Since the
question of how meaning arises from language, or even what it is we
are saying about a word when we say what it means, still awaits its
answer, it is hardly surprising that we encounter also conceptual
difficulties with the metaphorical use of semantic terminology in
genetic biology. It so happens, however, that some of the philo-
sophical contributions to the problem of linguistic meaning can
assist us also in the troublesome matter of the meaning of the
genetic information.

     One such philosophical contribution to semantics that helps in
the clarification of the meaning of "genome" is the distinction
between an ostensive and connotative definition. An ostensive definition of "phenome" is produced by pointing to an animal and saying

"this is what I mean by 'cat'", whereas a connotative definition is
produced by drawing up a list of necessary and sufficient properties
which an animal must have to qualify as a cat. Now, although our
ordinary, everyday notion of a cat has an ostensive basis, this
concept cannot serve as the phenome of whose relation to the feline
genome we can expect to be able to give a scientific account. The
reason for this is that the ostension-based Gestalt by which we
recognize any cat as a cat is so highly abstract that it lacks most
of the biological properties which are essential for even beginning
any attempt to explain its gene-directed embryological development.
If, in order to fill in these conceptual lacunae, we proceed to
examine an actual cat, we find that the animals presents us with such
a wealth of concrete detail that a full description of the phenome
would produce a virtually limitless catalogue of properties in want
of an explanation. Thus the conceptual endpoint of the feline epigenetic landscape must be the list of necessary and sufficient properties of a connotatively defined cat phenome, rather than an actual
cat. It follows, therefore, that the selection of a connotative
phenome for study is the first, and most crucial step in any embryological analysis. If the set of properties whose development one
sets out to explain is too simple, the explanation when eventually
found, may be of only trivial significance. If the chosen set is
too complex, the explanation, though it might be highly significant
if found, would probably be too difficult to fathom. Thus the art
of practicing developmental biology consists of defining an optimal
connotative phenome.

EXPLICIT AND IMPLICIT MEANING

     A second philosophical insight into semantics that can help us
to understand the meaning of the genome is the recognition that the
meaning of semantic structures usually depends on the context in
which they are produced. Thus it is useful to distinguish between
two different kinds of meaning, namely between explicit and implicit
meaning. The explicit meaning is that which a semantic structure has
by virtue of the syntactic relation of its elements. Hence, the
explicit meaning can be extracted from the structure by subjecting it
to a linguistic analysis. The implicit meaning, by contrast, is not
really contained in the structure itself and arises secondarily from
the explicit meaning by virtue of its context. For instance, the
explicit meaning of the sentence "John Smith is traveling to New
York", is that a particular individual is on his way to a particular
geographical location. However, depending on the context in which
the sentence is produced, it can also have a large number and variety
of implicit meanings. For instance, if it is produced at San Francisco airport, it would imply that Mr. Smith is about to board a
particular flight, that his suitcase is waiting to be loaded on a
particular baggage truck, that he cannot be reached by telephone
for the next six hours, and so on. The same sentence with the same
explicit meaning would carry a different set of implicit meanings

if it were produced at a roadside service station in Colorado.

Actually, it is difficult to draw a sharp line of demarcation between explicit and implicit meanings, since the extraction of even the explicit meaning is itself rarely context-free. For instance, in the example just given, the intrinsic ambiguity in the explicit meaning of whether "New York" refers to the state or the city is resolved by the San Francisco airport context under which the term can be safely assumed to refer to the city. Thus the distinction between explicit and implicit meaning is relative rather than absolute, with a meaning being the less explicit and the more implicit the more dependent it is on the context. Furthermore, because of its high degree of dependence on the context, the implicit meaning is open-ended, in that it can become ever more remote from the explicit meaning as the context is widened.

When we apply this distinction to the semantic relation between genome and phenome it becomes evident that the explicit meaning of the genetic information consists of the protein amino acid sequences encoded in the genes, and of the nucleotide sequences of the ribosomal and transfer RNA molecules encoded in other non-genic DNA sectors. The explicit meaning would include also those physicochemical properties of the non-genic control DNA segments that produce regulatory functions. These meanings are explicit in the sense that they can be extracted from an analysis of the DNA nucleotide base sequence itself, provided one knows that the DNA base sequence is transcribed into a complementary RNA base sequence, and one has access to the table of the genetic code. But these explicit meanings form only the basic skeleton of the functional relations that shape the epigenetic landscape. The bulk of these relations are merely implicit in the genetic information.

By way of an example of such an implicit meaning we may consider the three-dimensional conformation of protein molecules. Although it is in some sense true that the spatial conformation of a protein molecule is "genetically determined", this "determination" devolves from the DNA-encoded specification of the one-dimensional amino acid sequence of the molecule. Once assembled from its constituent amino acids, the protein molecule automatically folds to assume its functional three-dimensional structure. The physico-chemical principles which govern this folding are in part understood, although it is not yet possible (but soon may be) to predict the three-dimensional structure which a protein with a given amino acid sequence will assume. But it is important to note that these folding rules are nowhere represented in the DNA nucleotide base sequence, being part of the context rather than of the genetic informational structures. The enzymatic function of the protein molecule, which can also be said to be "genetically determined", has an even more purely implicit meaning of the genetic information than the spatial conformation. Once a protein molecule has been assembled specifically from

its constituent amino acids and <u>has</u> assumed its specific three-
dimensional structure, certain parts of that structure turn out to
possess the power to catalyze some particular chemical reaction.
The stereochemical principles which govern that catalysis are also
partly understood, although (to my knowledge, at least) it is not
yet possible to predict on the basis of the known three-dimensional
structure of a protein molecule the kind of reaction which that molecule can catalyze. It goes without saying that the principles of
chemical catalysis are not represented in the DNA nucleotide base
sequences either; they enter into the meaning of the genetic information at a second order level of a contextual hierarchy, at whose
first order level we found the protein folding process.

This procedure of identifying implicit meanings of the genetic
information can be continued almost indefinitely to higher and higher
levels of the contextual hierarchy. For instance, the physiological
function of a chemical substance whose formation is catalyzed by a
particular protein molecule can likewise be said to be "genetically
determined", as can be the overt behavioral feature to which that
physiological function gives rise. The nearly unlimited horizon of
implicit meanings of the genetic information shows that, as has long
been recognized (cf. Woodger, 1953), the notion of the "inborn
nature", or genetic determination of characters is so all inclusive
as to be nearly devoid of meaning. After all, there is no aspect of
the phenome to whose determination the genes cannot be said to have
made their contribution. Thus it transpires that the concept of
genetic information, which in the heyday of molecular biology was of
such great heuristic value for unraveling the structure and function
of the genes, i.e. the explicit meaning of that information, is no
longer so useful in this later period when the epigenetic relations
which remain in want of explanation represent mainly the implicit
meaning of that information.

DEVELOPMENT OF THE NERVOUS SYSTEM

Let us now consider the pertinence of these abstract semantic
discussions for the study of the development of the nervous system.
The nervous system is an especially suitable object for developmental investigations, because, it is the precise manner of the interconnection of the cellular network of that system to which the
organism's behavior is attributable. Thus here a connotative definition of a phenome in want of explanation can be provided in terms
of a network diagram of specified cellular elements. Although we
cannot be sure as yet that it <u>will</u> be possible to give an account of
the epigenetic landscape that produces the neural network, we can be
reasonably confident that the explanation, if found, would not be
trivial.

The general problem of the development of the nervous system
has been formulated by Seymour Benzer (1971) in the following
terms:

> When the individual organism develops from a fertilized
> egg, the one-dimensional information arrayed in the linear
> sequence of the genes on the chromosomes controls the
> formation of a two-dimensional cell layer that folds to
> give rise to a precise three-dimensional arrangement of
> sense organs, central nervous system and muscles. These
> elements interact to produce the organism's behavior, a
> phenomenon whose description requires four dimensions at
> least. Surely the genes, which so largely determine
> anatomical and biochemical characteristics, must also
> interact with the environment to determine behavior.
> But how?

AN INFORMATION-THEORETICAL FALLACY

One possible answer to the question of how the genes determine
behavior is that they, in fact, contain the information for the circuit diagram of the nervous system (Benzer, 1971). However, it has
been argued that the neuronal network cannot, in fact, be genetically
determined because the total amount of genetic information does not
suffice to specify the neuronal connections that need to be made
(Horridge, 1968). According to this argument, the linear sequence
of roughly 10^{10} DNA nucleotide bases in the genome of a higher vertebrate animal contains an upper limit of 2×10^{10} bits of information (since each base, being one of four possible types, embodies 2
bits). On the other hand, if each one of the roughly 10^{10} cells in
the nervous system of such an animal were connected to just two other
cells, then it would require of the order of $10^{10} \log_2 10^{10}$ or $3 \times$
10^{11} bits to specify this network. Thus even under the most absurdly
oversimplified view of the complexity of the nervous system, the
total information content of the genetic material, even if it had
no non-nervous determinative role, would be too low by an order of
magnitude to allow the specification of the network.

Although this anti-genetic argument has little merit, it is useful to examine it because it exemplifies two not uncommon errors of
thought which must be corrected before the relation of the genome to
the development of the neural phenome can be profitably considered.
The first of these errors derives from a spurious application of
information theory to biological problems. That is to say, it
derives from the failure to recognize that the quantitative concept
of information applies only to processes in which the probabilities
of realization of alternative outcomes are known or clearly defined.
To illustrate this point, we may consider a biological example which
bears some formal analogies to the problem of the neuronal network
but which is presently much better understood, namely the determi-

nation of the structure of protein molecules. A typical species of
protein molecule consists of about 300 amino acid building blocks,
or of about 4000 atoms held to each other in specific chemical
linkage, with each atom, on the average, being connected to about
two other atoms. We may ask how many bits of information are
needed to specify the chemical structure of that protein molecule.
If we were to proceed by the same calculation as that which was
just applied to the nervous system, we would reckon that about $4 \times 10^3 \log_2(4 \times 10^3)$ or about 5×10^4 bits are needed. But here we
encounter an apparent paradox, because the gene that encodes the
chemical structure of a 300-amino acid protein molecule consists
only of a sequence of about 900 nucleotide bases, and hence contains a maximum of $2 \times 900 = 1800$ bits of information. Thus the
information content of the gene would be too low by more than an
order of magnitude to encode the chemical structure it is known
to determine. The insights of molecular biology readily resolve
this apparent paradox: the protein molecule is not assembled by
soldering together a kit consisting of 4000 marked atoms of which
each atom is potentially connectable to every other atom. Instead the protein assembly proceeds by joining together a specific
sequence of 300 amino acid building blocks, each containing a dozen
or so atoms each, selected from a pool of 20 different kinds of amino
acids. Thus to specify this assembly process only $300 \times \log_2 20$, or
1300 bits of information are needed, or less than the maximum
information content of the correspondent gene. This example shows,
therefore that until the proceess is known by which the neural
network is assembled, or until some detailed credible algorithms
have been developed, it is impossible to form even a rough estimate
of the amount of genetic information that would be needed to specify
its structure. Hence, the possibility that the structure of the
nervous system is genetically determined cannot be ruled out on
purely information-theoretical grounds. In any case, it is obvious
that development of the network is not formally equivalent to
assembling a kit of 10^{10} individually labeled nerve cells, all potentially interconnectable, by soldering them together according to a
schematic supplied by the manufacturer. This is the second error
underlying the spurious antigenetic argument.

IDEOLOGICAL AND INSTRUMENTAL ASPECTS

     Before giving further consideration to how genes determine be-
havior, we should note that this question comes within the purview
of only one of two related, yet distinct conceptual aspects of the
genetic approach to developmental neurobiology, namely of the ideological aspect. The ideological aspect confronts us with the basic
belief that the structure and function of the nervous system, and
hence the behavior of an animal, is, in fact, determined by its
genes. And so the discovery of how genes play their determinative
role in the genesis of the nervous system and its behavioral output
would be the ultimate goal of developmental neurobiology. By con-

trast, as seen from its other, or _instrumental_ aspect, the genetic
approach does not necessarily entail a belief in genetic specification of the nervous system, or present as its goal the discovery of
how genes determine behavior. Instead, from the instrumental aspect
the genetic approach appears as the study of neural development by
probing differences in neurologic phenotype between animals of
various geno-types, without any particular interest (other than
methodologic) in the concept of genetic determination.

The many experimental findings inspired by the instrumental aspect indicates that the genetic approach to developmental neurobiology offers considerable strength. The results of such neurogenetic
studies have provided further support to (or placed on a more secure
basis) notions generally held by developmental neurobiologists.
Thus the detailed neuroanatomical comparisons of members of isogenic
clones of animals (Levinthal et al., 1975; White et al., 1976;
Macagno, 1980; Goodman, 1978; Pearson and Goodman, 1979) have brought
into clearer focus the quantitative aspects of developmental
"noise", of whose existence few embryologists could have had any
doubt (Waddington, 1957). Moreover, anatomical and physiological
comparison of normal and mutant specimens, such as the sound- and
wind-insensitive cricket mutants (Bentley, 1976), _Drosophilia_ eye
mutants (Meyerowitz and Kankel, 1978), and the visual cortex of the
Siamese cat (Hubel and Wiesel, 1971; Kaas and Guillery, 1973;
Shatz, 1977) have led to the general proposition that presynaptic
sensory neurons can play a morphogenetic or organizational role in
the development of postsynaptic sensory interneurons, which lies
squarely in the conceptual mainstream of developmental neurobiology.
They have led also to the converse proposition, applicable to the
development of motor systems that, as demonstrated by the case of
the granule cells in the _reeler_ (Caviness, 1977) and _staggerer_
(Landis and Sidman, 1978) mouse cerebellum, survival of the presynaptic neuron is contingent on contact with an appropriate target
cell. Finally, the conclusions that axons of peripheral sensory
neurons can make appropriate central terminations despite an abnormal
point of entry into the central nervous system as shown by _Drosophila_
homeotic mutants (Palka et al., 1979) and that at their cerebral terminus sensory cell axons are recognized according to their relative
positions of origin as shown by the innervation pattern of the LGN
of the Siamese cat (Guillery and Kaas, 1971), had also been previously reached on other grounds. However, study of the Purkinje
cells in the _reeler_ mouse mutants revealed a previously unknown
feature of histogenetic cell migration, namely that migrating cells
can be positioned individually by contact with a fine-grained, possibly cellular, mosaic rather than a homogeneous morphogenetic
field (Mullen and Herrup, 1979). It is difficult to see how this
insight could have been reached by any method other than genetic
mosaics. In any case, the neurologic mutants have been of great
value in unravelling the underlying mechanisms in the particular
cases to which they pertain and in providing working material for

the developmental neurobiologist. As for fate mapping, i.e., tracing the origin of the nervous system to specific sites of the blastula, this idea was first conceived and realized experimentally by direct observation of leech embryos more than a century ago by Whitman (1878). Nevertheless, the extension of genetic methodology to fate mapping in embryos of species such as Drosophila, whose complexity precludes direct observational methods, constitutes an important technical advance for developmental neurobiology.

One limitation of the instrumental aspect of the genetic approach to neural development should be noted, namely that, thus far at least, its contributions have furthered the understanding mainly of systems such as the arthropod compound eye or the mammalian visual system and cerebellum, for which prior neuroanatomical, neurophysiological, and behavioral investigations had already provided a fairly high level of understanding. The reason for this is that whereas for any approach to the nervous system, be it anatomical, physiological, or behavioral, the investigator must bring some preunderstanding to his material, this requirement is much more demanding in the case of the genetic approach.

Whereas the main strength of the genetic approach to neural development lies in its instrumental aspect, the main weakness derives from its ideological aspect. For the viewpoint that the structure and function of the nervous system and hence the behavior of an animal is determined by its genes provides too narrow a context for actually understanding developmental processes and thus sets a goal for the genetic approach that is unlikely to be reached. Here "too narrow" is not to mean that a belief in genetic determination of the nervous system necessarily implies a lack of awareness that in development there occurs an interaction between genes and environment, a fact of which all practitioners of the genetic approach are certainly aware. Rather, "too narrow" means that the role of the genes, which, thanks to the achievements of molecular biology, we now know to be the specification of the primary structure of protein molecules, is at too many removes from the processes that actually "build nerve cells and specify neural circuits which underlie behavior" to provide an appropriate conceptual framework for posing the developmental questions that need to be answered. Rather, the insights into developmental mechanisms thus far available suggest that the solution to the problem of development lies at a cellular and intercellular rather than a genetic level, although genes will undoubtedly figure in some crucial part, but only a part, of that solution.

WHAT IS A PROGRAM

Those who speak of a genetic determination of the nervous system, and hence of behavior, rarely spell out what it actually is that they have in mind. The genes obviously cannot embody a neuron-

by-neuron circuit diagram; and even if they did, the existence of
an agency that reads the diagram in carrying out the assembly of the
component parts of a neuronal Heathkit would still transcend our
comprehension. So a seemingly more reasonable view of the nature
of the genetic determination of behavior would be that the genes
embody, not a circuit diagram, but a program for the development of
the nervous system (Brenner 1973, 1974). But this view is rooted
in a semantic confusion about the concept of "program". Once that
confusion is cleared up, it becomes evident that development from egg
to adult is unlikely to be a programmatic phenomenon. Development
belongs to that large class of regular phenomena that share the
property that a particular set of antecedents generally leads, via
a more or less invariant sequence of intermediate steps, to a particular set of consequents; however, of the large class of regular
phenomena, programmatic phenomena form only a small subset, almost
all the members of which are associated with human activity. For
membership of a phenomenon in the subset of programmatic phenomena
it is a necessary condition that, in addition to the phenomenon itself, there exists a second thing, the "program", whose structure is
isomorphic with, i.e., can be brought into one-to-one correspondence
with, the phenomenon.   For instance, the on-stage events associated
with a performance of "Hamlet", a regular phenomenon, are programmatic
since there exists Shakespeare's text with which the actions of the
performers are isomorphic. But the no less regular off-stage events,
such as the actions of house staff and audience, are mainly nonpro-
grammatic, since their regularity is merely the automatic consequence
of the contextual situation of the performance. One of the very few
regular phenomena independent of human activity that can be said to
have a programmatic component is the formation of proteins. Here
the assembly of amino acids into a polypeptide chain of a particular
primary structure is programmatic because there exists a stretch of
DNA polynucleotide chain --- the gene --- whose nucleotide base
sequence is isomorphic with the sequence of events that unfolds at
the ribosomal assembly site. However, the subsequent folding of
the completed polypeptide chain into its specific tertiary structure lacks programmatic character, since the three-dimensional conformation of the molecule is the automatic consequence of its
contextual situation and has no isomorphic correspondent in the DNA.

When we extend these considerations to the regular phenomenon
of development we see that its programmatic aspect is confined mainly
to the assembly of polypeptide chains (and of various species of
RNA). But as for the overall phenomenon, it is most unlikely ---
and no credible hypothesis has as yet been advanced how this could
be the case --- that the sequence of its events is isomorphic with
the structure of any second thing, especially not with the genome.
The fact that mutation of a gene leads to an altered neurologic
phenotype shows that genes are part of the causal antecedents of
the adult organism, but does not in any way indicate that the mutant
gene is part of a program for development of the nervous system.

But, are not polemics about the meaning of words such as "program" just a waste of time for those who want to get on with the job of finding out how the nervous system develops? As J.H. Woodger (1952) pointed out, semantic confusion about fundamental terms, such as "gene", "genotype", "phenotype", and "determination", had become the bane of classical genetics. It would be well to avoid reconstituting that confusion in the context of developmental biology and to remember Woodger's advice that "an understanding of the pitfalls to which a too naive use of language exposes us is as necessary as some understanding of the artifacts which accompany the use of microscopical techniques."

DEVELOPMENT AS HISTORY

The notion of genetic determination of behavior is not only defective at the conceptual level but also represents a misinterpretation of the knowledge already available from developmental studies, including those that have resorted to the genetic approach. As Szekely (1979) has pointed out, we know enough about its mode of establishment already to make it most unlikely that neuronal network is, in fact, prespecified; rather, all indications (including those provided by the study of phenotypic variance reviewed here) point to stochastic processes as underlying the apparent regularity of neural development. That is to say, development of the nervous system, from fertilized egg to mature brain, is not a programmatic but a historical phenomenon under which one thing simply leads to another. To illustrate the difference between programmatic specification and stochastic history as alternative accounts of regular phenomena, we may consider the establishment of ecological communities upon colonization of islands (Simberloff, 1974), or growth of secondary forests (Whittaker, 1970). Both of these examples are regular phenomena, in the sense that a more or less predictable ecological structure arises via a stereotypic pattern of intermediate steps, in which the relative abundances of various types of flora and fauna follow a well-defined sequence. The regularity of these phenomena is obviously not the consequence of an ecological program encoded in the genome of the participating taxa. Rather it arises via a historical cascade of complex stochastic interactions between various biota (in which genes play an important role, of course) and the world as it is.

HERMENEUTICS

To fathom the complex interactions that produce a historical phenomenon, just as to fathom the meaning of the genome, it is necessary to understand the context in which it is embedded. And upon recognizing the importance of contextual relations for the problem of development, we move into a domain of phenomenological analysis to which conventional scientific methodology is no longer fully applicable. That domain bears a strong epistemological affinity

to the scholarly activity called "hermeneutics". This designation
was originally given by theologians to the theory of interpretation
of sacred texts, especially of the Bible. The name is derived from
that of Hermes, the divine messenger. In his capacity as an information channel linking gods and men, Hermes must "interpret", or
make explicit in terms that ordinary mortals can understand, the
implicit meaning that is hidden in the gods' messages. In recent
years, scholars have applied the term hermeneutics also to the
interpretation of secular texts, since there may be implicit meanings
hidden even in the literary creations of ordinary men that need to
be made explicit to their fellow mortals. But hidden meanings pose
a procedural difficulty for textual interpretation, because, as set
forth earlier in this article, one must understand the context in
which implicit meaning is embedded before one can uncover hidden
meanings in any of its parts. Here we face a logical dilemma, a
vicious hermeneutic circle. On the one hand, the words and sentences
of which a text is composed have no meaning until one knows the
meaning of the text as a whole. On the other hand, one can come to
know the meaning of the whole text only through understanding its
parts. To break this vicious circle --- which comes first, the
chicken or the egg? --- hermeneutics invokes the doctrine of pre-
understanding. As set forth by Rudolf Bultmann, hermeneutic pre-
understanding, or Vorverständnis, represents his life of experience
and insights that the subject must bring to the task of interpreting
a particular text.

In assessing the epistemological status of hermeneutic studies
we may ask to what extent the concept of objective validity is applicable to their results. An objectively valid interpretation would
presumably be one that has made explicit the "true" meaning hidden
in the text, i.e., the implicit meaning intended by the author. But
here we encounter the difficulty that the interpreter's preunderstanding is necessarily based on his own subjective historical,
social and personal background. Hence, agreement regarding the
validity of an interpretation could be reached only among persons
who happen to bring the same pre-understanding to the text. Thus,
because of the necessarily subjective nature of pre-understanding,
there cannot be such a thing as an objectively valid interpretation. It is this evident unattainability of universal and eternal
truth in interpretation that makes hermeneutics different from
science, for which the belief in the attainability of objectively
valid explanations of the world is metaphysical bedrock.

To what extent is this belief actually justified? According to
many contemporary philosophers of science, it is not really justified because resort is made also to subjective notions equivalent
to hermeneutic pre-understanding in the search for scientific explanations of phenomena. Thus, in judging the objective validity of
these explanations we must try to assess the degree to which pre-
understanding enters into their development. Such an assessment

can help us to understand why the belief in the attainability of
objectively valid explanations does seem to be more appropriate in
the "hard" sciences than in the "soft" human sciences, such as
economics, sociology and psychology.

One of the main reasons for this epistemological difference
between the "hard" and "soft" sciences is that the phenomena of
which the "soft" sciences seek to give an account are much more
complex than those addressed by the "hard" sciences. And the more
complex the ensemble of events that the scientist isolates concep-
tually for his attention, the more hermeneutic pre-understanding
must he bring to the phenomenon before he can break it down into
meaningful atomic components that are to be governed by the causal
connections of his eventual explanations. Accordingly, the less
likely is it that his explanations will have the aura of objective
truth. By way of comparing a pair of extreme examples --- one very
hard, the other very soft --- we may consider mechanics and psychoanalysis. There is an aura of objective truth about the laws of
classical mechanics because the phenomena which mechanics consider
significant, such as steel balls rolling down inclines, are of low
complexity. Because of that low complexity it is possible to
adduce critical observations or experiments about rolling steel
balls. By contrast, there is no comparable aura of truth about the
propositions of analytical psychology, because the phenomena of the
human psyche which it attends are very complex. Here there are no
critical observations or experiments because the failure of any
prediction based on psychoanalytic theory can almost always be explained away retrodictively, by considering additional factors or
by modifying slightly one's pre-understanding of the phenomenon.
Hence in psychoanalysis a counterfactual prediction rarely quali-
fies as negative evidence against the theory that generated it.

Neurobiology covers a broad range of this hardness-softness
scale. At the hard end, neurobiology is represented by cellular
electrophysiology whose phenomena, although more complex than those
associated with rolling steel balls, can still be acounted for in
terms of explanations that are susceptible to seemingly objective
proof. But at its soft end, neurobiology is represented by the study
of the function of large and complicated cellular networks as well
as by the developmental processes by which these networks arise.
As has long been realized of course, the output of neural networks
comprises phenomena whose complexity approaches that of the human
psyche --- in fact, that include the human psyche. Hence at its
soft end neurobiology takes on some of the characteristics of hermeneutics: the student of the function and development of a complex
neural network must bring considerable pre-understanding to the
system as a whole before attempting to interpret the function and
development of any of its parts. Accordingly, the functional and
developmental explanations that are advanced about complex neural
systems may remain beyond the reach of objective validation. Here,

to paraphrase my employer, Governor Edmund G. Brown, Jr., we may
have to be satisfied with less.

REFERENCES

Bentley, D., 1976, Genetic analysis of the nervous system. In:
    Simpler Networks and Behavior, ed. J.C. Fentress, Sunderland,
    Mass: Sinauer, Assoc., pp. 126-139.
Benzer, S., 1971, From gene to behavior, J. Amer. Med. Assoc.,
    218:1015-1022.
Brenner, S., 1973, The genetics of behavior, Brit. Med. Bull.,
    29:269-271.
Brenner, S., 1974, The genetics of Caenorhabditis elegans,
    Genetics, 77:71-94.
Caviness, V.S., Jr. and Rakie, P., 1978, Mechanisms of cortical
    development: A view from mutations in mice, Ann. Rev.
    Neurosci., 1:297-326.
Goodman, C.S., 1978, Isogenic grasshoppers: Genetic variability in
    the morphology of identified neruons, J. Comp. Neurol.,
    182:681-705.
Guillery, R.W. and Kaas, J., II, 1971, A study of normal and
    congenitally abnormal retinogeniculate projections in cats,
    J. Comp. Neurol., 143:73-100.
Horridge, G.A., 1968, Interneurons, Freeman, San Francisco, p. 321.
Hubel, D., II. and Wiesel, T.N., 1971, Aberrant visual projections
    in the Siamese cat, J. Physiol. (Lond.), 218:33-62.
Jacob, F., 1973, The Logic of Life, Pantheon, New York.
Kaas, J., II., and Guillery, R.W., 1973, The transfer of abnormal
    visual field representations from dorsal lateral geniculate
    nucleus to visual cortex in Siamese cats, Brain Res.,
    59:61-95.
Landis, D.M.D. and Sidman, R.L., 1978, Electron microscopic analysis
    of postnatal histogenesis in the cerebellar cortex of staggerer
    mutant mice, J. Comp. Neurol., 179:831-864.
Levinthal, F., Macagno, E.R. and Levinthal, C., 1975, Anatomy and
    development of identified cells in isogenic organisms,
    Cold Spring Harbor Symp. Quant. Biol., 40:321-331.
Macagno, E.R., Lopresti, V. and Levinthal, C., 1973, Structure and
    development of neuronal connections in isogenic organisms,
    Variations and similarities in the optic system of Daphnia
    magna., Proc. Natl. Acad. Sci. USA, 70:57-61.
Meyerowitz, E.M. and Kankel, D.R., 1978, A genetic analysis of
    visual system development in Drosophila melanogaster,
    Develop. Biol., 62:63-93.
Mullen, R.J. and Herrup, K., 1979, Chimeric analysis of mouse cere-
    bellar mutants. In Neurogenetics: Genetic Approaches to the
    Nervous System, ed. X. Breakefield, New York: Elsevier/North
    Holland, 175-196.

Palka, J., Lawrence, P.A. and Hart, S., II., 1979, Neural projection
    patterns from homeotic tissue of Drosophila studied in bithorax
    mutants and mosaics, Develop. Biol., 69:549-575.
Pearson, K.G. and Goodman, C.S., 1979, Correlation of variability in
    structure with variability in synaptic connection of an identi-
    fied interneuron in locusts, J. Comp. Neurol., 184:141-165.
Sagan, C., 1973, Communication with Extraterrestrial Intelligence,
    M.I.T. Press, Cambridge, Mass., p. 331.
Schrödinger, E., 1945, What is Life?, Cambridge University Press,
    New York.
Shatz, C.J., 1977, A comparison of visual pathways in Boston and
    Mid-western Siamese cats, J. Comp. Neurol., 171:205-228.
Simberloff, D.S., 1974, Equilibrium theory of island biogeography and
    ecology, Ann. Rev. Ecology Syst., 5:161-182.
Stent, G.S., 1977, Explicit and implicit semantic content of the
    genetic information. I. Genetic information. In: Foundational
    Problems in the Special Sciences, R. Butts and J. Hintikka, eds.
    131-149. D. Reidel, Dordrecht. Reprinted in Paradoxes of
    Progress (G.S. Stent) W.H. Freeman & Co.: San Francisco, 1978.
Stent, G.S. (1981a), Strength and weakness of the genetic approach to
    the development of the nervous system, Ann. Rev. Neurosci.,
    4:163-194.
Stent, G.S. (1981b), Cerebral hermeneutics, J. Soc. Biol. Struct.,
    4:107-124.
Szekely, G., 1979, Order and plasticity in the nervous system,
    Trends in Neurosci., 2(10):245-248.
Waddington, C.H., 1957, The Strategy of the Genes, Allen and Unwin,
    London.
White, J.G., Southgate, E., Thomson, J.N. and Brenner, S., 1976, The
    structure of the ventral nerve cord of Caenorhabditis elegans,
    Philos. Trans. R. Soc. London Ser. B., 275:327-348.
Whitman, C.O., 1878, The embryology of Clepsine, Q. J. Micros. Sci.,
    18:215-315.
Whittaker, R.H., 1970, Communities and Ecosystems, MacMillan, New
    York, pp. 158.
Woodger, J.H., 1952, Biology and Language, Cambridge University Press
    Cambridge, Mass., 364 pp.
Woodger, J.H., 1953, What do we mean by inborn?, Brit. J. Phil. Sci..
    3:319.

DEVELOPMENTAL NEUROBIOLOGY OF THE LEECH

Gunther S. Stent

Department of Molecular Biology
University of California
Berkeley, California

LEECH NERVOUS SYSTEM

The leech CNS consists of a ventral chain of 32 segmentally
iterated ganglia. The first four and last seven segmental ganglia
are fused, constituting a rostral and caudal ganglionic mass, respectively. The rostral ganglionic mass, or subesophageal ganglion, is
connected at its anterior end to a dorsally situated supraesophageal
ganglion. Each segmental ganglion contains about 400 bilaterally
paired neurons, as well as a few unpaired neurons. Their somata form
a cortex around the outer surface of the ganglion. The neurons are
monopolar; their processes project into a central neuropil, where
they make synaptic contacts. From there, the processes of some
neurons project to other ganglia via a connective nerve. Sensory
and effector neurons project their processes to targets outside the
CNS via segmental nerves, whose roots emerge from the lateral edge
of the ganglion. In each ganglion, the neuronal somata are distributed over six cell packets, of which two form an anterior and two
a posterior pair of lateral packets. The remaining two packets are
unpaired, one lying anterior and the other posterior on the ventromedial aspect. Each cell packet contains one giant glial cell,
whereas two giant glial cells are associated with the ganglionic
neuropil. Additional giant glia are present in the interganglionic
connective nerves.

The anatomy of the leech ganglion is sufficiently stereotyped
that a large fraction of its neurons are identifiable. That is,
after characterizing a particular neuron in a particular ganglion
of a particular specimen according to such criteria as soma size

161

and position, axonal and dendritic branching patterns, synaptic connectivity, or electrophysiological and histochemical properties,
homologous neurons can usually be found on the other side of that
same ganglion, in other ganglia of that same specimen, in the
ganglia of other specimen of the same species, and even in other
leech species, families or orders. Despite this high degree of
neural sterotypy, there do occur some systematic variations in the
number of cells among different segmental ganglia within the same
nerve cord, and among corresponding ganglia in the nerve cords of
different leech species. For instance, in the hirudinid leech
Hirudo medicinalis, the ganglia in the two (clitellar) body
segments containing the male and female reproductive organs of the
hermaphrodite leech have nearly twice as many cells as the other
ganglia. Although the corresponding clitellar ganglia in the glossiphoniid leech Haementeria ghilianii also contain more cells than
the other segmental ganglia, here the excess is only of the order
of 5%. Moreover, there is some slight variation in the exact number
of neurons per ganglion between corresponding ganglia of different
specimens of the same species. This "developmental noise" amounts
to a variance of about 1% in the total number of neurons per corresponding ganglion (Macagno, 1980).

    Roughly one-quarter of the neurons of the segmental ganglia of
Hirudo medicinalis have been identified according to various
criteria, including function. Thus, many cells have been classified
as sensory, motor, or interneurons, and their connectivity has been
elucidated. These surveys have culminated in the description of
sensory pathways and of neuronal networks controlling various behaviors, such as body shortening, heartbeat and swimming. Thanks to
this detailed knowledge of its functional elements, the leech nervous
system presents developmental neurobiologists with a clearly defined
conceptual endpoint in the search for understanding how a complex
ensemble of specifically interconnected neurons develops from the
fertilized egg. (For a detailed account of the leech nervous system,
cf. Muller et al., 1981).

    It should be noted that most investigations of the adult leech
nervous system were carried out with species belonging to the family
of Hirudinidae (order Gnathobdellidae). By contrast, most investigations of leech embryology were carried out with species belonging to
the family of Flossiphoniidae (order Rhyncobdellidae)(Schleip, 1936;
Fernandez, 1980; Stent and Weisblat, 1982). Fortunately the nervous
systems of leeches belonging to these two different orders are sufficiently similar that much of the neurophysiological and neuroanatomical knowledge available from the study of the Hirudinidae is
applicable to the Glossiphoniidae (Kramer and Goldman, 1981;
Kramer, 1981).

LEECH EMBRYOGENESIS

Glossiphoniid leeches are well-suited for developmental studies because their eggs are large and undergo stereotyped cleavages that produce an early embryo consisting of large identifiable cells, or blastomeres. The embryos can be observed, manipulated and cultured to maturity in simple media. Moreover, development from egg to adult is direct, without passage through larval forms (Whitman, 1878; Schleip, 1936). The development studies to be presented here were carried out with two glossiphoniid leech species, maintained as continuously breeding laboratory colonies since 1976. One of these is the dwarf species, Helobdella triserialis, which reaches an adult length of about 1 cm and propagates with an egg to egg generation time of about six weeks. The other is the giant species Haementeria ghilianii, which can reach an adult length of up to 50 cm and has an egg to egg generation time of about 10 months. Its short generation time and robust embryo make Helobdella a favorable material for developmental studies, but its small size renders it less favorable for neurophysiology. By contrast the enormous size of Haementeria makes its adult and embryonic nervous systems both accessible to intracellular electrical recording and other techniques that require penetration of single cells, but the long generation time, more demanding breeding conditions and less hardy embryo also present drawbacks compared to Helobdella. Despite their disparate sizes, both species are sufficiently similar in adult body plan and embryonic development that they can be considered as interchangeable for many developmental studies, thus providing greater scope for experimentation than would either species alone.

Helobdella and Haementeria lay yolk-rich eggs about 0.5 mm and 2.5 mm in diameter, respectively. The eggs are laid in clutches, enclosed in transparent, fluid-filled cocoons, that remain attached to the ventral body wall of the brooding parent. Embryonic development begins as soon as the eggs are laid, and, at a temperature of 25°C, two weeks later (Helobdella), or a month later (Haementeria), a juvenile leech has arisen whose form differs from the adult mainly by its smaller size. The eggs can be removed from the cocoon at any stage of development and cultured to maturity in a saline whose composition resembles that of the cocoon fluid. The egg yolk provides the nutrients needed for this development. Upon exhaustion of the yolk, the juvenile leech takes its first meal from a host animal. Subsequent, post-embryonic growth and maturation of the juvenile leech represents both an increase in cell size, and to a lesser degree, cell number.

Figure 1 presents the generalized staging system that has recently been devised for the embryonic development of glossiphoniid leeches, based on studies carried out with Helobdella (Weisblat et al., 1980a) and with Theromyzon rude (Fernandez, 1980; Fernandez and Stent, 1980). Figure 2 presents the cell lineage pedigree which

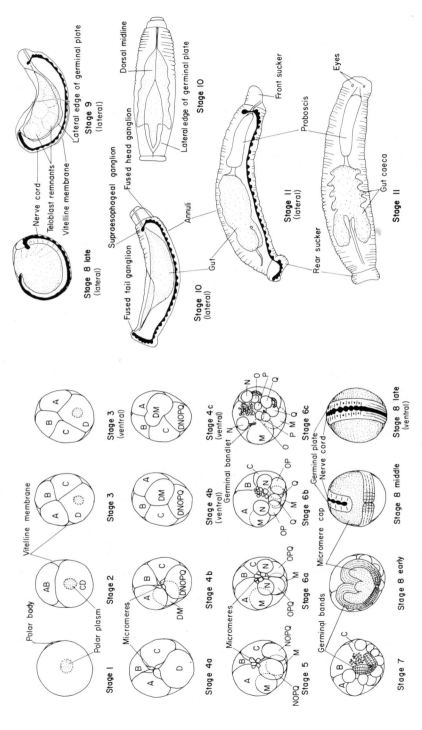

Figure 1. The 11 stages of development of glossiphoniid leeches, beginning with the uncleaved egg (stage 1) and ending with the juvenile leech (stage 11). All drawings, unless otherwise noted, are views of the future dorsal aspect of the embryo.

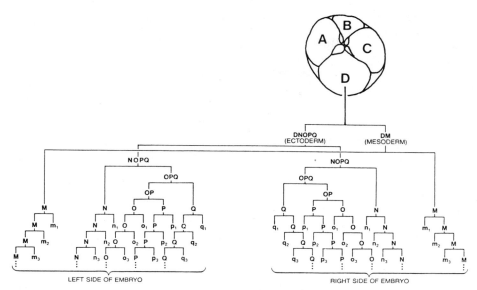

Figure 2. Cell pedigrees during stages 4 to 7 of glossiphoniid leech development.

results from the stereotyped cleavage pattern during the first 7 of
the 11 developmental stages (Schleip, 1936). As the glossiphoniid
egg approaches its first cleavage there becomes visible at each of
its two poles a region of colorless cytoplasm, or teloplasm, as
distinct from the colored yolk that fills most of the egg. One of
these poles marks the future dorsal and the other the future ventral
surface of the embryo. The first cleavage divides the egg into two
large cells AB and CD, with all of the teloplasm passing into CD. The
second cleavage gives rise to four cells, A,B,C and D, of which D
receives all of the teloplasm. Cell D cleaves to yield two cells,
one designated DNOPQ, which lies more dorsally and receives the teloplasm from the dorsal pole, and another designated DM, which lies
more ventrally and receives the teloplasm from the ventral pole. At
this stage separation of the embryo into the three germinal tissue
layers has been accomplished: the progeny cells of A, B and C will
give rise to endoderm, the progeny of DNOPQ to ectoderm, and the
progeny of DM to mesoderm. The next two cleavages establish the
bilateral symmetry of the embryo: DM divides to yield the pair of
right and left M cells and DNOPQ divides to yield the pair of NOPQ
cells lying on either side of the future midline. Three further
cleavages of the NOPQ cell pair produce four bilateral cell pairs
designated as N, O, P and Q.

The paired M, N, O, P and Q cells, among which the teloplasm of
the egg has now been partitioned, are referred to as teloblasts. As
soon as it has been formed, each teloblast begins to carry out a
series of highly unequal divisions. These divisions produce a bandlet of small blast cells, to which most of the teleoplasm, but little
of the yolk, of the teloblast is eventually distributed. The blast
cell bandlets produced by the five teloblasts on each side grow and
merge on either side of the midline to form a prominent pair of cell
ridges, the right and left germinal bands. The blast cell bandlet
produced by M lies under the other four ectodermal bandlets. With
ongoing production of more and more blast cells, right and left
germinal bands advance frontward along a crescent-shaped path over the
future dorsal surface of the embryo and converge at the site of the
future head. The mid-portions of the still lengthening germinal
bands move circumferentially and enter the future ventral surface.
Eventually right and left germinal bands meet on the ventral midline,
where they coalesce. Coalescence begins at the future head and continues zipper-like in a rearward direction. When coalescence has
gone to completion the coalesced germinal bands have given rise to
the germinal plate lying on the ventral midline. In the course of
subsequent development, the cells of the germinal plate divide to
produce the precursor cells of the adult tissues. This cell proliferation results in a gradual thickening and circumferential expansion of the germinal plate over the surface of the embryo back into
dorsal territory. Eventually, right and left leading edges of the
expanding germinal plate meet and coalesce on the future dorsal
midline, thus closing the leech body.

Early in this expansion process, the germinal plate becomes
partitioned into a series of tissue blocks, separated by transverse
septa. Each of these blocks corresponds to a future body segment.
Segmentation starts at the front, progresses rearward, and is complete upon formation of the hindmost 32nd segment, by which time
the expanding germinal plate covers about one third of the ventral
surface. Meanwhile formation of the embryonic gut, derived from
the endodermal precursor cells A, B and C, is under way. The gut
first appears as a long cylinder (filled with yolk provided by
cells A, B and C), and then becomes segmented as a result of a series
of annular constrictions of the yolk-filled cylinder in register
with (and possibly produced by growth of) the septa. This gives
rise to paired gut expansions, or caeca, in register with the abdominal body segments. Gut segmentation is completed concurrently
with body closure; the embryo now has the general shape of the
juvenile leech.

DEVELOPMENT OF THE NERVOUS SYSTEM

The progressive segmentation of the germinal plate is manifest
also in the formation of the nervous system, which similarly follows
the general front-to-rear developmental sequence of the germinal

plate. The first indication of the presence of nervous tissue is the
appearance of paired hemispheric cell masses on either side of the
germinal plate midline. Each of these cell mass pairs corresponds
to the primordium of a segmental ganglion. The paired primordia
coalesce sequentially on the ventral midline to form intact, globular
ganglia which already contain the approximate adult number of neurons. When the expanding germinal plate covers about half of the
ventral surface of the embryo, all 32 ganglia are present. Initially, the nascent ganglion lies in direct contact with its neighboring
ganglia of the next anterior and posterior segment. Later the
ganglion becomes separated from its neighbors by a short connective
nerve which grows in length to accommodate the gradual increase in
inter-ganglionic distance with progressive elongation of the whole
embryo.

My colleague, Andrew Kramer, has been able to dissect the developing nervous system from Haementeria embryos and to penetrate its
neurons with microelectrodes. This has allowed him to take intracellular recordings from embryonic neurons and inject fluorescent
dyes into them. Kramer found, in collaboration with John Kuwada
(Kuwada and Kramer, 1982) that when segmental ganglia first appear
in their globular form, their neurons have not yet grown any of the
extensions -- axons and dendrites -- characteristic of adult neurons.
Groups of these immature neurons are coupled via junctions that permit the passage from cell to cell of injected dye molecules. Later,
the neurons begin to grow axons, and their earlier coupling largely
disappears. However the embryonic neurons do not yet show the
electrical activities characteristic of adult neurons such as action
potentials. These electrical activities appear at a still later
stage, when the growing axons have begun to enter the connective
and the segmental nerves. Finally, by the time of body closure,
the embryonic nervous system has taken on the general properties of
the adult. The neurons now show transient changes in electrical
potential resembling inhibitory and excitatory synaptic potentials,
which suggests linkage of the neurons via synaptic connections.

Since the function of synaptic connections depends on the
release of neurotransmitters, it would follow that by the time of
body closure, the embryonic neurons must be sufficiently mature to
be able to carry out neurotransmitter synthesis. Studies by my colleague, Duncan Stuart, have shown that this is indeed the case. To
ascertain the time course of the development of the capacity for
synthesis of the neurotransmitter acetylcholine, Stuart dissected
the nerve cord from leech embryos of various ages and placed it
into a solution containing ^{3}H-labeled choline, the metabolic precursor of acetylcholine. The rate of formation of ^{3}H-labeled
acetylcholine in this preparation then provides a quantitative
index of the level of enzymes that catalyze the uptake of choline
and its conversion to acetylcholine. Stuart found that the capacity
for acetylcholine synthesis is still very low when the ganglia are

already morphologically intact and their neurons have begun to grow
axons. The synthetic capacity begins to rise rapidly however, once
the neurons have sent axons into the connective and segmental nerves
and have begun to produce action potentials. By the time of body
closure the capacity of the nerve cord for acetylcholine synthesis
has increased more than 25 times over its initial value. Two other
neurotransmitters studied by Stuart are dopamine and 5-hydroxytryp-
tamine (5-HT, or serotonin) contained by some identified leech neurons. Upon treatment of adult ganglia with glyoxylic acid, the
5-HT-containing neurons and the dopamine-containing neurons can be
readily identified under the microscope by their greenish fluorescence. By exposing the nervous system of embryos of various ages to
glyoxylic acid, Stuart found that the 5-HT-and dopamine-containing
neurons first take on glyoxylic acid-induced fluorescence, i.e.,
start accumulating their neurotransmitter, at about the same time
at which other neurons gain the capacity for acetylcholine synthesis
and at which acetylcholine esterase makes its appearance in the
ganglionic neuropil (Fitzpatrick-McElligott and Stent, 1981).

     This morphological, electrical and biochemical maturation of
the leech nervous system is paralleled by a behavioral evolution of
the embryo, which begins at an early stage and proceeds via a stereotyped sequence of motor acts. Analyses by Kramer of videotape
recordings of Haementeria embryos have shown that embryonic behavior
progresses from simple, irregular twitching to complex, concatenated
movement patterns. Simple movements of early embryos form part of
more complex movements displayed at later stages. These more complex
movements are, in turn, components of locomotory routines of the
juvenile and adult animals. Some of these embryonic movements may
fulfill a physiological function at the stage at which they occur,
such as circulation of nutrients or hatching from the egg membrane,
but others might be no more than preludes to adult behavior, inci-
dental to the formation of functional connections between the components of the developing central nervous system. Overt movements
begin with a peristaltic constriction wave as coalescence of the
germinal plate goes to completion. Since as yet there is no nervous
system, the peristaltic wave is likely to represent a myogenic
rhythm (i.e., one originating in the musculature rather than in the
nervous system) of contractile cells that already gird the embryo.
Peristalsis eventually results in hatching from the egg membrane,
in which, up to then the embryo is still enclosed. After hatching,
peristalsis tapers off and the embryo begins intermittent lateral
bending movements, effected by contraction and distension of the
longitudinal muscles on right or left sides. By this time, maturation of the ventral nerve cord has progressed far enough to permit
execution of neurogenic movements (i.e., those originating in the
nervous system). After body closure, the lateral bending movements
give way to a more complicated motion cycle, which is evidently the
prelude to the inchworm crawling of the juvenile leech. Later,
after front and rear suckers have developed, the precrawling cycle

of the embryo ripens into actual walking. Upon reaching the status
of juvenile, the mini-leech can also perform the coordinated contractile rhythm of its longitudinal muscles underlying the swimming movement. Thus the juvenile Haementeria is able to seek its first
blood meal by either walking or swimming towards a prospective host.

CELL LINEAGE TRACERS

        Nearly a century ago, C.O. Whitman (1887) inquired into the
embryonic origins of the leech nervous system. To that end, Whitman
followed the lines of descent from cells A, B and C and of the
teloblasts and their blast cell bandlets by direct microscopic examination of early embryos. But with the increase in cell number at
later developmental stages the method of direct observation becomes
too cumbersome for following the further fate of individual cells.
Hence in order to make possible more detailed developmental cell
pedigrees in the developing leech nervous system, we devised a new
cell lineage tracer technique (for review, see Stent et al., 1982).
This technique consists of injection of a tracer molecule through a
micropipette into an identified cell of the early embryo. After
tracer injection, embryonic development is allowed to progress to a
later stage, whereupon the distribution pattern of the tracer within
the tissues is visualized. This method proved feasible because the
tracers we use satisfy three essential conditions: 1) embryonic
development continues normally after intracellular injection of the
tracer; 2) the injected tracer remains intact and is not diluted too
much in the developing embryo; and 3) the tracer does not pass
through the junctions that link embryonic cells; thus it is passed
on exclusively to direct descendants of the injected cell.

        One of the tracers we used for this purpose is the red-fluores-
cing dye rhodamine, coupled to a tailor-made polypeptide carrier
molecule of amino acid sequence glu-ala-glu-ala-lys-ala-glu-ala-
glu-lys-gly (Weisblat et al., 1980b). David Weisblat, in collaboration with Janice Young, synthesized this polypeptide from amino acids
in the unnatural D-configuration, so as to render it resistant to
digestion by proteolytic enzymes. The rhodamine-polypeptide, to
which we refer as RDP, has proven particularly useful for visualizing
the development of the germinal plate. For this purpose, a teloblast
(or teloblast precursor cell) is injected with RDP and the embryo is
later fixed, cleared of yolk by a method invented by Juan Fernandez
(1980), and treated with the blue-fluorescing, DNA-specific stain
Hoechst 33258 (Sedat and Manuelides, 1977). The resulting blue
fluorescence of the cell nuclei and the red fluorescence of the
RDP-labeled cytoplasm can then be viewed and photographed under a
fluorescence microscope. In one such experiment one mesodermal precursor or M teloblast, was injected with RDP during stage 5 and the
embryo examined at stage 8. The large red M teloblast could be seen
to lie deep in the embryo and the bandlet of red blast cells descended from it projecting upwards. On reaching the surface, the

bandlet made a sharp turn and joined the crescent-shaped germinal
band. Most importantly, at its front end, the mesodermal blast
cell bandlet was subdivided into iterated clusters of labeled cells.
Such subdivision is the first overt sign of segmentation of the mesodermal tissue, which occurs even before the coalescence of right
and left germinal bands. Closer examination of these labeled blast
cell clusters showed that adjacent clusters are isomorphic, i.e,
that their cells are in topographical and morphological correspondence. This isomorphism suggests that the early development of the
mesoderm of each body segment proceeds, as does cleavage and teloblast formation in the whole early embryo, by a sequence of stereotyped cell divisions. More recent experiments by Saul Zackson (1982)
have shown that each of these cell clusters is, in fact, derived
from a single M-teloblast progeny stem cell and that a single cluster is the precursor of a mesodermal segment on that side. Hence
it would follow that each of the 32 mesodermal body segments is
founded by a bilateral pair of M-teloblast progeny stem cells.

     The other tracer that we have used for establishing embryonic
cell lineage is the enzyme horseradish peroxidase, or HRP (Weisblat
et al., 1978; 1980a). For this purpose, one blastomere is injected
with HRP at an early stage of development and at a later stage, the
embryo is treated with hydrogen peroxide and benzidine. As a result
of this treatment, those, and only those cells containing HRP, i.e.,
having descended from the injected blastomere, turn black. In order
to ascertain the origin of the leech nervous system, we injected one
of the ectodermal precursor N, O, P or Q teloblasts with HRP and
allowed development to proceed to the stage at which expansion of the
germinal plate covers nearly all of the ventral surface and all 32
segmental ganglia of the nerve cord are present. Upon treatment of
such embryos with H_2O_2 and benzidine, HRP stain was seen in segmentally repeated structures. The size, shape and location of some of
these structures indicated that they are within the half-ganglia on
the same side of the ventral nerve cord as the injected teloblast.
Hence each of the ectodermal precursor teloblasts is the progenitor
of a characteristic part of the ipsilateral nervous system. However,
another part of the HRP stain forms a characteristic segmentally
repeated pattern in the ipsilateral epidermis of the germinal plate.
Hence the blast cells derived from the N, O, P and Q teloblasts give
rise to both neural and non-neural ectoderm.

     The cellular distribution of HRP stain can be ascertained in
much finer detail in serial histological sections of embryos. Sections through the nerve cord of embryos in which the N, O, P or Q
teloblasts had been HRP-injected individually, have shown that the
descendents of each teloblast give rise to characteristic patterns
of neuronal clusters in each segmental ganglion. The size and position of each of these clusters is quite invariant from segment to
segment and from specimen to specimen. This finding suggests that
the four different developmental cell lineages represented by the

neuronal progeny of each of the four teloblast pairs correspond to four distinct neuronal sibs. Moreover, in view of the known positional invariance of identified neurons in the segmental ganglia of the leech, it would appear that each identified neuron is the lineal descendant of a given teloblast (Fig. 3).

BLASTOMERE ABLATIONS

These cell lineage analyses, or fate maps, thus show that leech neurogenesis is highly determinate, in the sense that a particular teloblast regularly gives rise to a given part of the nervous system during normal development. Another aspect of this determinacy is that upon death or malfunction of a teloblast, its normal developmental role is not taken over fully by any other cell. Thus killing or ablating a teloblast of the early embryo leads to characteristic developmental aberrations. Seth Blair (1982) and Blair and Weisblat (1982) examined the neuroanatomical consequences of killing identified teloblasts, or teloblast precursor cells, by intracellular injection of toxic enzymes, such as proteases or deoxyribonucleases. They found, in accord with the cell lineage analyses, that killing an N teloblast during stage 6 results in formation of an embryonic nervous system whose segmental ganglia show anatomical deficits on the ablated side. However, the pattern of these deficits is not as regular as one might have expected; the half-ganglia on the ablated side vary greatly in size within the same specimen, ranging from a nearly normal cell number to a total absence of segmental neurons. Half-ganglia that are nearly normal in size contain the cells normally provided by the O, P and Q teloblasts on the same side, and, in addition, they contain some cells that are derived from the (non-ablated) N teloblast on the other side; these latter cells have made an abnormal crossing of the midline of the germinal plate during formation of the ganglionic primordia. That some half-ganglia are entirely absent in these specimens, i.e., do not receive any cells even from the (non-ablated) O, P and Q teloblasts on the same side, suggests that the abnormal midline crossing of N-derived cells is subject to considerable fluctuation and that the N-derived cells play some organizing role for the O-, P- and Q-derived cells in founding the ganglionic primordia.

As would have been expected, killing of an M-teloblast results in an embryo that lacks all mesodermal segmental structures on the ablated side. However, in addition, the ablated side also lacks a recognizable nervous system, including any half-ganglia. Here the (non-ablated) N, O, P and Q teloblasts still produce their bandlets of stem cells, but in the absence of the segmental mesodermal tissue blocks, the normal precursor cells of the nervous system are not organized into ganglionic primordia. These deficits produced by ablation of teloblasts show the importance of interactions between cells of different lines of descent in shaping the normal development of the leech nervous system.

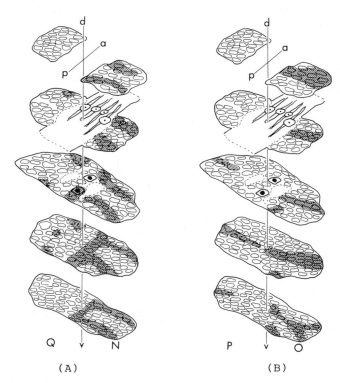

Figure 3.   Embryonic origins of the cells of the Helobdella segmental
ganglion.   The drawing shows 5 horizontal sections through a midbody
segmental ganglion of the embryo at mid-stage 10.   (Dorsal aspect at
the top; front edge facing away from the viewer.)   The 2 pairs of
dark, elongated contours in the center of the second section from
the top represent identifiable muscle cells in the longitudinal nerve
tract.   They are descendants of the M teloblast pair.   The two dark,
circular contours in the center of the middle section represent
2 identifiable glial cells, each of which is a descendant of one N
teloblast.   The faint contours do not correspond to actual cells
but are shown to indicate the approximate size, disposition and
number of neurons in the ganglion.   In each half-ganglion, domains
are shown crosshatched that contain descendants of the teloblast,
designated at the bottom of the figure.

CODA

As is evident from this account, studies of the development of the leech nervous system have thus far provided information of a mainly descriptive nature. But many fairly narrowly focused questions pertaining to developmental mechanisms can now be asked. For instance, how is the precise morphogenetic succession of alternating cell cleavage planes, first during early embryogenesis and later during formation of the mesodermal segments, actually determined? This determination probably reflects the replication and positioning of the elements of the embryonic cytoskeleton whose orientation governs the cleavage planes in cell division. A related question concerns the developmental role of the teloplasm that is passed on only to Cell D, of which the ventral part is given to cell DM and its mesodermal precursor cells, and which is eventually parcelled out by the teloblasts to their blast cell descendants. What kind of counting mechanism is at work which assures that exactly 32 - never 31 or 33 -stem cells descended from the M teloblast found a segmental block of mesodermal tissue on each side of the embryo? How do the cells descended from the ectodermal precursor teloblasts N, O, P and Q lying within such a tissue block assemble to form the neurons of the ganglionic primordia? Is the morphological, electrical and chemical maturation of the neurons dependent on interaction of their growing axons with target cells or tissues? Does the development of the motor neurons and their connections that underlies the gradual perfection of the walking and swimming movements require practice, or does locomotory behavior arise autonomously during embryogenesis without need of any functional feedback? Finally, does its line of descent govern the ultimate character of a neuron because it has received a particular set of intracellular determinants that were distributed in some regular fashion over the daughter cells in successive embryonic cell divisions, or because the cell occupies a particular topographic position in the embryo thanks to the regular cleavage pattern through which it arose? We hope that our studies of leech development will allow us to answer some of these questions before too long by means of experimental techniques already at hand.

ACKNOWLEDGEMENTS

The work summarized in this article was supported by NIH research grant NS 12818, by NIH training grants GM-07232 and GM-07048, by NSF grant BN577-19181 and by a research grant from the March of Dimes Birth Defects Foundation.

REFERENCES

Blair, S.S., 1982, Interactions between mesoderm and ectoderm in segment formation in the embryo of a glossiphoniid leech, Develop. Biol., 89:389-396.

Blair, S.S. and D.A. Weisblat, 1982, Ectodermal interactions during
    neurogenesis in the Glossiphoniid leech Helobdella
    triserialis, Develop. Biol., 76:245-262.
Fernandez, J., 1980, Embryonic development of the glossiphoniid
    leech Theromyzon rude: Characterization of developmental
    stages, Develop. Biol., 76:245-262.
Fernandez, J. and G.S. Stent, 1982, Embryonic development of the
    glossiphoniid leech Theromyzon rude: Structure and development
    of the germinal bands, Develop. Biol., 78:407-434.
Fitzpatrick-McElligott, S. and G.S.Stent, 1981, Appearance and local-
    ization of acetylcholinesterase in embryos of the leech,
    Helobdella triserialis, J. Neurosci., 1:901-907.
Kramer, A.P. and J.R. Goldman, 1980, The nervous system of the glossi
    phoniid leech Haementeria ghilianii. I. Identification of
    neurons, J. Comp. Physiol., 144:435-448.
Kramer, A.P., 1981, The nervous system of the glossiphoniid leech
    Haementeria ghilianii. II. Synaptic pathways controlling body
    wall shortening, J. Comp. Physiol., 144:449-457.
Kuwada, J.Y. and A.P. Kramer, 1982, Embryonic development of
    identified leech neurons, submitted for publication.
Macagno, E.R., 1980, The number and distribution of neurons in leech
    segmental ganglia, J. Comp. Neurol., 190:283-302.
Muller, K.J., J.G. Nicholls and G.S. Stent, eds., 1981, Neurobiology
    of the Leech, Cold Spring Harbor Laboratory, Cold Spring Harbor,
    New York.
Schleip, W., 1936, Ontogonie der Hirudineen, in: Klassen und
    Ordnungen des Tierreichs, Vol. 4, Div. III, Book 4, Part 2,
    1-121, H.G. Bronn, ed., Akad. Verlagsgesellschaft, Leipzig.
Sedat, S. and M. Manuelides, 1977, A direct approach to the structure
    of eukaryotic chromosomes. Cold Spring Harbor Symp. Quart.
    Biol., 42:331.
Stent, G.S. and D.S. Weisblat, 1982, Cell lineage in the development
    of the leech nervous system, Trends in Neurosciences, 4(10):
    251-255.
Stent, G.S., D.A. Weisblat, S.S. Blair and S.L. Zackson, 1982,
    Cell lineage in the development of the leech nervous system,
    Neuronal Development, N. Spitzer, Ed., Plenum, New York,
    pp. 1-44.
Weisblat, D.A., G. Harper, G.S. Stent and R.T. Sawyer, 1980a,
    Embryonic cell lineages in the nervous system of the glossi-
    phoniid leech Helobdella triserialis, Develop. Biol.,
    76:58-78.
Weisblat, D.A., R.T. Sawyerand G.S. Stent, 1978, Cell lineage
    analysis by intracellular injection of tracer, Science,
    202:1295-1298.
Weisblat, D.A., S.L. Zackson, S.S. Blair and J.D. Young, 1980b,
    Cell lineage analysis by intracellular injection of fluores-
    cent tracers, Science, 209:1538-1541.
Whitman, C.O., 1878, The embryology of Clepsine, Quart. J. Microscop.
    Sci. (N.S.), 18:215-315.

Whitman, C.O., contribution to the history of germ layers in
    Clepsine, J. Morphol., 1:105-182.
Zackson, S.L., 1982, Cell clones and segmentation in leech develop-
    ment, submitted for publication to Cell.

DEVELOPMENT OF NEUROTRANSMITTER SYSTEMS IN THE GOLDFISH RETINA

S.C. Sharma and R. Petrucci

Dept. of Opthalmology
New York Medical College
Valhalla, N.Y. 10595

In the adult vertebrate retina, aminobuteric acid (GABA),
glycine and dopamine have been localized in particular cell types
and their role implicated as neurotransmitter for those cells. The
cells have been shown to contain high concentrations of neurotransmitter and its synthetic enzymes and they accumulate the putative
transmitter or its precursors. These retinal neurons are also
capable of releasing the transmitter in response to an appropriate
stimulus (Hall et al., 1974; Robert et al., 1976, for review). In
the retina of adult Xenopus laevis, GABA accumulates predominantly
in horizontal cells and in certain amacrine cells of the inner
nuclear layer (Hollyfield et al., 1979). Similar cell types in the
adult goldfish retina also contain GABA; specifically, GABA has
been localized in H-1 type cone horizontal cells and Ab type pyriform amacrine cells (Marc et al., 1978).

Glycine uptake and its release in response to light have been
observed in some amacrine cells of the rabbit retina (Brunn and
Ehinger, 1972; Ehinger and Lindberg-Bauer, 1976). In Xenopus
laevis, glycine is accumulated by cells in the inner nuclear layer,
and these cells have terminals which are located both in the inner
and the outer plexiform layers (Rayborn et al., 1981). Furthermore,
Marc and Lam (1981) reported the uptake of glycine in Aa type amacrine
cells and I-2 interplexiform cells of the adult goldfish retina.

Dopaminergic neurons have been localized in the inner plexiform
layer of rabbit (Dowling and Ehinger, 1978; Hedden and Dowling,
1978) and in the goldfish retina by Marc (1980) who further characterized these cells as I-1 type interplexiform cells.

A recent series of papers (Hollyfield et al., 1979; Rayborn et al., 1981; Sarthy et al., 1981) described development of GABA, glycine and dopamine in <u>Xenopus laevis</u>. The appearance of high affinity uptake systems for GABA, glycine and dopamine occurs at a different stage of development in a particular order. The GABA system appears first, followed by the glycine system and then the dopamine system. For GABA and glycine, the uptake systems emerge prior to synpatic formation of these cells (Sarthy et al., 1981). The release mechanisms for these transmitters, which are K+ stimulated and Ca++ dependent, develops last and is linked to the appearance of synaptic formations (Sarthy et al., 1981). Thus, there is a precise temporal sequence in the appearance of specific properties for these neurotransmitters. Initial studies of GABA and glycine accumulation in the human retina show results similar to those seen in amphibians and lower vertebrates (Lam and Hollyfield, 1980).

The role of GABA and glycine has also been implicated in the "red" cone mechanism in the adult goldfish retina (Marc, 1980; Marc and Lam, 1981). Since the goldfish retina has been extensively used in investigations of synaptic circuitry (Stell, 1967; Stell and Lightfoot, 1975; Marc and Sperling, 1976), we felt it important to study the development of the properties associated with neurotransmitters in the goldfish retina. Here we report the emergence and localization of GABA-ergic, glycinergic and dopaminergic transmitter systems in the developing goldfish retina.

The present study encompasses retinae of animals at stage late 23/early 24 (80 hours after spawning), stage 25 (hatching) and thereafter every 24 hours after hatching for 9 days (designated as stage 25+1 day, 25+2 days, etc.). The cornea of stage 23 and subsequent stage embryos was pierced with a fine tungsten electrode. In the later stage embryos (after stage 25), the lens was also removed. The embryos were transferred to vials containing 100 μCi/ml of ^{3}H-GABA, ^{3}H-glycine, or ^{3}H-dopamine (specific activity 60 Ci/mmole, 12.3 Ci/mmole, and 48 Ci/mmole respectively) and were allowed to swim freely in it for 20 minutes. The embryos were then washed in aerated goldfish ringers and fixed in 3% glutaraldehyde in 0.1 M phosphate buffer pH 7.4. Optimal exposure time for ^{3}H-GABA autoradiography was 5 days, for ^{3}H-glycine 6 days, and for ^{3}H-dopamine 4 days. K$^+$ stimulated ^{3}H-GABA release was measured using a procedure similar to Sarthy and Lam (1979).

^{3}H-GABA uptake was seen in the earliest developmental stages (late stage 23), although distinct cellular layers do not start to appear until stage 25. By stage 25+2, large numbers of silver grains were observed over the horizontal cell layer (Fig. 1). Two days later (stage 25+4) the outer plexiform layer was identifiable (Fig. 1). It was at this stage that specific uptake of ^{3}H-GABA could be clearly seen in the most distal horizontal cells.

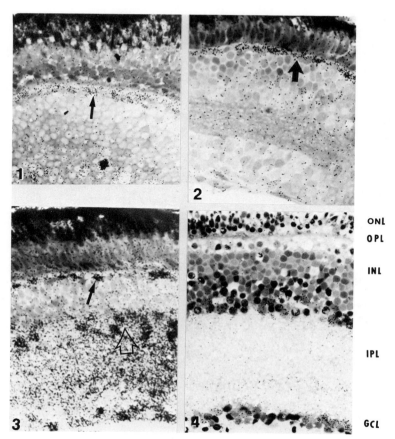

Figure 1. Retinae of developmental stages incubated in the presence
of ^{3}H-GABA and processed for autoradiography: 1) 2 days post hatching (2, P.H.); 2) 4 P.H.; and 3) 6 P.H. At early stage no high affinity uptake was evident. In (1) certain cells have higher concentration of grains indicating the development of the properties of high
affinity uptake. Arrow in (1) indicates such cells in the horizontal
cell layer. In (2 and 3) accumulation of grains becomes evident onto
inner nuclear layer cells (see arrow). (3) Certain cells in the
ganglion cell layer are heavily labelled. These cells may represent
displaced amacrine cells which are GABA-ergic. All micrographs are
of the same magnification. Autoradiograph of retina (6 P.H.) following K$^+$ stimulated release of GABA. (4) Compare it to (3). ONL,
outer nuclear layer; OPL, outer plexiform layer; INL, inner nuclear
layer; IPL, inner plexiform layer; GCL, ganglion cell layer.

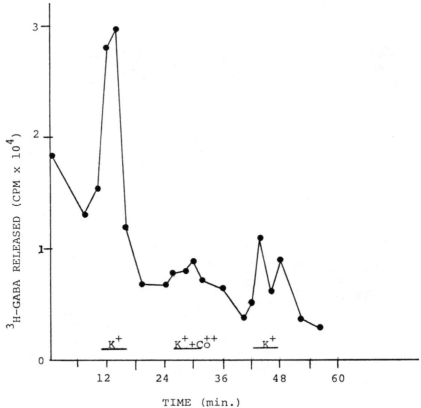

TIME (min.)

Figure 2. Potassium (K^+) stimulated release of ^{3}H-GABA from
retinas of stage 25+6 eyes and the effect of 5 mM Co^{++}. 20 eyes
were incubated for 15 minutes with ^{3}H-GABA, washed with goldfish
ringers and transferred to 2 ml ringer solution, K^+ medium (56 mM)
or K^+ medium containing Co^{++} (5 mM) every two minutes. Radioactivity in each incubation medium was measured by scintillation
counting. Similar results were obtained in 10 other experiments.

These cells were similar in their location to those seen in
the adult goldfish retina and were designated as H-l type cone
horizontal cells (Marc et al., 1978). Silver grains also begin to
appear within the amacrine cell layer at about stage 25+5. By
stage 25+6 (Fig. 1) GABA was incorporated specifically in the
proximal (vitread) amacrine cells, which were designated as Ab type
amacrine cells by Marc (1980).

Release of GABA was studied for 2 stages (25+5 and 25+6) of
retinal development. Release of GABA by a K^+ stimulated and Ca^{++}
dependent mechanism is a property of functional GABA-ergic synapse.

The GABA can be released by increasing the K^+ concentration in the medium (Fig. 2). Presence of 5 mM concentration of Co^{++} into the medium inhibits the release of GABA, suggesting that the release may be Ca^{++} dependent. However, when Co^{++} is removed from the medium and replaced by K^+, a release is again stimulated. Auto-radiography on these retinas showed no grains on the horizontal cells. Grain counts on amacrine cells after K^+ stimulated release were reduced to 10% of the count before K^+ treatment (Figs. 1 - 3 and 4). These data suggest that K^+ stimulated release of GABA was from horizontal and amacrine cells.

^{3}H-glycine uptake was first observed at late stage 23/early stage 24 in neuroepithelial cells, but could not be localized to any specific cell types. At stages 25+2 - 25+4, the specific glycine uptake appeared in distally located amacrine cells. By stage 25+6 and 25+8 this uptake was clearly established and localized to Aa type amacrine cells (Fig. 3). Marc and Lam (1981) have localized glycine uptake to this cell layer in the adult goldfish retina as well as to I-2 type cells of the interplexiform cells of the inter-nuclear layer. Silver grains can also be found within this layer.

Dopaminergic uptake systems appear last in the developing goldfish retina. Little or no specific dopamine uptake was seen at stage 25+3 embryos. Dopamine labelling starts at stage 25+4 (Fig. 4) in the inner nuclear layer. Specific dopamine uptake was seen at stage 25+6 to 25+8 and was localized in a few large cells between the inner nuclear layer and the inner plexiform layer.These cells have been described by Dowling and Ehinger in the goldfish retina (1975, 1978). In goldfish these cells have been referred to as dopaminergic interplexiform cells in the adult retina (Marc, 1982).

At the earliest stage (late stage 23), neuroepithelial cells, with no apparent stratification, show evenly distributed grains throughout the retinal epithelium. The cells which take up the GABA are positioned at most levels except the future ganglion cells in the center. In the subsequent histogenesis of the retina, most of the labelled cells occupy positions along the border of the inner nuclear layer, which is the future horizontal cell layer of the adult retina. The outer plexiform layer is not yet evident. Other GABA labelled cells of the neuroepithelium occupy the inner-most layer of the inner nuclear layer, which in the adult retina is composed of amacrine cells. The specific label on amacrine cells does not appear until 5 days after hatching. These results suggest that GABA uptake occurs much earlier, but perhaps specific release of the transmitter does not occur until the appropriate synapses are formed. At present, we cannot substantiate such a claim as there are no developmental studies, concerning synaptogenesis, available in the goldfish retina. The pattern of cessation of mitotic activity in the developing goldfish retina proceeds in a vitread to sclerad pattern (Sharma and Ungar, 1980). The ganglion

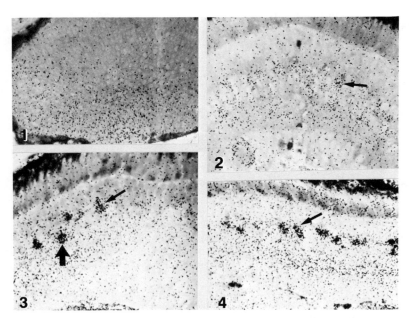

Figure 3. Autoradiographs of the developing retinas from stages
(1) 23/24; (2) 25+2; (3) 25+6; and (4) 25+8 which were incubated
for 20 minutes in ^{3}H glycine. Diffuse labelling in (1) is
evident. The emergence of heavy labelled cells appears in (2). In
(3) the arrow points to probable Aa amacrine cells. The labelled
cell above, especially the more medial one, is a probable I-2
interplexiform cell. Punctate labelled area below the labelled
cells in (4) is near the ganglion cell layer. All micrographs are
of the same magnification.

cells become post-mitotic first at the center of the retina at stage
20, followed by the inner nuclear layer cells at stage 21. By
stage 23 most cells in the central retina are post-mitotic except
for a few horizontal cells and receptor nuclei. Our results,
showing that high affinity uptake system for GABA in differentiating
horizontal cells first appears at stage 23, suggests that these
cells have become post-mitotic. These results confirm earlier
observations of Hollyfield et al (1979) in the developing Xenopus
retina.

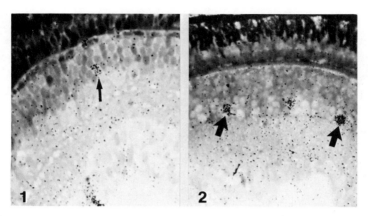

Figure 4.   Autoradiographs of the developing retinas from stages
(1) 25+4; and (2) 25+8 which were incubated for 20 minutes in ^{3}H
dopamine.   Accumulation of radioactive grains first appears at
stage 25+4.   There was no indication of any specific label up to
stage 25+3.   At the inner border of the inner nuclear layer,
specific dopamine accumulating neurons appear in (2).   The cells
probably are future I-1 interplexiform cells (arrow).   Figures are
at the same magnification.

Glycine has been suggested as a possible neurotransmitter for
certain amacrine cells (Aa) and interplexiform cells (I-2) by Marc
and Lam (1981) in the adult goldfish retina.   They have further
suggested that glycinergic cells are involved in "red" coding
circuits in the retina.   Retinas at embryonic stage late 23/early
24 show the development of high affinity uptake mechanism for
glycine.   In later stages of development (2 days after hatching),
the accumulation of ^{3}H glycine becomes evident in the cells of the
inner nuclear layer.   Two distinct laminae containing labelled
cells can be easily distinguished in retinas of stage 25+3.   The
question of whether sclerad layer cells are I-2 cells of the interplexiform layer and virtread layer cells are Aa amacrine cells is
not clear.

^{3}H-dopamine uptake in the adult goldfish retina occurs in
interplexiform cells.   I-1 type cells are comparatively fewer in
number and their somas are situated in the amacrine cell layer with
some processes in the inner plexiform and external horizontal cell
layer (Sarthy and Lam, 1979; Marc, 1980).   The synthesis of
dopamine first becomes evident at 3 days post-hatching but with no
specific label on any retinal cells.   The first specific localiza-

tion of ^{3}H-dopamine appears in animals 4 days after hatching and
becomes progressively distinct in later stages. The distinct band
of label in external horizontal cells and the inner plexiform layer
probably appears after 8 days post-hatching and perhaps is correlated with the development of synaptic connectivity.

It appears that the high affinity uptake system becomes
evident first in interneurons of the sclerad region of the retina
(horizontal cells) and continues towards the vitread side. This
pattern of uptake system suggests a spatial order and also holds
true for the differentiation of uptake, synthesis and release of
neurotransmitters in the developing retinae of Xenopus laevis
(Sarthy et al., 1981). K$^+$ stimulated Ca^{++} dependent GABA release
is present in goldfish retinae at 6 days post-hatching. Since
Sarthy et al. (1981) suggested that differentiation of the release
mechanism correlates well with synaptic formation in Xenopus, we
presume, at least for the GABA, that the specific synaptogenesis is
well under way by this time (6 days post-hatching) in goldfish
retina as well.

GABA, glycine and dopamine are implicated as transmitters for
interneurons involved in long wave length information (Marc, 1980).
Red color processing connectivity involves cones, H-1 cone
horizontal cells, Aa and Ab amacrine cells and I-1 inner plexiform
cells (Marc, 1980). The order of the emergence of different transmitters is identical to that of interneurons involved in red color
processing. It has been further proposed (Chen and Witkovsky,
1979) that as light stimulation of photoreceptors proceeds, it may
stimulate synaptic formation. Hence, the differentiation of
neuronal properties may be dependent upon light stimulation, while
the order and direction of differentiation might determine the
precise connectivity. This could account for the retinal neuronal
differentiation from sclerad to vitread direction in spite of the
fact that retinal cells become post-mitotic (Sharma and Unger,
1980) from vitread to sclerad direction.

References

Brunn, A. and Ehinger, B., 1972, Uptake of the putative neurotrans-
    mitter, glycine, into the rabbit retina. Invest. Ophthalmol.,
    11:191-198.
Chen, F. and Witkovsky, P., 1979, the formation of photoreceptor
    synapses in the retina of larval Xenopus. J. Neurocytol.,
    7:721-740.
Chin, C.A. and Lam, D.M.K., 1980, The uptake and release of ^{3}H-
    Glycine in the goldfish retina. J. Physiol. (Lond),
    308:185-195.

Dowling, J.E. and Ehinger, B., 1975, Synaptic organization of the
    amine-containing interplexiform cells of the goldfish and Cebus
    monkey retinas. Science, 188:270-273.
Ehinger, G. and Lundberg-Bauer, B., 1976, Light evoked release of
    Glycine from cat and rabbit retina. Brain Res., 113:535-549.
Hall, Z.W., Hildebrand, J.G. and Kravitz, E.A., 1974, Chemistry of
    synaptic transmission, Chiron Press, Newton, Mass.
Hedden, W.L. and Dowlilng, J.E., 1978, The interplexiform cell
    system, II. Effects of dopamine on goldfish retinal neurons.
    Proc. Roy. Soc. B., 201:27-55.
Hollyfield, J.G., Rayborn, M.E., Sarthy, P.V. and Lam, D.M.K.,
    1979, The emergence, localization and maturation of
    neurotransmitter systems during development of the retina in
    Xenopus laevis. I. γ-Aminobutyric acid. J. Comp. Neur.
    188:587-595.
Kajishima, T., 1960, The normal developmental stages of the
    goldfish Carassius auratus. Japan. J. Ichthylology. 8:20-28.
Lam, D.M.K. and Hollyfield, J.G., 1980, Localization of putative
    amino acid neurotransmitters in the human retina.
    Exp. Eye Res. 31:729-732.
Marc, R.E., 1980, Retinal colour channels and their neurotransmit-
    ters. In Colour Deficiencies V, Institute of Physics, London.
    Adam Hilger, Ltd., London. pp. 15-29.
Marc, R.C., 1982, Spatial organization of neurochemically
    classified interneurons of the goldfish retina-1. Local
    patterns. Vision Research, 22:589-608.
Marc, R.E. and Lam, D.M.K., 1981, Glycinergic pathways in the
    goldfish retina. J. Neuroscience. 1:152-165.
Marc, R.E. and Sperling, H.G., 1976, Color receptor identities of
    goldfish cones. Science, 191:487-489.
Marc, R.E. and Summerall, R.D., 1980, Development of the
    transmitter systems in the teleost retina. Suppl. Inv.
    Ophthal. Visual Sci., 20:247.
Rayborn, M.E., Sarthy, P.V., Lam, D.M.K. and Hollyfield, J.G.,
    1981, The emergence, localization and maturation of neuro-
    transmitter systems during development of the retina in
    Xenopus laevis. II. Glycine. J. Comp. Neur. 195:585-593.
Roberts, E., Chase, T. and Tower, D.B., 1976, Gaba in nervous
    system function. Raven Press, New York.
Sarthy, P.V. and Lam, D.M.K., 1979, The uptake and release of ³H-
    dopamine in the goldfish retina. J. Neurochem., 32:1269-1277.
Sarthy, P.V., Rayborn, M.E., Hollyfield, J.G. and Lam, D.M.K., The
    emergence, localization and maturation of neurotransmitter
    systems during development of the retina in Xenopus laevis.
    III. Dopamine. J. Comp. Neur., 195:595-602.
Sharma, S.C. and Ungar, F., 1980, Histogenesis of the goldfish
    retina. J. Comp. Neur., 191:373-382.
Stell, W.K., 1967, The structure and relationships of horizontal
    cells and photoreceptor-bipolar synaptic complexes in goldfish
    retina. Am. J. Anat., 121:401-423.

Stell, W.K. and Lightfoot, D.O., 1975, Color-specific interconnec-
    tions of cones and horizontal cells in the retina of goldfish.
    J. Comp. Neur., 159:473-502.

POSTNATAL NEUROCHEMICAL DEVELOPMENT OF THE RAT VISUAL SYSTEM

Viggo M. Fosse, Ivar Kvale, Ragnar Lund-Karlsen
and Frode Fonnum

Norwegian Defense Research Establishment
Division for Toxicology
Kjeller, Norway

INTRODUCTION

The visual system of many animal species is well described anatomically and physiologically. For this reason it is well suited for neurochemical as well as developmental investigations.

In many lower mammals the visual centers are immature at birth although the main visual pathways are already formed at this time. During early postnatal life the lateral geniculate body, superior colliculus and visual cortex will develop mainly by the formation of synaptic contact zones, integration of their neuronal circuitry and neurochemical maturation (Karlsson, 1966, 1976; Lund and Lund, 1971; Lund, 1978; Cragg, 1975; De Groot and Vrensen, 1978; Holländer et al. 1979), concomitant with the development of retinal function and response to light in subcortical visual centers (Hollander and Distel, 1978). Neurochemical development must include aquisition of the ability for synthesis, storage, release, re-uptake and degradation of the appropriate neurotransmitter.

The retinotectal as well as the corticofugal fibers from layer VI of visual cortex to lateral geniculate body have already innervated their target tissues at birth (Lund, 1978). In contrast, the corticofugal fibers from layer V of visual cortex to superior colliculus have not completed their innervation until postnatal day 3 (Lund, 1978, this volume). A certain amount of plasticity is retained however in the corticotectal projection of the rat until postnatal day 20 (Mustari and Lund, 1976). Furthermore, between postnatal week 1 and 2 there appears to be a marked alteration in the distribution of synaptic input from visual cortex to the upper 3 laminae of superior colliculus, in rats and rabbits (Lund, 1978; Holländer et al., 1979).

In our laboratory we have for some time been engaged in studies aimed at the localization of neurotransmitters in the main visual pathways as well as of interneurons in visual structures of the albino rat. Furthermore, putative neurotransmitters in retinal neurons have been identified also (Lund-Karlsen, 1978; Lund-Karlsen and Fonnum, 1978; Fonnum et al., 1979, 1981). Recently we have become interested in and monitored the postnatal development of several neurotransmitter marker enzymes, high affinity uptake acti- vities and release mechanisms in the visual system of the newborn rat. These results will be presented here and discussed in relation to previously observed anatomical changes, e.g. synaptogenesis, in lateral geniculate body, superior colliculus and visual cortex.

Neurotransmitters in the Visual System

First, a brief account of putative neurotransmitters in the visual system will be presented: Taurine may be a transmitter or "trophic factor" released from receptor cells in the retina (Pasantes-Morales et al., 1973; Lund-Karlsen, 1978). Calcium may also be a transmitter for some of these cells. In the goldfish aspartate is the putative transmitter of red and green cones, while the rods may employ glutamate (Mark and Lam, 1981). For unknown reasons the blue cones specifically accumulate the dye lucifer yellow (I. Thompson, pers. communication) which presumably mimics a hitherto unknown transmitter in these cells. In some species there is a specific localization of GABA in the horizontal cells, while the bipolar cells probably employ glutamate/aspartate as transmitter (Redburn, 1981). The amacrine cells, on the other hand, contain a wide array of neurotransmitters but apparently each transmitter species is confined to only a subset of the amacrine cell population. Both GABA, acetylcholine, glycine, dopamine and serotonin are trans- mitter candidates for these cells (Lund-Karlsen, 1978; McGeer et al., 1978). Also, these cells show immunoreactivity for a wide variety of neuroactive peptides, i.e., enkephalin, β-endorphin, glucagon, neuortensin, substance P, thyroid releasing hormone (TRH) and vasoactive intestinal peptide (VIP). The different peptides are contained in different amacrine cells with distinct lamination and stratification patterns of their terminals (N. Brecha, this volume). Glutamate/aspartate appears to be the neurotransmitter of at least a fraction of the retinal ganglion cells projecting to the pigeon optic tectum (Cuenod et al., 1981) and rat superior col- liculus (Fosse and Fonnum, in preparation). However, there is no evidence to suggest which is the transmitter employed by retinal ganglion cells projecting to the lateral geniculate body. Neither is there any evidence for the transmitter of the projection to visual cortex from lateral geniculate body. On the other hand,

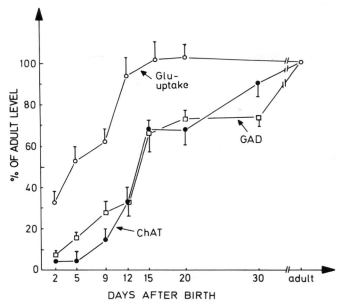

Figure 1. Postnatal development of high affinity uptake of glutamate, glutamic acid decarboxylase and choline acetytransferase in
rat visual cortex. Each point is expressed as percent of adult level,
and represents the mean value from 5-7 experiments. Adult levels
were (mean ±SD): 86.5 ± 10.5 pmole/mg protein/3 min for glutamate
uptake, 100.1 ± 5.4 nmole/mg protein/hr for glutamic acid decarboxylase and 52.4 ± 1.2 nmole/mg protein/hr for choline acetyltransferase.

glutamate and/or aspartate are strong candidates as neurotransmitters
of the corticofugal fibers from visual cortex to lateral geniculate
body (Lund-Karlsen and Fonnum, 1978; Baughman and Gilbert, 1980;
Fosse and Fonnum, in preparation), superior colliculus (Lund-Karlsen
and Fonnum, 1978; Fosse and Fonnum, in preparation) and to pulvinar
(Fosse and Fonnum, in preparation). Glutamate, aspartate, β-alanine
and GABA may also be transmitters of intrinsic neurons in superior
colliculus (Lund-Karlsen, 1978; Fonnum et al., 1979; Sandberg and
Jacobson, 1981; Fosse and Fonnum, in preparation). Also, GABA is
the transmitter-candidate for the nigrotectal pathway to deeper
layers of superior colliculus (Fonnum et al., 1979; Fosse and
Sandberg, unpublished results), and acetylcholine for the fibers
from the parabigeminal nucleus to the superior colliculus (Fonnum et
al., 1979). Finally, intrinsic neurons in visual cortex may use
glutamate, aspartate and GABA as their transmitters (McGeer et al.,
1978; Fonnum et al., 1981; Baughman and Gilbert, 1980; Fosse and
Fonnum, unpublished results).

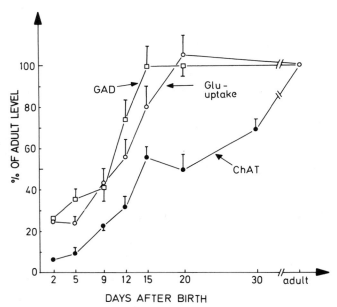

Figure 2. Postnatal development of high affinity uptake of glutamate, glutamic acid decarboxylase and choline acetyltransferase in
lateral geniculate body of the rat. Each point is expressed as
percent of adult level, and represents the mean value from 5-7
experiments. Adult levels were (mean ± SD): 180.7 ± 44.8 pmole/mg
protein/3 min for glutamate uptake, 79.81 ± 8.4 nmole/mg protein/hr
for glutamic acid decarboxylase and 56.1 ± 4.0 nmole/ng protein/hr
for choline acetyltransferase.

METHODS

     Surgical operations, dissection and preparation of tissue will
be described elsewhere (Kvale et al., 1982; Fosse and Fonnum, in
preparation). High affinity uptake studies were performed with both
sucrose homogenates and resuspended pellets containing synaptosomes
(Kvale et al., 1982). Choline acetyltransferase was determined as
described by Fonnum (1975), and glutamate decarboxylase as described
by Fonnum et al. (1970).

     K+-evoked release of endogenous and preloaded transmitters
from slices of superior colliculus and visual cortex were performed
essentially as described by Baughman and Gilbert (1980), with some
modifications (Fosse et al., in preparation). The measurement of
released L-glutamate was performed by a novel, highly sensitive
bioluminescent method (Fosse et al., in preparation), with the LKB
luminometer Model 1250 and 1251.

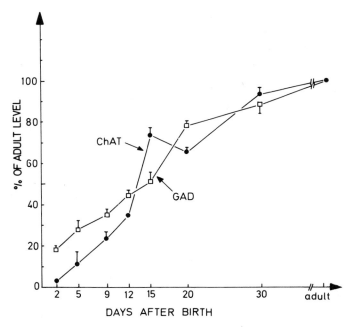

Figure 3. Postnatal development of glutamic acid decarboxylase and
choline acetyltransferase in rat superior colliculus. Each point
is expressed as percent of adult level, and represents the mean
value from 5-7 experiments. Adult levels were (mean ± SD):202.6 ±
9.7 nmole/mg protein/hr for glutamic acid decarboxylase and
49.4 ± 7.2 nmole/mg protein/hr for choline acetyltransferase.

RESULTS

High Affinity Uptake of Glutamate

In visual cortex and lateral geniculate body we observed a
continuous increase in high affinity uptake of L-glutamate and
D-aspartate until postnatal days 15 and 20, respectively (Figures 1
and 2). Thereafter the activity remained at adult level in both
structures. In superior colliculus, however, the high affinity
uptake was higher in neonates than in adults (Figure 4) with a small
but significant peak on postnatal day 12. The activity equalled
adult level from day 20 onwards. Unilateral aspiration of visual
cortex, i.e. areas 17, 18 and 18a (Krieg, 1946), was performed in
order to study the maturation of the corticotectal projection in
neonatal rats. We found only a marginal decrease in the uptake of
L-glutamate/D-aspartate ipsilateral to the lesion when introduced
on either postnatal day 5 or 8. Removal of visual cortex after

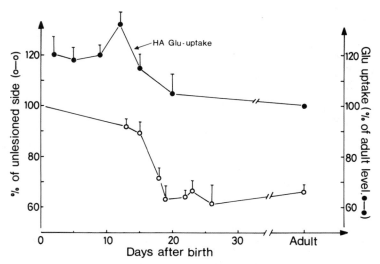

Figure 4.   Postnatal development of high affinity uptake of glutamate, and the effect of visual cortex ablation in rat superior
colliculus.   The upper curve describes the development of glutamate
uptake (---). The adult level was 37.3 ± 5.4 pmole/mg protein/3 min
with L-glutamate as substrate and 68.4 ± 6.2 pmole/mg protein/3 min
with D-aspartate as substrate. The lower curve (---) describes the
effect of visual cortex ablation on glutamate uptake in superior
collliculus in newborn rats. Each represents day on which uptake
was measured. Lesions were introduced 6 or 7 days prior to this.
Each is expressed as percent of the activity on the unlesioned side,
and represents the mean value from 6 animals.

postnatal day 9-10 resulted in a dramatic decrease in glutamate
crude sucrose homogenates or resuspended pellets (not shown).

Kinetic parameters (K_m and V_{max}) were also determined for the
high affinity uptake of L-glutamate in neonatal and adult rats (Table
I). We did not observe any significant changes in the K_m values.
Alterations in V_{max} were to a great extent similar to the changes
shown in Figures 1 and 2, for lateral geniculate body and visual
cortex. In superior colliculus, however, V_{max} was 207% of adult
level on pastnatal day 2 (Table I) as compared to 120% when measured
at 0.1 μl substrate (Figure 4).

TABLE I.

		2 DAYS	ADULT
K_m	LGB	7.1	5.2
	SC	5.6	3.5
	VC	2.6	3.9
V_{max}	LGB	376	3535
	SC	642	310
	VC	337	2312

K_m and V_{max} determined for high affinity uptake of L-glutamate in lateral geniculate body (LGB), superior colliculus (SC) and visual cortex (VC). The values are obtained from Lineweaver-Burk plots, and are based on 5 separate experiments, each using 5 different substrate concentrations. K_m is expressed in μM, V_{max} as cpm/μg protein. S D never exceeded 12%.

TABLE II.

	2 DAYS	15 DAYS	ADULT
SC	20 ± 2	59 ± 5	17 ± 1
LGB	7 ± 2	24 ± 2	8 ± 1
VC	9 ± 1	30 ± 3	18 ± 3

The high affinity uptake of GABA (final substrate concentration 10^{-7} M) measured on postnatal day 2 and 15, and in adult rats (2 1/2 months) in lateral geniculate body (LGB), superior colliculus (SC) and visual cortex (VC).

The results represent mean ± S D from 5 separate experiments, and are expressed as pmole/mg protein/3 min.

Release of Endogenous Glutamate

Potassium (K+)-evoked release of endogenous L-glutamate (Figures 5 and 6) and preloaded D-aspartate (not shown) from slices of superior colliculus and visual cortex were studied as well, in neonatal rats. L-glutamate was measured by a novel and very sensitive bioluminescent method which was developed recently in our laboratory (Fosse et al., in preparation). The evoked release developed differently from the high affinity uptake in the two structures. In both the release was 20%, or less, of adult level until postnatal day 15. Thereafter we observed a rapid increase in release from superior colliculus between postnatal days 16 and 18. The increase was less dramatic in visual cortex in which the evoked release of L-glutamate was only 30% of adult level on postnatal day 21.

Choline Acetyltransferase

Choline acetyltransferase, which is considered the best marker for cholinergic neurons, demonstrated a gradual increase postnatally

in all three regions (Figures 1,2 and 3). Between postnatal days 15
and 20 there was a transient plateau, however, It may also be worth
noting that adult level was not fully reached before 30 days after
birth.

Glutamic Acid Decarboxylase

Glutamic acid decarboxylase, the best marker for GABAergic
neurons, increased progressively after birth in all three structures
(Figures 1,2 and 3). In the lateral geniculate body, adult level was
reached on postnatal day 15, whereas in the superior colliculus and
visual cortex this was not reached even after 30 days.

High Affinity Uptake of GABA

Both neurons and glia cells have high affinity transport systems
for GABA (Fonnum et al., 1980). The GABA uptake was measured on
postnatal days 2 and 15, and in adults. Its development differed
from the postnatal changes in glutamic acid decarboxylase activity
(Table II). In all three structures we observed a significantly
(2-3 fold) higher GABA uptake on day 15 compared to postnatal day 2
and adults. K_m for the GABA uptake increased 3-4 times in lateral
geniculate body, whereas no significant change was found in the other
two structures (Table III). Based on V_{max} measurements the transport activity was lower in the day 2 animals than that found at the
fixed substrate concentration of 0.1 μm.

High Affinity Uptake of β-Alanine

High affinity uptake of β-alanine was higher in neonates than
in adults, in all three regions (Table IV). The difference was
least in visual cortex and largest in superior colliculus. Since
the uptake of β-alanine is assumed to reflect GABA uptake into glial
cells (Schon and Kelly, 1975) this finding may indicate a relatively
lesser importance of glial GABA uptake in the adult visual system.

DISCUSSION

Our findings confirm previous anatomical observations that the
visual system of the newborn rat is immature. It is noteworthy that
the corticotectal and corticogeniculate pathways do not appear to
follow the same innervation and maturation pattern during postnatal
development. Furthermore, the difference in developmental time-
course between glutamate uptake and release is remarkable.

Lateral Geniculate Body

In rabbits the corticofugal fibers have innervated the lateral
geniculate body at birth (Holländer et al., 1979). Few synapses are
found in the lateral geniculate body however (Karlsson, 1966, 1967).

During development different subsets of synapses are thought to mature at different stages in this structure (Frost and Schneider, 1979; Poppe et al., 1973), and the synapses are believed to be axo-dendritic (Brückner et al., 1972; Karlsson, 1967). More than 50% of the glutamate uptake in lateral geniculate body is localized at the terminals of the corticogeniculate projection as judged by visual cortex ablation studies (Lund-Karlsen and Fonnum, 1978; Fosse and Fonnum, unpublished). Ablation of visual cortex in neonates does not reduce glutamate uptake in lateral geniculate body however (I. Kvale, unpublished). This may indicate that the terminals of this pathway have not yet formed mature synapses before postnatal day 5. The uptake activity observed in newborns is probably due to interneurons possessing fully developed high affinity uptake mechanisms for glutamate. It is therefore reasonable to assume that the increase in glutamate uptake which we observe is largely due to the maturation of synapses formed by the corticogeniculate projection. Our findings that the glutamergic, cholinergic and GABAergic increased from birth onwards correlate with the synaptogenesis in this structure. A postnatal increase in glutamic acid decarboxylase has also been observed by others (McDonald et al., 1980)

Visual Cortex

In cerebral cortex of rabbits (DeGroot and Vrensen, 1978; Vrensen et al., 1977), cats (Cragg, 1975) and rats (Caley and Maxwell, 1968; Jones and Cullen, 1979) a postnatal increase in synaptic density has been shown. At the end of gestation cortical synapses are scarce, and largely confined to the molecular layer deep in the cortical plate (Peters and Feldman, 1973). In addition marked postnatal changes are found in all layers of rat visual cortex (Wolff, 1977; Wolff and Bar, 1977). Therefore, development of synapses and terminal sprouting seem to play a dominating role in the maturation of visual cortex, rather than neuronal proliferation (Vrensen et al., 1979). In agreement with this we observed a gradual increase in glutamate uptake which reached adult level on postnatal day 15. In other brain regions glutamergic fibers develop differently. After 30 days synaptosomal glutamate uptake in striatum is 80% of adult level (Compachiaro and Coyle, 1978; Wong and McGeer, 1981). Furthermore, in homogenates from whole rat cortex glutamate uptake develops differently in different subgroups of synaptosomes (Hitzemann and Loh, 1978). The aquisition of mature release mechanisms for glutamate is evident only after high affinity uptake for the transmitter has reached adult level in the visual cortex (Figure 5), i.e., after postnatal day 15. Thereafter we found a slow development of glutamate release which may reflect an abeyant fine-tuning and/or high turnover rate of cortical synapses at this developmental stage (Ruffolo et al., 1978). Unexpectedly, neither glutamic acid decarboxylase nor choline acetyltransferase were fully developed 30 days after birth, although the

TABLE III

		2 DAYS	ADULT
K_m	LGB	1.5	5.4
	SC	2.1	2.4
	VC	1.4	2.2
V_{max}	LGB	120	295
	SC	488	510
	VC	33	592

K_m and V_{max} determined for high affinity uptake of GABA in lateral geniculate body (LGB), superior colliculus SC) and visual cortex (VC).

The values are obtained from Lineweaver-Burk plots, and are based on 5 separate experiments, each using 5 different substrate concentrations. K_m is espressed in μM, V_{max} as cpm/μg protein. S D never exceeded 15%.

TABLE IV

	2 DAYS	ADULT
LGB	1.03 ± 0.16	0.28 ± 0.03
SC	1.48 ± 0.20	0.32 ± 0.04
VC	0.40 ± 0.06	0.21 ± 0.03

The high affinity uptake of β-alanine (final substrate concentration 10^{-7} M) measured in 2 days old and adult (2 1/2 months) rats in lateral geniculate body (LGB), superior colliculus (SC) and visual cortex (VC).

The results represent mean ± S D from 5 separate experiments, and are expressed as pmole/mg protein/3 min.

increase in cortical synaptic density appears to have culminated at this stage. Both the homolateral cortical association fibers and the corticocortical callosal projection (Nauta and Bucher, 1954; Hughes and Wilson, 1969; Hollander et al., 1979) may be responsible for glutamate uptake in visual cortex (Fonnum et al., 1981). Interneurons may contribute to this uptake as well (Baughman and Gilbert, 1980; Fosse and Fonnum, unpublished).

Superior Colliculus

Apparently, the superior colliculus develops differently from visual cortex and lateral geniculate body. In the rabbit there seems to be a transient overshoot of input from visual cortex between post-natal days 10 and 15 (Lund, 1978). Neuronal death occurs in the optic layers of superior colliculus until 8 days after birth (Giordano et al., 1980). There is also evidence which suggests a transient increase of excitatory terminals in the rat superior colliculus (Lund and Lund, 1971). These observations inter-digitate with our findings that the high affinity uptake of gluta-mate is higher in neonates than in adults. Furthermore, there is a small but significant peak on postnatal day 12. We have previous-ly shown that about 40% of the glutamate uptake is confined to ter-minals of the cortico-tectal projection (Figure 4; Lund-Karlsen and Fonnum, 1978; Fosse and Fonnum, in preparation). However, the excess uptake is not due to this input since ablation of visual cortex before postnatal day 10 has no effect on glutamate uptake in superior colliculus (Figure 4). These terminals do not appear to mature until after postnatal day 12, which correlates with the peak of glutamate uptake as well as the onset of retinal function. Sensi-tivity to kainic acid, which exerts toxic action on cell bodies and dendrites receiving glutamergic input (Coyle et al., 1978; McGeer et al., 1978), and retinal ablation studies suggests interneurons and retinotectal fibers to account for the remaining glutamate uptake in superior colliculus of the rat (Fosse and Fonnum, in preparation). Hence, interneurons and possibly the retinotectal neurons seem to acquire their potential for high affinity glutamate uptake far earlier than the corticofugal fibers in superior colliculus. The possibility that glial cells might influence uptake of glutamate in the immature superior colliculus cannot be excluded however. In contrast, the ability to release endogenous glutamate or preloaded D-aspartate is not manifested until after postnatal day 16 (Figures 5 and 6). This cannot be accounted for by a higher concentration of transmitter in the adult (I. Kvale, unpublished). Development of high affinity uptake mechanisms prior to the acquisition of mechanisms for transmitter release therefore seems to be a general feature of neuronal development in the retina (Bader et al., 1978; Baughman and Bader, 1977; Thompson, 1982), cerebellum (G.A. Foster, personal communication), visual cortex and superior colliculus (this work). The same developmental time-course is found whether endogenous or preloaded neurotransmitters are measured (not shown). Both choline acetyltransferase and glutamic acid decarboxylase de-monstrated a gradual increase after birth. We interpret this as maturaton of cholinergic and GABAergic nerve terminals in superior colliculus.

High Affinity Uptake of GABA and β-Alanine

In all 3 structures high affinity uptake of GABA showed a marked peak on day 15 after birth, which is in contrast to the development of glutamic acid decarboxylase. This has been observed in synaptosomal preparations from other brain regions also (Coyle and Enna, 1976; Wong and McGeer, 1981), but not when measured in cortical slices (Johnston and Davies, 1974). High affinity uptake of β-alanine, which apparently is associated with the glial GABA up-take (Schon and Kelly, 1975; Wong and McGeer, 1981) was higher in neonates than in adults. This is also the case in striatum but not

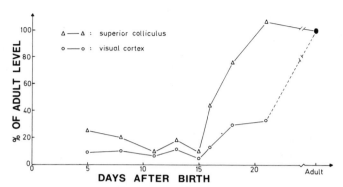

Figure 5. Postnatal development of K+-evoked glutamate release from
visual cortex and superior colliculus. Essentially, release experiments were performed by incubation of slices in 1 ml of Krebs-Ringer
solution, which was replaced every 5 minutes. Slices were depolar-
ized by 50 mM KCl, in the presence of 2 mM CaCl$_2$ and 1 mM MgCl$_2$.
"Calcium-free" pulse-medium contained 0.1 mM CaCl$_2$ and 10 mM MgSO$_4$.
Small aliquots of each fraction were assayed for radioactivity, and
for released endogenous L-glutamate by a novel and very sensitive
bioluminescent method (Fosse, Iverson and Fonnum, in preparation).
Adult levels were: 1.43 nmole/mg protein/5 min for visual cortex
and 1.07 nmole/mg protein/5 min for superior colliculus.

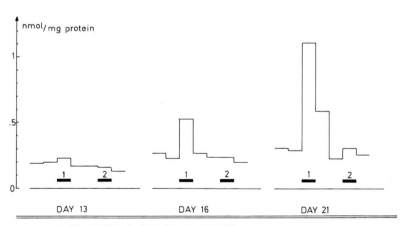

1: 50 mM KCl, 2 mM CaCl$_2$, 1 mM MgSO$_4$
2: 50 mM KCl, 0.1 mM CaCl$_2$, 10 mM MgSO$_4$

Figure 6. Postnatal development of K+-evoked glutamate release
from superior colliculus, and its calcium dependency. Release experiments were performed as described in Figure 5.

frontal cortex (Wong and McGeer, 1981). Hence, glial cells are
probably responsible for most of the early postnatal changes in the
high affinity uptake of GABA. In superior colliculus GABA is mainly localized in interneurons in the superficial layers (Okada,
1974) and in terminals of the nigrotectal projection (Di Chiara et
al., 1979; Fonnum et al., 1979). Both will probably contribute to
the development of GABA uptake and glutamic acid decarboxylase
activity in superior colliculus. In the rat visual cortex specific
GABA neurons have been identified (Ribak, 1977) and GABA may be an
interneuronal inhibitory transmitter (Baughman and Gilbert, 1980;
Chronwall and Wolff, 1978; Fosse and Fonnum, unpublished).

Conclusions

    In conclusion, the postnatal development of neurotransmitter
markers in superior colliculus, visual cortex and lateral geniculate body parallels previously observed morphological maturation
of nerve terminals. The temporal sequence in which high affinity
uptake mechanisms develop before the ability for transmitter
release seems to be a general feature of neuronal development.
It is also worth noting the correlation between neurochemical
maturation and onset of retinal function.

ACKNOWLEDGEMENTS

    The authors are grateful to Dr. Didima de Groot for helpful
discussions concerning morphological development of the visual
cortex. Also, the skillful and enthusiastic technical assistance
of Mrs. Evy Iversen is appreciated.

REFERENCES

Bader, C.R., Baughman, R.W. and Moore, J.L. , 1978, Different time
    course of development for high affinity choline uptake and
    choline acetyltransferase in the chick retina, Proc. Natl.
    Acad. Sci. USA, 75, 2525-2529.
Baughman, R.W. and Bader, C.R. , 1978, Biochemical characterization
    and cellular localization of the cholinergic system in the
    chick retina, Brain Research, 183, 469-485.
Baughman, R.W. and Gilbert, C.D. , 1980, Aspartate and glutamate as
    possible neurotransmitters of cells in layer 6 of the visual
    cortex, Nature, 287, 848-850.
Bennet, J.P., Jr., Logan, W.J. and Snyder, S.H., 1973, Amino acids
    as central nervous transmitters: The influence of ions, amino
    acid analogues and onotogeny of transport systems for L-glutamic
    and L-aspartic acids and glycine into central nervous synapto-
    somes of the rat, J. Neuorchem., 21, 1533-1550.

Brückner, G., Baer, H. and Biesold, D., 1972, Zur ultrastruktur den
    synaptischen kontakte im corpus geniculatum laterale der ratte,
    Z. Mikrosk. Anat. Forsch., 86, 513-530.
Caley, D.W. and Maxwell, D.S., 1968, An electronmicroscopic study of
    neurons during postnatal development of the rat cerebral
    cortex, J. Comp. Neurol., 133, 17-44.
Compachiaro, P. and Coyle, J.T., 1978, Ontogenetic development of
    kainate neurotoxicity: Correlates with glutamergic innervation,
    Proc. Natl. Acad. Sci. USA, 75, 2025-2029.
Chronwall, B.M. and Wolff, J.R., 1978, Classification and location
    of ^{3}H-GABA in the visual cortex of rats. In: Amino Acids as
    chemical transmitters, F. Fonnum, ed., Plenum Press, New York,
    pp. 297-303.
Coyle, J.T. and Enna, S.J., 1976, Neurochemical aspects of the onto-
    genesis of GABAergic neurons in the rat brain, Brain Research,
    111, 119-133.
Coyle, J.T., Molliver, M.E. and Kuhar, M.J., 1978, In situ injection
    of kainic acid: A new method for selectively lesioning neuronal
    cell bodies while sparing axons of passage, J. Comp. Neurol.,
    180, 301-324.
Cuénod, M., Beaudet, A., Canzek, V., Streit, P. and Reubi, J.C.,
    1981, Glutamatergic pathways in the pigeon and the rat brain.
    In: Glutamate as a neurotransmitter, G. Di Chiara and G.L.
    Gessa, eds., Raven Press, New York, pp.57-68.
Cragg, B.G., 1975, The development of synapses in the visual system
    of the cat, J. Comp. Neurol., 160, 147-166.
De Groot, D. and Vrensen, G., 1978, Postnatal development of
    synaptic contact zones in the visual cortex of rabbits, Brain
    Research, 147, 362-369.
Di Chiara, G., Porceddu, M.L., Morelli, M., Mulas, M.L., and Gessa,
    G.L., 1979, Evidence for GABAergic projections from the
    substantia nigra to the ventromedial thalamus and to the
    superior colliculus of the rat, Brain Research, 176, 273-284.
Fonnum, F., 1975, A rapid radiochemical method for determination of
    choline acetyltransferase, J. Neurochem., 24, 407-409.
Fonnum, F., Storm-Mathison, J. and Walberg, F., 1970, Glutamate de-
    carboxylase in inhibitory neurons. A study of the enzyme in
    Purkinje cells, Brain Research, 20, 259-275.
Fonnum, F., Lund-Karlsen, R., Malthe-Sorenson, D., Skrede, K.K. and
    Walaas, I., 1979, Localization of neurotransmitters, particular-
    ly glutamate in hippocampus, septum, nucleus accumbens and
    superior colliculus, Progr. in Brain Res., 51, 167-191.
Fonnum, F., Lund-Karlsen, R., Malthe-Sorenssen, D., Sterri, S. and
    Walaas, I., 1980, High affinity transport systems and their
    role in transmitter action. In: The cell surface and their
    role in transmitter action, G. Poste, C. Cotman and G.
    Nicholson, eds., Cell Surface Reviews, 6, 455-504.
Fonnum, F., Soreide, A., Kvale, I., Walker, J., and Walaas, I.,
    1981, Glutamate in cortical fibers. In: Glutamate as a neuro-

transmitter, G. Di Chiara and G.L. Gessa, eds., Raven Press, New York, pp. 29-41.

Frost, D.O. and Schneider, G.E., 1979, Postnatal development of retinal projections in Syrian hamsters: A study using auto-radiographic and anterograde degeneration techniques, Neuroscience, 4, 1649-1677.

Giordano, D.L., Murray, M. and Cunningham, T.J., 1980, Naturally occurring neuron death in the optic layers of the superior colliculus of the postnatal rat, J. Neurocytol., 9, 603-614.

Gosavi, V.S. and Dubey, P.N., 1972, Projection of striate cortex to the dorsal lateral geniculate body in the rat, J. Anat., 113, 75-82.

Hitzemann, R.J. and Loh, H.H., 1978, High affinity GABA and gluta-mate transport in developing nerve ending particles, Brain Research, 159, 29-40.

Holländer, H. and Distel, H., 1978, Postnatal development of the projection from the striate cortex to the superior colliculus in the rabbit, Arch. Ital. Biol., 116, 402-405.

Holländer, H., Tietze, J. and Distal, H., 1979, An autoradiographic study of the subcortical projection of the rabbit striate cortex in the adult and during postnatal development, J. Comp. Neurol., 184, 783-794.

Hughes, A. and Wilson, M.E., 1969, Callosal terminations along the boundary between visual areas I and II in the rabbit, Brain Research, 12, 19-25.

Johnston, G.A.R. and Davies, L.P., 1974, Postnatal changes in the high affinity uptake of glycine and GABA in the rat central nervous system, J. Neurochem., 22, 101-105.

Jones, D.G. and Cullen, A.M., 1979, A quantitative investigation of some presynaptic terminal parameters during synaptogenesis, Exp. Neurol., 64, 245-259.

Karlsson, U., 1966, Observations on the postnatal development of neuronal structures in the lateral geniculate nucleus of the rat by electron microscopy, J. Ultrastruct. Res., 17, 158-175.

Karlsson, U., 1967, Three-dimensional studies of neurons in the lateral geniculate nucleus of the rat. III: Specialized neuronal contacts in the neuropil, J. Ultrastruct. Res., 18, 137-157.

Krieg, W.J.S., 1946, Connections of the cerebral cortex. I: The albino rat. A. Topography of the cortical areas, J. Comp. Neurol., 84, 221-275.

Kristt, D.A. and Molliver, M.E., 1976, Synapses in newborn rat cerebral cortex: A quantitative study. Brain Research, 108, 180-186.

Kvale, I., Fosse, V.M. and Fonnum, F., 1982, Development of neuro-transmitter parameters in lateral geniculate body, superior colliculus and visual cortex of the albino rat, Dev. Brain Res., in press.

Lund, R.D., 1966, The occipitotectal pathway in the rat, J. Anat., 100, 51-62.

Lund, R.D., 1978, Development and plasticity of the brain. An intro-
    duction. Oxford University Press, New York.
Lund, R.D. and Lund, J.S., 1971, Modifications of synaptic patterns
    in the superior colliculus of the rat during development and
    following deafferentiation, Vis. Res. Suppl., 3, 281-298.
Lund-Karlsen, R., 1978, Neurotransmitters of the mammalian visual
    system. In: Amino acids as chemical transmitters, F. Fonnum,
    ed., Plenum Press, New York, pp. 241-256.
Lund-Karlsen, R. and Fonnum, F., 1978, Evidence for glutamate as a
    neurotransmitter in the corticofugal fibers to dorsal lateral
    geniculate body and the superior colliculus in rats,
    Brain Research, 151, 457-467.
Marc, R.E. and Lam, D.M.K., 1981, Uptake of aspartic and glutamic
    acid by photoreceptors in goldfish retina, Proc. Natl. Acad.
    Sci. USA, 78, 7185-7189.
McDonald, J.K., Speciale, S.G. and Parnavelas, J.G., 1981, The
    development of glutamic acid decarboxylase in the visual cortex
    and the dorsal lateral geniculate nucleus of the rat, Brain
    Research, 217, 364-367.
McGeer, P.L., Eccles, J.C. and McGeer, E.G., 1978,. Molecular neuro-
    biology of the mammalian brain, Plenum Press, New York.
Mustari, J.M. and Lund, R.D., 1976, An aberrant crossed visual
    corticotectal pathway in albino rats, Brain Research, 112,
    37-44.
Nauta, W.J.H. and Bucher, V., 1954, Efferent connections of the
    striate cortex in the albino rat, J. Comp. Neurol., 100,
    257-258.
Okada, I., 1974, Distribution of γ-aminobutyric acid (GABA) in the
    layers of superior colliculus of rabbits, Brain Research, 75,
    363-365.
Pasantes-Morales, H., Urban, P.F., Klethi, J. and Mandel, P., 1973,
    Light stimulated release of ^{35}S-taurine from chicken retina,
    Brain Research, 51, 375-378.
Peters, A. and Feldman, M., 1973, The cortical plate and molecular
    layer of the late rat fetus, Z. Anat. Entwickl. Gesch., 141,
    3-37.
Poppe, H., Bruckner, G. and Biesold, D., 1973, Postnatale entwicklung
    der synaptischen kontaktzonen im dorsalen geniculatum laterale
    der ratte, Z. Mikrosk. Anat. Forsch. (Leipzig), 87, 457-464.
Redburn, D.A., 1981, GABA and glutamate as retina neurotransmitters
    in rabbit retina. In: Glutamate as a neurotransmitter,
    G. Di Chiara and G.L. Gessa, eds., Raven Press, New York,
    pp. 79-89.
Ribak, C.E., 1977, The immunocytochemical localization of GAD within
    stellate neurons of rat visual cortex, Anat. Rec., 187,
    692-693.
Ruffolo, R.R., Jr., Eisenbarth, G.E., Thompson, J.M. and Nirenberg,
    M., 1978, Synapse turnover: a mechanism for acquiring synaptic
    specificity, Proc. Natl. Acad. Sci. USA, 75, 2281-2285.

Sandberg, M. and Jacobson, I., 1981, β-alanine, a possible neuro-transmitter in the visual system? J. Neurochem., 37, 1353-1356.

Thompson, J.M., 1982, Increase in acetylcholine release from chick embryo retina during development, Dev. Brain Research, 4, 259-264.

Vrensen, G., De Groot, D. and Nunez-Cordoza, J., 1977, The postnatal development of neurons and synapses in the visual and motor cortex of rabbits: a quantitative light and electron micro-scopic study, Brain Research Bulletin, 2, 405-416.

Wolff, J.R., 1977, Quantitative analysis of topography and develop-ment of synapses in the visual cortex, Exp. Brain Res. Suppl. I.

Wolff, J.R. and Bär, Th., 1977, Morphometrie der postnatalen synapto-genese in occipital cortex der ratte, Ver. Anat. Ges., 71, 89-91.

Wong, P. T-H. and McGeer, E.G., 1981, Postnatal changes of GABAergic and glutamergic parameters, Dev. Brain Research, 1, 519-529.

DEVELOPMENT OF PEPTIDE IMMUNOREACTIVITY IN THE HIPPOCAMPUS, VISUAL

CORTEX AND RETINA

Christine Gall[1], Nicholas Brecha[2],
and John G. Parnavelas[3]

[1]Department of Anatomy
University of California at Irvine
Irvine, California

[2]Center for Ulcer Research and Education
V.A. Medical Center-Wadsworth
Los Angeles, California

and

Department of Medicine
Brain Research Institute and Jules Stein Eye Institute
School of Medicine
University of California at Los Angeles
Los Angeles, California

[3]Department of Anatomy and Embryology
University College London
London, England

INTRODUCTION

During the last several years many studies have reported that biologically active peptides have an extensive distribution within the nervous system. At least twenty peptides have been described in the brain and periphery, each belonging to seemingly morphologically distinct systems and each presumably playing distinct functional roles (Emson, 1979; Hokfelt et al., 1980; Walsh, 1981). The majority of studies have examined adult tissues; there are relatively few studies which have examined the ontogeny of peptide-containing systems (Gash et al., 1980; Brecha et al., 1981B; De Vries et al.,

1981; McDonald et al., a,b,c,d; Inagaki et al., 1982; Shiosaka et
al., 1982; Gall et al., 1983).

An analysis of the ontogeny of neuropeptides is likely to be
helpful in understanding the physiological significance of these
substances both during development and in the adult. The possibility
that biologically active peptides participate in migration, differentiation, and synaptogenetic activities of cell populations, such
as has been suggested for catecholamines in the development of the
cerebral cortex (Coyle and Molliver, 1977; Blue and Parnavelas,
1982; Felten et al., 1982), can be examined. A clue to a particular
peptide's function might also be gained by examining the correlation
between the developmental appearance of the peptide within a defined
anatomical system and the onset of distinct physiological activities.
In addition, several studies have made the empirical observation
that, immature and young tissues stain better than older tissues
(Gall et al., 1983; Emson et al., 1979). This observation may be
due to several factors. The concentration of neuropeptides are often
reported to be greater in young tissue than in the adult tissue
(Martino et al., 1980; McGregor et al., 1982; Cilluffo et al., 1983)
and this would likely result in better staining. There may also be
certain factors in the mature brain, such as myelination, that
interfere with the penetration of the immunohistochemical reagents
into the tissue (Jones and Hartman, 1978). Thus, a developmental
study could strengthen and clarify conclusions drawn from the
analysis of adult material, as well as to provide a more detailed
description of those cells which are immunoreactive in the adult.

In this chapter, we will describe the developmental appearance
of peptide immunoreactivity in three well studied, stereotypically
organized brain regions: hippocampus, visual cortex and retina.
These systems are well suited to developmental analysis of this
type for several reasons. The normal morphology of these structures, their major cell types, afferent and efferent innervation
patterns and ultrastructural characteristics are reasonably well
known in the adult. The neurogenesis and morphogenesis of each area
have been characterized. Moreover, biochemical and physiological
studies have also focused on these systems, providing information
on the developmental onset of various biochemical and physiological
processes which may reflect functional maturation.

Several basic questions will be addressed, whenever possible,
in presenting this developmental data. Specifically, we will consider what relationship there may be between the time course for
the appearance of peptide immunoreactivity and 1) neurogenesis of
the parent neuron, 2) the outgrowth of dendritic and axonal processes and 3) physiological activity. Finally, and most importantly, we will consider whether there are common developmental
features across these model systems that are of general relevance
for understanding the biology of peptides in the nervous system.

Hippocampus

     The hippocampal formation is a simply organized cortical
structure characterized by the exclusive lamination of its major
cell types and axonal system (Figure 1). As illustrated in Figure
1, there are two compact curving neuronal cell layers. The larger,
stratum pyramidale, contains pyramidal shaped neurons whose apical
dendrites radiate toward the center of the curve and whose shorter
basal dendrites radiate toward the outside of the curve. The Nissl
and Golgi appearance of these neurons have been used to subdivide
the cell layer into regions CA1 through CA3. On the basis of
pyramidal cell morphology and the lamination of afferent systems,
the hippocampal molecular layers are further subdivided into strata,
the boundaries of which lie parallel to the pyramidal cell layer
(Blackstad, 1956; Figure 1). These strata are continuous throughout
the hippocampus with the exception of stratum lucidum which is restricted to the proximal apical dendritic zone of region CA3 and
possibly CA2. This distinction is the basis of the frequently used
radial segregation of the hippocampus proper into the regio superior
(region CA1, lacking the stratum lucidum) and regio inferior
(regions CA2 and CA3, containing stratum lucidum).

     The dentate gyrus is made up of a curving layer of granule cells
(stratum granulosum) and the overlying molecular layer of the granule
cell dendritic arborizations. The area immediately below the granule
cells, the hilus, contains scattered polymorph projection neurons,
interneurons, and granule cell axons.

     There are numerous interneurons scattered throughout the hippo-
campal formation. No simple description can adequately summarize
the wide variety of morphological types that have been described
(Amaral, 1978; Cajal, 1911; Lorenté de Nó, 1934). However, some
general statements can be made. There are pyramidal shaped interneurons found within stratum pyramidale such that one cannot distinguish on the basis of cell shape and dendritic arborization patterns,
whether an individual cell is an interneuron or a projection neuron.
Most of the neurons lying within the molecular layers of the dentate
gyrus and hippocampus proper are interneurons or locally arborizing
cells. The granule and pyramidal cells receive somatic innervation
from interneurons whose somata lie in the deeper aspects, or below,
each principal cell layer. Finally, within the hippocampus proper
there are interneurons whose axonal arborizations remain confined
to specific strata of the pyramidal dendritic field thus limiting
their direct influence to the zone dominated by specific principal
afferent systems (Lorenté de Nó, 1934).

     The principal afferents to both the granule and pyramidal
cells terminate in a discretely laminated fashion. Mention of the
distribution of two of these axonal systems, the lateral entorhinal
afferents and the mossy fibers, is particularly pertinent here in

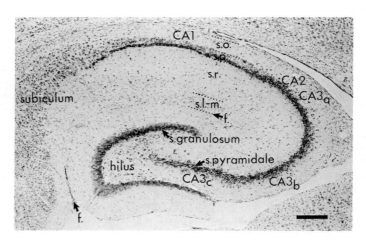

Figure 1. Nissl section of the rat hippocampal formation cut in a
horizontal plane illustrating its laminated cytoarchitecture as
described in the text. The stratification of the hippocampus
proper is indicated in region CAl. Abbreviations: f., hippocampal
fissure; s.o., stratum oriens; s.p., stratum pyramidale; s.r.,
stratum radiatum; s.l.-m, stratum lacunosum-moleculare. Calibration
bar, 300 μm.

that they both contain peptide-like immunoreactivity. The entorhinal
cortex is the principal region giving rise to extrinsic hippocampal
afferents. These afferents terminate within the dentate gyrus
molecular layer in a highly topographic fashion such that the lateral
entorhinal cortex innervates the distal third and the medial entorhinal cortex innervates the middle third of the granule cell
dendritic field (Hjorth-Simonsen, 1972; Steward, 1976). The lateral
entorhinal afferents contain enkephalin-like (ENK) immunoreactivity.
The mossy fiber axons of the dentate gyrus granule cells also contain
ENK immunoreactivity. These axons emerge from the basal (hilar)
side of the granule cell body, collect within the hilus, and course
radially through stratum lucidum of regio inferior. The mossy
fibers warrant their descriptive title because of the unusually
large synaptic boutons with which they terminate on the proximal
dendrites of regio inferior pyramidal cells (Laatsch and Cowan,
1965).

Various aspects of development of the rat hippocampal formation
have been extensively studied using ^{3}H-thymidine autoradiography
(Bayer et al., 1980), amino acid autoradiography (Fricke and Cowan,
1977; Loy et al., 1977), Golgi impregnation and electron microscopic

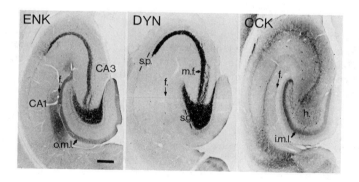

Figure 2. Horizontal sections through the rat hippocampal formation processed by the peroxidase anti-peroxidase (PAP) technique for the immunohistochemical localization of enkephalin-(ENK), dynorphin-(DYN), or cholecystokinin-like (CCK) immunoreactivity. Abbreviations: f., hippocampal fissure; h., hilus; m.f., mossy fibers; o.m.l., outer molecular layer; s.g., stratum granulosum; s.p., stratum pyramidale. Calibration bar, 300 μm.

techniques. Thus, data is available on the gradients in hippocampal neurogenesis, the elaboration of hippocampal neuron dendritic morphology, and the time-course of extrinsic and intrinsic afferent ingrowth. This is particularly helpful in evaluating the ontogenetic immunohistochemical material and is discussed in that context in the subsequent sections of this chapter.

Enkephalin-like Immunoreactivity in the Adult

    A complex pattern of ENK immunoreactivity is seen in the hippocampal formation of the adult rat (Figure 2). ENK immunoreactivity is localized within sparsely distributed and morphologically diverse interneurons in all fields of the hippocampus proper as well as within granule cells of the dentate gyrus. In addition, immunoreactivity has been localized within two highly recognizable projection systems: the lateral entorhinal/perirhinal afferents to the outer molecular layer of the temporal dentate gyrus and the mossy fiber axons of the dentate gyrus granule cells (Gall et al., 1981; McGinty et al., 1983; Khachaturian et al., 1983). Although species differences have been noted in the distribution of other hippocampal neuropeptides, the same basic ENK immunoreactive staining patterns seen in the hippocampus of the adult rat have been observed in the hippocampus of guinea pig (Stengaard-Pederson et al., 1981; Tielen et al., 1983), tree shrew (Fitzpatrick and Johnson, 1981), cat, mouse, hamster and squirrel monkey (Gall, unpublished observations).

Ontogeny of Enkephalin-like Immunoreactivity in the Rat Hippocampus

     In the neonatal rat, from the day of birth to postnatal day 3,
no intrinsic hippocampal elements are found to be immunoreactive.
However, ENK immunoreactive axons are scattered within the fimbria
and the alveus and are seen crossing the depth of the retrohippocampal cortex.

     At about four days of age, ENK immunoreactivity begins to
appear within perikarya in the hippocampus proper and in the distal
dentate gyrus molecular layer. The latter pattern, consisting of a
very fine granular band of staining within the outer molecular
layer, is inconsistently observed at days 3 and 4 but is always
present at later time points. At its earliest appearance, this outer
molecular layer immunoreactive band is limited to the suprapyramidal
extreme of the rapidly developing granule cell dendritic field.
From 6 to 10 days of age, the immunoreactive staining of the outer
molecular layer becomes evenly dense and seems as intensely stained
as in the mature hippocampal formation (Figures 3 and 4). This
band corresponds with the terminal field of afferent axons which
originate within the ipsilateral lateral entorhinal/perirhinal
cortices (Gall et al., 1981).

     Immunoreactive hippocampal perikarya are first observed around
day 4 within stratum radiatum of hippocampal field CA3. By day 6
very sparsely stained perikarya are consistently observed in the
central portions of the hilus as well. After day 6, there is a
conspicuous increase in the incidence and staining intensity of
immunoreactive perikarya within the hippocampus. By day 8, cells
exhibiting ENK immunoreactivity are found sparsely scattered within
the hilus, within both the pyramidal cell and molecular layers of
region CA3, less frequently within the apical dendritic field of
region CA1, and in the subiculum (Table 1). Moreover, on day 8
intensely immunoreactive perikarya are occasionally seen. At this
age, these extremely well stained cells are only observed within
the hilus or hippocampal regio inferior: those areas in which
immunoreactive perikarya first appear. Unlike the perikaryal
staining seen in younger animals or in the adult, these intensely
immunoreactive neruons are stained sufficiently well to permit a
detailed characterization of the dendritic and most probably axonal
arborizations (Figure 4).

     In the 10 day old rat, immunoreactive cells are observed in
all areas containing ENK immunoreactive perikarya in the adult. As
at day 8, very intensely immunoractive neurons are observed in
regio inferior, although by day 10 a few are also seen in regio
superior and the subiculum. At this time, immunoreactive neurons
within the apical dendritic field of regio superior begin to assume
the distribution of ENK immunoreactive neurons seen in this area in
the adult rat. Specifically, labeled multipolar neurons are present

Table 1.

Age of peak of neurogenesis and the appearance of perikaryal ENK

immunoreactivity in the principal subfields of the rat hippocampus

Subfield	Peak in Neurogenesis*	Appearance of Immunoreactive Perikarya	Delay (days)
CA3 - Molecular Layers	E15	P4, P6	12-14
CA3 - Stratum Pyramidale	E17	P6, P8	12-14
Subiculum	E16	P8	15
Hilus	E17	P6	12
CA1 - Stratum Pyramidale	E17-E19	P10	13-15
Dentate Gyrus - Stratum Granulosum	E19-P6 (70% by P8)	P8, P10, P14	

*   Neurogenesis data from Bayer, 1980
E = Embryonic Day
P = Postnatal Day - Day of Birth considered to be both P0 and E 23

---

in a loose band across the middle of the CA1 apical dendritic field;
between this "band" and the pyramidal cell layer, bipolar immunoreactive neurons are frequently observed.

Prior to day 11, ENK immunoreactivity is not consistently observed in mossy fiber axons or boutons of the dentate gyrus granule
cells (Figure 5). At day 11, faint immunoreactive staining is
present deep within the hilus and CA3a stratum lucidum although no
distinctly labeled structures can be resolved. By postnatal days
13 and 14, the zone of immunoreactive staining clearly extends
throughout stratum lucidum of regio inferior. At these time points,
ENK immunoreactivity has a punctate appearance, remaining confined
to distinct spherical swellings of approximately 5 μm in diameter

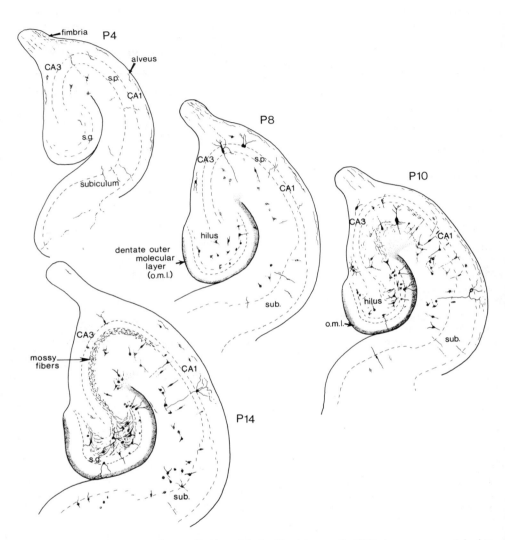

Figure 3. Illustration of the distribution of ENK immunoreactivity
in the hippocampal formation of rats sacrificed on postnatal days
4, 8, 10 and 14.

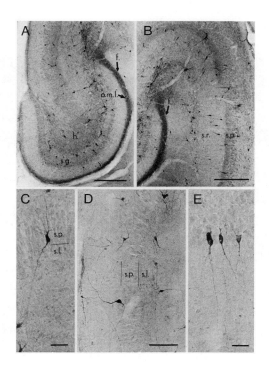

Figure 4. ENK immunoreactivity in the developing rat hippocampus.
The low power photomicrographs in A and B show the localization of
immunoreactive staining in the dentate gyrus (A) and region CA1 (B).
C, D, and E show examples of intensely immunoreactive neurons in
tissue from rats sacrificed at postnatal days 8, 12 and 19. Note
the absence of immunoreactive staining in stratum lucidum (s.l.) at
8 days postnatal (C) and the very scanty immunoreactive varicosities
seen in this zone at postnatal day 12 (D). Abbreviations: f.,
hippocampal fissure; h., hilus; o.m.l., outer molecular layers;
s.l., stratum lucidum; s.p., stratum pyramidale; s.r., stratum
radiatum. Calibration bars: A, B, D, 100 μm; C, 40 μm; E, 30 μm.

in region CA3a. This pattern suggests that the immunoreactive
material first appears within somewhat mature (i.e. already
enlarged) mossy fiber boutons (Amaral et al., 1981). Only at later
date, after 14 days postnatal, are the thin mossy fiber axons
observed to be immunoreactive.

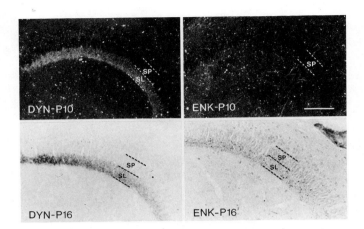

Figure 5. Dark and light field photomicrographs of DYN and ENK immunoreactive staining within hippocampal region CA3 at postnatal days 10 and 16. Note the presence of mossy fiber DYN immunoreactivity --- and the absence of mossy fiber ENK immunoreactivity --- in stratum lucidum at postnatal day 10. By postnatal day 16 both immunoreactivities are present within the mossy fiber zone although ENK immunoreactive staining is still quite sparse and granular. SP, stratum pyramidale. Calibration bar, 100 µm.

     All systems that exhibit ENK immunoreactivity in the adult rat hippocampal formation are present and exhibit some immunoreactivity in the 14 day old rat. There are, however, changes in the distribution and intensity of staining after this age: 1) ENK immunoreactivity within the mossy fiber system increases considerably and is still somewhat less intense at day 19 when compared to the adult; 2) the incidence of extremely well labeled cells decreases with age, being virtually absent in the adult; 3) the midmolecular layer band of immunoreactive neurons in the apical dendritic field of CA1 becomes narrower and shifts to a proportionally more distal point in this dendritic field; 4) the density of neurons seen to be immunoreactive decreases dramatically from the juvenile to the adult rat; and 5) this immunoreactive perikaryal density loss is more severe in hippocampal regio inferior than in regio superior such that a relatively higher numbr of immunoreactive somata are seen in the latter region in the adult (Gall et al., 1983).

Several comments can be made about the emergence of hippocampal ENK immunoreactivity when evaluated in conjunction with what is known about the time of hippocampal neurogenesis, morphogenesis and afferent ingrowth. First, from the data summarized on table one, it can be seen that the spatial order in the appearance of ENK immunoreactive perikarya follows the order of hippocampal neurogenesis by about two weeks. The post-mitotic delay to the appearance of ENK immunoreactivity is much more difficult to determine for the dentate gyrus granule cells due to the very broad proliferative period of these neurons. There are, however, distinct spatial gradients in the neurogenesis of stratum granulosum such that, by position, one can more closely approximate the age of neurons within a given sector of that cell layer (Bayer, 1980). In a previous quantitative study (Gall et al., 1983) the time of appearance and final distribution of stratum granulosum ENK immunoreactive neurons was compared to these neurogenetic gradients. From this work two conclusions were drawn. First, by the position of ENK immunoreactive neurons within stratum granulosum it was evident that early as well as late forming granule cells exhibit ENK immunoreactivity. Second, the spatial distribution, and time of emergence of perikaryal immunoreactivity followed the order of neurogenesis and, as in other hippocampal subfields, followed the age of last division by several days, possibly up to two weeks.

The two ENK immunoreactive axonal systems, the afferent axons from the lateral enorhinal cortex and the mossy fibers, differ sharply in their maturity at the time immunoreactivity appears. The lateral entorhinal afferents occupy the outer molecular layer of the suprapyramidal dentate gyrus as early as day 4 and grow around the curve of the dentate gyrus over the next few days. ENK immunoreactivity associated with the lateral entorhinal afferents is also first seen in the suprapyrmidal molecular layer on day 4 and in the infrapyramidal zone at later time points. The precise fit between the time of ingrowth (Fricke and Cowan, 1977; Loy et al., 1977) and the development of immunoreactivity (Gall et al., 1983) within this afferent system indicates that enkephalin is either already present in the axons growing into the molecular layer or becomes present in axons very soon after contact between afferent and target is made.

In contrast, the appearance of ENK immunoreactivity within the hippocampal mossy fibers occurs "late" relative to the morphological and functional maturation of these axons. Smooth mossy fiber axons grow into stratum lucidum as early as day 3 and begin a slow elaboration of their large terminal expansions only after synaptic contact is established with dendrites of CA3 pyramidal cells (Amaral et al., 1981). By day 7, small bouton expansions can be seen in Golgi material. The mossy boutons acquire about half of their adult cross-sectional size by day 9 but do not achieve adult dimensions until approximately day 21 (Amaral et al., 1981). Physiologically the mossy fibers become functional in the earliest phases of this protracted morphological development. Stimulation of the mossy fiber plexus can "drive" the CA3 pyramidal cells as early as day 5. Using the same test, a much stronger functional synaptic connection is observed on day 10 (Gall, unpublished observations; Bliss et al., 1974). In this context, it is interesting that mossy fiber ENK immunoreactivity is not consistently seen until day 11, and by day 13 or 14 is clearly localized within enlarged mossy fiber boutons. From data on the appearance and distribution of immunoreactive perikarya within the developing stratum granulosum, we are quite confident that immunoreactivity is present within early, as well as, late forming granule cells and is, consequently, present within early and late forming mossy fibers. Therefore, one must conclude that ENK immunoreactivity appears within morphologically elaborated mossy fiber boutons well after the formation of mossy fiber/pyramidal cell synaptic contact and the establishment of functional synapses.

Dynorphin-like Immunoreactivity in the Adult

In addition to enkephalin, the opioid peptide dynorphin has been localized to the hippocampal mossy fiber system (Watson et al., 1982; McGinty et al., 1983). When first reported, this observation raised uncertainty as to which opioid, enkephalin or dynorphin, was being identified by the antibodies in this system. Most antisera directed to enkephalin exhibit some degree of cross reactivity with the various forms of dynorphin, all of which contain the leu^5-enkephalin amino acid sequence at their amine terminus (Goldstein et al., 1979; Gall et al., 1981). However, immunohistochemical studies localizing dynorphin fragments ($dynorphin^{7-17}$) which do not contain leu^5-enkephalin and enkephalin precursor fragments (Bam 22) have demonstrated that both ENK and dynorphin-like (DYN) immunoreactivities are present within mossy fibers (Khachaturian et al., 1982; Watson et al., 1982). This is the only hippocampal system in which DYN immunoreactivity is found (Figure 2).

Ontogeny of Dynorphin-like Immunoreactivity in Hippocampal Mossy Fibers

The ontogeny of hippocampal DYN immunoreactivity was evaluated using an antiserum directed to $dynorphin^{1-17}$ provided by L. Terenius. This antiserum has no reported cross reactivity to the pentapeptide enkephalins (McGinty et al., 1983). Absorption tests for the specificity of immunohistochemical staining show no apparent reduction in hippocampal DYN immunoreactive staining following preabsorption of the antisera with 50 µM leu^5-enkephalin, met^5-enkephalin, $dynorphin^{1-8}$, or $dynorphin^{1-13}$ but show complete elimination of hippocampal DYN immunoreactive staining following preabsorption with 50 µm $dynorphin^{1-17}$.

DYN immunoreactivity is not seen in the hippocampal formation
of rat pups sacrificed prior to 6 days postnatal. Although at
these ages, strong staining is present in other brain areas
including the substantia nigra, caudate, and globus pallidus. At
day 6, very faint DYN immunoreactivity is present within the suprapyramidal hilus and by day 8, lightly stained processes fill the
hilus and stratum lucidum. At this age occasional immunoreactive
bouton-like profiles are seen in CA3a-stratum lucidum but most of
the staining in this zone is not associated with distinct structures. By day 13, immunoreactivity in the stratum lucidum has
increased and some is clearly localized to spherical swellings. A
further increase in mossy fiber DYN content is indicated by the
denser immunoreactive staining seen in older rats but, as with
later stages in the ontogeny of ENK immunoreactivity in this zone,
the age at which adult DYN concentrations are reached cannot be
determined using immunocytochemistry.

Clearly the time course of the appearance of DYN immunoreactivity in the mossy fibers stands in sharp contrast to that established for ENK immunoreactivity in the same system (Figure 5). ENK
immunoreactivity is first detected on day 13 in relatively mature,
morphologically elaborated mossy fiber boutons well after the
establishment of functional synaptic contact in region CA3. In
contrast, mossy fiber DYN immunoreactivity is first seen on day 6,
one day after the earliest age mossy fiber evoked potentials have
been recorded (Bliss et al., 1974). It is worth emphasizing that
stratum lucidum DYN immunoreactivity is not first seen within
enlarged mossy bouton-like structures, although DYN is present in
enlarged boutons at later time points. These observations indicate
that mossy fiber contained DYN immunoreactivity is appearing prior
to the elaboration of mossy terminal boutons. Therefore, by
comparing both the age of first detection and the morphological
appearance of ENK and DYN immunoreactivities in the mossy fiber
system, we must conclude that these two opioids arise at different
points in the maturation of individual mossy fiber axons; DYN
immunoreactivity appears relatively early, ENK immunoreactivity
appears relatively late. It is not known at present whether ENK
and DYN immunoreactivities are co-localized within individual mossy
fibers but at least for the mossy fiber "system" the ontogenies of
the two endogenous opioids contained therein are separate phenomena.

Cholecystokinin-like Immunoreactivity in the Adult

The immunohistochemical distribution of cholecystokinin-like
(CCK) immunoreactivity in the rat hippocampus has been described
(Greenwood et al., 1981; Handelmann et al., 1981). CCK immunoreactivity is localized to interneuronal perikarya clustered around
stratum pyramidale of both regio inferior and regio superior and
within the polymorph zone of hilus. These cells appear to give
rise to varicose axons which arborize within and around stratum

pyramidale of the hippocampus proper and within the supragranular region of the dentate gyrus molecular layer. In the temporal half of the hippocampus there is, in addition, a band of fine granular immunoreactive staining within the inner molecular layer (commissural afferent zone) of the dentate gyrus (Figure 2). The source of this seemingly terminal-contained CCK immunoreactivity is unknown, but transection studies by ourselves and others (Handelmann et al., 1981), as well as negative findings in double label (fluorescent dye transport/immunocytochemistry) preparations indicate that, like other intrahippocampal axonal CCK immunoreactivity, this system is of intrinsic origin (Gall et al., in preparation).

Ontogeny of Cholecystokinin-like Immunoreactivity in Rat Hippocampus

CCK immunoreactive neurons are present in the hippocampal formation at one day postnatal, the earliest time point examined. At this age, a few faintly stained neurons are seen within the apical aspect of the subicular cell layer, the suprapyramidal hilus and stratum radiatum of the hippocampus proper. Occasional varicose axons are also present in these areas and in stratum oriens.

A dramatic increase in both the number of immunoreactive perikarya and the density of immunoreactive axons is observed on postnatal day 3. In the hippocampus proper (CA1-CA3), the labeled axons and cell bodies are found in the proximal one third of the apical dendritic field, stratum oriens, the hilus and the alveus. With occasional exceptions, the neurons observed at days 1 through 3 are morphologically immature (Figure 6). Generally they have one or two short stick-like processes which are frequently coarse and noded in their proximal aspect. Although numerous immunoreactive axons are seen, these axons constitute a small fraction of the number present in the adult and are distributed across broad fields unlike the predominantly pericellular distribution of CCK immunoreactive axons seen in the adult hippocampus.

From day 3 to 6 there are further increases in the number of immunoreactive axons within the hippocampus (Figure 7). Varicose CCK-containing axons fill the hilus. Immunoreactive axons also loosely outline stratum pyramidale neurons located in regions CA1 and CA3 and cross stratum pyramidale in region CA2 making this somewhat obscure cytoarchitectonic zone quite visible in the PAP material. From days 6 to 8 there is a much more dramatic change in the number and distribution of immunoreactive axons. CCK immunoreactive axons of the hippocampus proper assume their adult pattern; CCK-containing axons tightly outline the apical edge of stratum pyramidale in field CA1 and more loosely arborize within and around the less densely packed pyramidal cells of region CA3. In addition, between days 6 and 8, CCK immunoreactivity appears in a plexus of axons in the proximal dentate gyrus molecular layer (Figure 7). It is worth noting that unlike the narrow 'supragranular' field of CCK

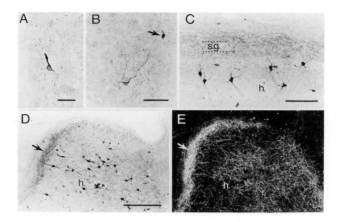

Figure 6. Perikaryal CCK immunoreactivity in the developing rat
hippocampal formation. At postnatal day 3 immunoreactive neurons
typically lack well elaborated processes (A, cell with arrow) in
B) although occasionally more fully differentiated neurons are seen
(B). By postnatal day 10 (C and D) most of the immunoreactive
neurons have numerous slender branching processes. Panels D and E
illustrate the very different appearance of the same hilar field
when seen using either light-field (D) or dark field (E) illumination: the arrow in both D and E indicates comparable positions in
the supragranular immunoreactive plexus in the two micrographs.
Immunoreactive perikarya are best visualized in light field whereas
immunoreactive fibers are best seen in dark field. Abbreviations:
h., hilus; s.g., stratum granulosum. Calibration bars: A, 25 μm;
B, 50 μm; C, 100 μm; D,E, 200 μm.

immunoreactive axons seen by ourselves and others (Greenwood et
al., 1981; Handelmann et al., 1981) in the rostral hippocampus, the
proximal molecular layer plexus observed in the temporal dentate
gyrus of the young rat clearly exceeds both the supragranular zone
and the "inner molecular layer" (defined by the terminal field of
commissural afferent axons).

   From day 8 to day 19, CCK immunoreactive axonal systems exhibit
the same general distribution seen in the adult. There is, however,
a change in the appearance of the immunoreactive staining of the
dentate gyrus inner molecular layer after day 19 (Figure 8). In
the adult, this region of the molecular layer is filled with a fine
granular band of immunoreactive staining; distinctly labeled axons
that cannot be resolved. In contrast, at day 19 this same region

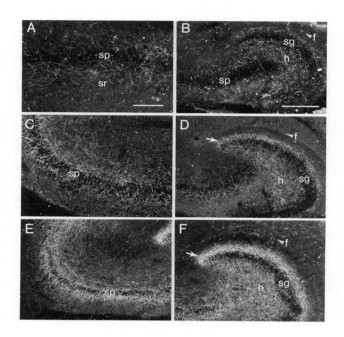

Figure 7. Dark field photomicrographs of PAP labeled CCK immunoreactivity in region CA1 (A) and the dentate gyrus of a rat pup
sacrificed at day 5; in region CA3b (C) and the dentate gyrus of a
rat sacrificed at day 8; and in region CA3 (E) and the dentate
gyrus (F) of a rat sacrificed at day 10. Note the absence of an
immunoreactive supragranular axonal plexus at day 5 (B) and the
increasing prsence of such a plexus at days 8 and 10 (indicated by
arrows in panels D and F). Abbreviations: f., hippocampal fissure;
h., hilus; s.g., stratum granulosum; s.p., stratum pyramidale;
s.r., stratum radiatum. Calibration bars in A, 100 µm for A and C;
in B, 200 µm for B, D, E and F.

is filled with fine varicose axons coursing parallel to stratum
granulosum.

    The number of CCK-containing perikarya seems to increase
gradually through day 8. Over this same interval labeled neurons
appear to mature morphologically; the noded stick-like processes
seen at earlier time points decrease in frequency and more long,
slender, branching processes are seen. By day 8 immunoreactive
neurons, not clearly of the granule cell type, are seen within
stratum granulosum. After day 8 the only striking change seen in

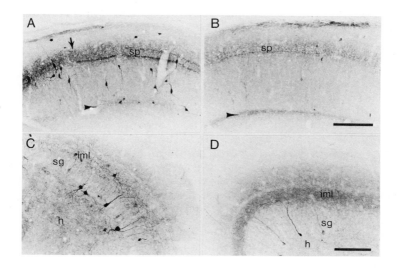

Figure 8. CCK immunoreactive neurons in the hippocampus of postnatal day 19 (A and C) and adult (B and D) rats. Panels A and B
show the region CA1; panels C and D show an aspect of the dentate
gyrus. In each area there is much more intense and extensive perikaryal labeling at the earlier time point. In addition one can see
the difference in the character of the immunoreactive staining of
the dentate gyrus molecular layer at these ages. At day 19 (C)
distinctly labeled axon-like processes can be seen in the inner
molecular layer (i.m.l.) whereas in the adult the zone is filled
with a finely granular band of staining. Abbreviations: s.p.
stratum pyramidale; s.g., stratum granulosum; h., hilus. The arrowhead in panels A and B indicates the band of immunostaining along
the stratum radiatum/stratum locumosum-moleculare interface.
Calibration bars: in B, 100 μm for A and B; in D, 200 μm for C and
D.

the distribution of CCK-containing neurons is the appearance,
between days 13 and 19, of labeled perikarya scattered along the
stratum radiatum/stratum lacunosum-molecular interface in region
CA1. Neurons are present in this apical dendritic field at earlier
time points but do not, at those ages, appear in register with the
known lamina of the field. Finally, immunoreactive perikarya are
much more intensely labeled in young tissues than in untreated
adult material. As can be seen in Figure 8, the relatively mature

neurons of the day 19 hippocampus are sufficiently well labeled to permit detailed camera lucida analysis of the dendritic and, in some cases, the proximal axonal arborizations.

In summary, perikaryal CCK immunoreactivity appears very early in the developing hippocampus being localized to morphologically immature appearing neurons as early as day 1. Axonal immunoreactivity also appears very early in most areas and, as with the perikaryal staining, slowly elaborates into the adult form. In contrast to the early appearance and gradual development of immunoreactive elements in the hippocampus proper, in the dentate gyrus CCK immunoreactivity appears late, about day 8, in relatively mature non-granular appearing neurons and in an inner molecular layer fiber plexus. Although all CCK immunoreactive systems seen in the adult hippocampus exhibit some immunoreactivity by day 8, the addition of and morphological elaboration of immunoreactive elements continues through day 19.

It is difficult to use the literature on hippocampal morphogenesis to extend our interpretation of the ontogeny of CCK immunoreactivity in hippocampus. The majority, if not all CCK immunoreactivity is present within interneurons and their axonal ramifications. Autoradiographic studies indicate that neurons located within the dendritic fields of the hippocampus proper, where a large proportion of the CCK immunoreactive neurons are found, arise between embryonic days 15 and 18 (Bayer, 1980). Since immunoreactive perikarya are observed within these fields at post-natal day 1, there may be a delay of three to six days between neurogenesis and the appearance of immunoreactivity. However, one should not hastily accept this conclusion. The period of neuro-genesis and the appearance of perikaryal immunoreactivity are both fairly broad. There is a heterogeneity of interneuronal types within the hippocampal molecular layers and, as yet, we do not know which subpopulation(s) contain CCK immunoreactivity and whether the distinct interneuronal types arise at different ages. Finally, CCK immunoreactive perikarya were seen at the youngest time point examined in the present study and they may, in fact, arise much earlier. Therefore, although we can quite confidently state CCK immunoreactivity is present in hippocampal perikarya within one week of their last division, we cannot determine the true length of this interval. The latter step will require the combined use of ^{3}H-thymidine autoradiography and immunohistochemistry; studies of this type are currently in progress.

The emergence of axonal CCK immunoreactivity is similarly difficult to interpret. The early appearance and slow increase in the number of labeled axons seen in most areas suggests immunoreactivity is present either during or soon after axonal outgrowth. The one possible exception to this interpretation is the immuno-reactive plexus present in the proximal molecular layer of the dentate gyrus. This population of axons develops immunoreactive staining so rapidly that one is inclined to conclude that these axons grew into this field at some point prior to the immunohisto-chemical appearance of CCK immunoreactivity. Until the origin of this axonal population is identified, further interpretation is not possible.

Summary of the Ontogeny of Peptide Immunoreactivity in Rat Hippocampus

In the preceding sections the emergence of hippocampal ENK, DYN, and CCK immunoreactivities have been described. Peptide-like immunoreactivity has been localized within interneuronal perikarya, projection neurons (granule cells), interneuronal axonal networks and intrinsic and extrinsic afferent systems. No general pattern was observed in the first appearance of either perikaryal or axonal immunoreactivity. Although a lengthly delay from neurogenesis to immunoreactivity was observed for all hippocampal cell types exhibit-ing ENK immunoreactivity, perikaryal CCK immunoreactivity was very close to the neurogenesis of some neurons, and well after the last division of others. Very dramatic differences were seen in the maturational age at which axonal immunoreactivity first appeared as well. ENK immunoreactivity was detectable within lateral entorhinal axons as they first grew into the dentate gyrus while it was not detected within the mossy fiber system until at least one week after synaptogenesis. In contrast, mossy fiber DYN immunoreactivity was detected much closer to the age of mossy fiber synaptogenesis.

There are some common characteristics in the later stages of development of these three peptidergic systems. Once fully present, all three immunoreactive staining patterns very slowly shifted toward the adult staining pattern. In all three cases neither the density or character of the labeling seen was identical to the adult pattern as late as postnatal day 19, the last time point ex-amined. Finally, CCK and ENK immunoreactive perikarya are much more heavily stained in the juvenile than is generally observed in the adult.

VISUAL CORTEX

The primary visual cortex (area 17) of the rat is located in the occipital region of the cerebral hemisphere. Six layers can be distinguished in Nissl-stained coronal sections through area 17, a feature common to the neocortex of other mammals. In the rat visual cortex, individual layers are clearly distinguished with the exception of layers II and III which are not delineated by a discrete border.

Based on observations of Golgi preparations, two main types of neurons have been described in the mammalian cerebral cortex:

pyramidal and nonpyramidal neurons. Pyramidal cells, present in all cortical layers except layer I, comprise the majority of neurons in the cerebral cortex. Their perikarya are typically pyramidal in shape and their dendrites display consistent morphological features which include: 1) a rich complement of spines, 2) prominent apical dendrite and 3) basal dendrites (see reviews, Parvavelas et al., 1977; Parnavelas and McDonald, 1983). The axons of cortical pyramidal neurons descend towards the white matter and appear to project to subcortical structures or to cortical areas of the same or opposite hemisphere (Parnevalas and McDonald, 1983).

Nonpyramidal neurons, which are present in all cortical layers, comprise a heteromorphic group of cells whose axons are distributed, for the most part, within the rat visual cortex. Feldman and Peters (1978) have classified nonpyramidal neurons into three categories on the basis of dendritic geometry: multipolar, bitufted and bipolar (see Parnavelas and McDonald, 1983; Parnavelas, 1984, for reviews). The preponderance of nonpyramidal cells encountered in the rat visual cortex are multipolar. Their perikarya, which are present in all layers, vary considerably in size and shape and their dendrites extend in various directions. Bitufted cells are most frequently present in layers IV and V. The dendrites typically arise from each pole of a vertically elongated soma and branch to form superficial and deep dendritic tufts. Finally, bipolar cells are predominantly present in layers II, III and IV. Most bipolar cells possess vertically elongated perikarya and dendrites which extend vertically and branch only sparsely.

The axons of multipolar and bitufted cells have been observed to form type II synaptic contacts with pyramidal and nonpyramidal neurons in the visual cortex (Peters and Fairne, 1978; Parnavelas and McDonald, 1983). However the axons of some bipolar cells have been reported to form type I synapses with perikarya and dendrites of other cortical neurons (Peters and Kimerer, 1981).

Radioimmunoassay and immunohistochemical studies describe vasoactive intestinal polypeptide (VIP)-, somastatin (SRIF)-, CCK-, avian pancreatic polypeptide (APP)- and corticotropin releasing factor (CRF)-like immunoreactivities in cortex (Fuxe et al., 1977; Lorén et al., 1979b; Brownstein et al., 1975; Finley et al., 1978; Besson et al., 1979; Fahrenkrug et al., 1979; Dockray, 1980; Bennett-Clarke et al., 1980; Shiosaka et al., 1982; Emson, 1979; Beinfeld et al., 1980; Beinfeld and Palkovits, 1981, 1982; Beinfeld et al., 1981; Greenwood et al., 1981; Bockden et al., 1981; Handelmann et al., 1981; Emson et al., 1982; Merchenthaler et al., 1982; Swanson et al., 1983). VIP immunoreactivity has been localized to cortical non-pyramidal cells whose cell bodies are distributed in layers II through VI (Fuxe et al., 1972; Lorén et al., 1979b; Emson et al., 1979; Sims et al., 1980; McDonald et al., 1982b). The majority of these immunoreactive neurons are bipolar

in form and are concentrated in layers II and III (Figure 9). SRIF
immunoreactive neurons are present in layers II through VI with the
majority situated in layers II and III. These cells exhibit morphologies typical of multipolar or bitufted forms of non-pyramidal
neurons (Bennet-Clark et al., 1980; Krisch, 1980; Takatsuki et al.,
1981; McDonald et al., 1982a)(Figure 10). Most CCK immunoreactive
cells in the rat central cortex are of the bitufted variety of non-
pyramidal neurons although a substantial number of multipolar cells
and a small number of bipolar neurons are also present (Emson et
al., 1980; Emson and Hunt, 1981; McDonald et al., 1982c; Peters et
al., 1983)(Figure 11). Labeled APP cells are predominantly non-
pyramidal neurons (multipolar, bitufted and bipolar forms) but a
very small number exhibit morphologies typical of pyramidal neurons
(Lorén et al., 1979a; McDonald et al., 1982d)(Figure 12). We have
recently observed an identical distribution of neuropeptide Y-like
(NPY) and APP immunoreactive neurons in the rat visual cortex.
This observation and other studies demonstrating 1) similarities in
amino acid sequence between neuropeptide Y and several of the
sequenced pancreatic polypeptides (Tatemoto, 1982), 2) the high
concentration of NPY in nervous tissues (Tatemoto, 1982) and 3) the
cross reactivity of APP antisera with synthetic neuropeptide Y
(Tatemoto, 1982) suggest that neuropeptide Y is likely the immunoreactive substance localized in the cortex (Sunder et al., 1983).
Interestingly, a subpopulation of APP/NPY-containing neurons have
been observed to also contain SRIF immunoreactivity (McDonald et
al., 1982a; Vincent et al., 1982). Finally, CRF immunoreactivity
has been localized in bipolar cells whose cell bodies are situated
in layers II through VI but primarily in layers II and III
(Merchenthaler et al., 1982; Swanson et al., 1983).

Ontogeny of Vasoactive Intestinal Polypeptide-like Immunoreactivity
in the Rat Visual Cortex

     VIP immunoreactive neurons first appear in the visual cortex
at postnatal day 4. These cells, mainly bipolar in appearance, are
faintly stained and are concentrated in layers V and VI. They
possess small, elongated perikarya and primary dendrites which
branch sparsely. Between days 4 and 7 some labeled cells appear in
progressively more superficial layers and by day 8 they are
primarily present in layers II and III (Figure 13a).

     These observations suggest that at least some of the immuno-
reactive cells identified in the lower cortical layers during the
first postnatal week are in the process of migration to their final
positions in the more superficial layers (Emson et al., 1979;
McDonald et al., 1982b). The simultaneous application of [3H]-
thymidine autoradiography and immunohistochemistry is required to
fully examine the generation and pattern of migration and differentiation of VIP immunoreactive neurons in the cerebral cortex.
Labeled cells appear considerably more mature during the second

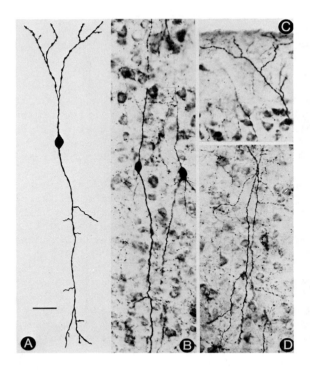

Figure 9.   VIP labeled neurons in the visual cortex of the adult
rat.   (A)   Drawing made from photomicrographs of a typical VIP
immunoreactive bipolar bell in layer III.   Scale: 50 μm.
(B) Bipolar cells in layer IV of the adult rat.   X625.   (C) Portion
of a subpial tuft focused by the ascending process of a bipolar
cell in layer I.   X625.   (D) Descending processes of bipolar cells
displaying characteristic branching pattern in layers IV and V.
X625.

postnatal week due to a marked increase in the complexity of their
dendritic fields. A gradual increase in the resemblance of VIP
immunoreactive neurons to their adult counterparts occurs during
the third postnatal week and both bipolar and multipolar forms
acquire their adult morphology by the middle of the fourth week of
postnatal life (McDonald et al., 1982b). This pattern of maturation is in agreement with radioimmunoassay analysis of VIP development in the rat posterior cortex (Emson et al., 1979).

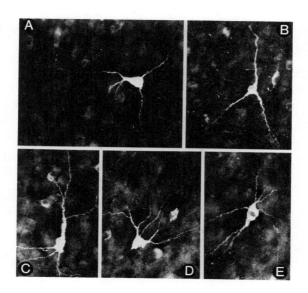

Figure 10. Photomicrographs of SRIF labeled neurons in the visual cortex of the rat. X625. (A) Postnatal day 10. Multipolar neuron in layer V. (B) Postnatal day 12. Multipolar neuron in layer VI. (C) Postnatal day 14. Bitufted cell in layer V. (D) Postnatal day 21. Multipolar neuron in layer II. Arrowhead points to an axon. (E) Postnatal day 21. Bitufted cell in layer V.

Ontogeny of SRIF Immunoreactivity in the Rat Visual Cortex

Well stained SRIF immunoreactive neurons are present in the "subplate" region of the visual cortex on the first postnatal day. They are either immature multipolar neurons or neurons with dendrites emerging from opposite poles of the perikaryon. With the exception of an occasional cell in layer IV, labeled neurons remain concentrated in layers V and VI throughout the first postnatal week. Their appearance in the more superficial layers begins in the second postnatal week and their adult distribution is attained at the end of this period (McDonald et al., 1982a)(Figure 13b). The late appearance of labeled cells in layers II and III, where they are predominantly found in adult animals, suggests that the immunoreactivity exhibited by most of these neurons develops several days after they complete their migration and assume their

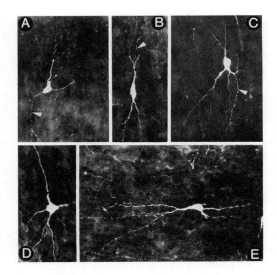

Figure 11. Photomicrographs of CCK immunoreactive non-pyramidal
neuron in the visual cortex of the rat. X625. (A, B) Postnatal
day 14. Bitufted neurons in layers II and III displaying large
perikarya and extensive dendritic fields. Arrowheads point to
axons. (C) Postnatal day 14. Multipolar neuron in layers II and
III. (D) Postnatal day 14. Cell in layer I displaying an overall
horizontal orientation.

positions in the visual cortex (Berry, 1974). During the second
week of postnatal development, the dendrites of SRIF labelled cells
are longer and more branched than at earlier ages. This difference
is more pronounced in the cells present in layers V and VI which
appear more mature and intensely stained than the labeled cells
identified in the superficial layers. The differentiation of SRIF-
containing neurons continues during the third week and at day 21
they appear indistinguishable from the adult forms (McDonald et
al., 1982a). Radioimmunoassay analysis of SRIF confirms the
presence of this peptide in rat and human fetal cortex (Aubert et
al., 1977; McGregor et al., 1982). McGregor et al. (1982), using
pooled samples of cortex and basal ganglia, reported a rapid period
of development in the second week but noted a decline in the concentration of SRIF immunoreactivity during the third postnatal week
which continued into adulthood. This finding suggests that the
cellular concentration of SRIF immunoreactivity decreases with age.

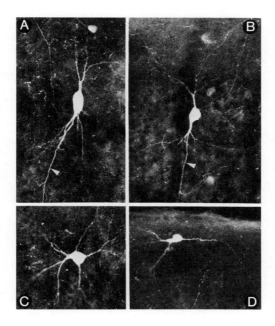

Figure 12. Photomicrographs of APP labeled non-pyramidal neuron in the rat visual cortex. Arrowheads point to axons. X625. (A) Postnatal day 3. Immature multipolar neuron in layer V. (B) Postnatal day 8. Bitufted neuron in layer IV. (C, D) Postnatal day 12. Multipolar neurons in layer V. (E) Postnatal day 12. Multipolar neuron with horizontally oriented dendrites in layer VI.

Summary of the Ontogeny of Peptide Immunoreactivity in Rat Visual Cortex.

From the foregoing description of the ontogeny of VIP and SRIF immunoreactivity it is evident that in visual cortex, as in hippocampus, each peptide follows a distinct developmental schedule (Figure 13). VIP is first detected as faint perikaryal staining restricted to the deeper layers (V, VI) of cortex on postnatal day 4 and is seen predominantly in perikarya of the more superficial layers by postnatal day 8. This early shift to the superficial layers suggests that the immunoreactive substance is present in immature neurons actively migrating from deep to superficial cortex (McDonald et al., 1982b; Emson et al., 1979). Perikaryal SRIF immunoreactivity

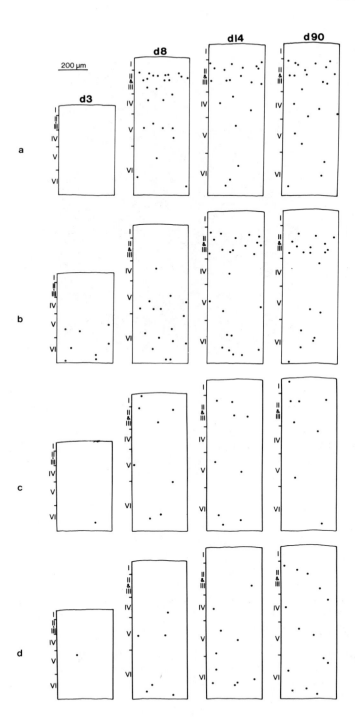

is also first seen in deep (layers V, VI) cortical neurons but, in contrast to VIP immunoreactive neurons, is not detected in the more superficial layers until week two. At this time the SRIF immuno- reactive neurons of the deep cortex appear morphologically more mature than those found more superficial. Thus, for the SRIF immunoreactive neurons it seems we have immunoreactivity appearing first in deep cortical neurons fated to remain in their lamina and then in more superficially located cortical neurons after their final migration.

In addition to VIP and SRIF, the ontogeny of CCK and APP has been studied using immunohistochemical techniques. The emergence of perikaryal CCK bears similarity to the pattern observed for VIP in that immunoreactivity is first detected in deep layers on day 4 and becomes detectable in neurons of the more superficial layers by day 8. The ontogeny of APP immunoreactivity is strikingly similar to that of VIP in that it appears sufficiently late in the super- ficial cortical layers so as to suggest the peptide does not become present until migration is complete.

In summary, there appears to be a heterogeneity in these peptide-containing cell populations in both the time of their appearance and their relative location in the cortex. Until double label ^{3}H-thymidine autoradiography and immunohistochemical studies are complete, it is difficult to comment on the histogenesis of these different cortical interneuronal cell populations.

RETINA

The retina is a thin sheet of tissue characterized by a dis- tinct laminar organization of its neurons and their processes (Cajal, 1893)(Figure 14). The retina contains six neuronal cell types: photoreceptor (rods and cones), bipolar, horizontal, amacrine, interplexiform and ganglion cells. The identifying characteristics of each of these cell types is the location of its somata within the nuclear layers and the distribution of its processes to one or both of the plexiform layers. For many of these major cell types a wide variety of morphological subtypes have been described. In the case of amacrine and ganglion cells, as many as 20 or 25 distinct types have been described (Cajal, 1893;

Figure 13. Distribution of VIP (a), SRIF (b), CCK (c) and APP (d) immunoreactive neurons in strips of visual cortex extending from the pia to the white matter at 3, 8, 14 and 90 days of postnatal life.

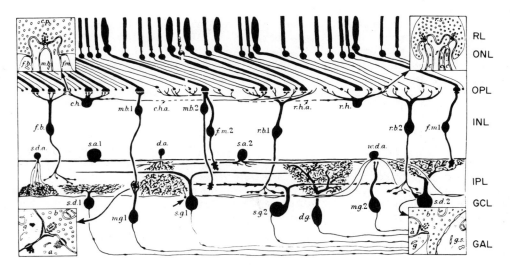

Figure 14.   Schematic representation of the retina from Boycott
and Dowling (1969).   Abbreviations: PRL, photoreceptor layer; ONC,
outer nuclear layer; OPL, outer plexiform layer; INL, inner nuclear
layer; IPL, inner plexiform layer; GCL, ganglion cell layer; OAL,
optic axon layer.

Kolb et al., 1981).   Recent studies have demonstrated that many of
these amacrine cell types closely match histochemically identified
amacrine cells (Brecha, 1983; Brecha et al., 1983).

      In chick retina, ^{3}H-thymidine studies demonstrate a central to
peripheral gradient for retinal cell neurogenesis.   Golgi studies
demonstrate that ganglion cells have elaborated many of their processes by embryonic day 13 (Nishimura, 1980).   Amacrine cells begin
to elaborate their processes as early as embryonic day 9 and many
cells may be morphologically mature by embryonic day 14 (Castro,
1966).   Therefore, most retinal cells seem to be in their final
position and their processes have undergone considerable elaboration
by embryonic day 14, 6 to 7 days before hatching.

      Bioassay, immunoassay and immunohistochemical studies have
firmly established the presence of at least fifteen peptide-like
substances in the vertebrate retina (Brecha, 1983; Brecha and Karten,
1983; Brecha et al, 1983)(Table 2).   The best evidence suggests
that several neuropeptides are present in the retina of any one
species.   However, not all of the neuropeptides that have been

Table 2

Peptide activity or immunoreactivity in the vertebrate retina

	Bioassay	Radioimmuno-assay	Chromatography	Immunohisto-chemistry
APP				x
CCK		x	x	x
CRF				x
ENK		x	x	x
β-END		x		x
FMRF				x
GLU		x	x	x
LRF		x		x
NT		x		x
NPY				x
PHI				x
SP	x	x	x	x
SRIF	x	x	x	x
TRH		x	x	
VIP		x		x

found to be present in the retina of one vertebrate species will necessarily be found in the retina of another.

Using the bird retina as a model system, detailed studies of the presence and distribution of ENK, SRIF, VIP, glucagon- (GLU), neurotensin- (NT), and substance P- (SP) like immunoreactivity by radioimmunoassay and immunohistochemistry have been reported (Brecha et al., 1979; Brecha et al., 1980; Brecha et al., 1981A; Buckerfield et al., 1981; Karten and Brecha, 1980; Osborne et al., 1982; Brecha et al., 1982, 1983; Cilluffo et al., 1983; Kuwayama et al., 1982). Immunohistochemical studies have identified at least six specific peptide-containing amacrine cell populations in chicken and pigeon retinas (Brecha et al., 1983). These studies have clearly established the presence of unistratified SP and multi-stratified ENK, NT and SRIF immunoreactive cell populations. In addition, it is likely that there are at least two VIP- and three GLU-containing multistratified cell populations (Brecha et al., 1983). Each of these immunoreactive substances appear to be present in morphologically distinct amacrine cells. Preliminary studies on the ontogeny of the ENK- and GLU-containing amacrine cell populations are described below (Brecha et al., 1980; Cilluffo et al., 1983).

Enkephalin-like Immunoreactivity in the Avian Retina

ENK immunoreactivity is present in what appears to be a
specific group of multistratified amacrine cells in both the pigeon
and chicken retina (Brecha et al., 1979)(Figure 15D). In chicken
retina, these multistratified amacrine cells are characterized by a
single process which descends to the border of the inner plexiform
layer (IPL) before arborizing into several secondary processes in
lamina 1. Some of these processes in turn descend to and ramify
within laminae 3 and 4 of the IPL. ENK immunoreactive somata
usually are located within the 2nd and 3rd tier of cells from the
border of the inner nuclear layer (INL) and IPL.

Ontogeny of Enkephalin-like Immunoreactivity in Amacrine Cells

Radioimmunoassay and chromatographic studies indicate that ENK
immunoreactivity is present in chick retina at embryronic day 11,
about 10 days prior to hatching (Humbert et al., 1979). However,
by immunohistochemistry, very faint staining ENK immunoreactive
somata are not detected until embryonic day 13 or 14. These immunoreactive somata are scattered through the proximal INL in central
retinal regions (Figure 15) and are characterized by a round shape
and a sparse distribution of immunoreactivity within their cytoplasm.
At this age, no ENK immunoreactive processes are observed. Not
until embryonic day 18 or 19 are more heavily labeled perikarya
observed in all retinal regions within the proximal INL. At this
age, poorly labeled, discontinuous immunoreactive processes are
present within the distal IPL. However, within several hours after
hatching, ENK immunoreactivity is clearly visualized throughout the
entire cell and its processes. These cells appear to be identical
in morphology to ENK-containing amacrine cells present in the adult
retina. That is, their somata are located in the proximal INL and
their processes are distributed in a laminar manner within the IPL.
Interestingly, for several days following hatching, these ENK-
containing amacrine cells are observed to be more intensely stained
than are the same cell types in the adult retina (Figure 15). This
increased staining might be due to an elevated concentration of
enkephalin or enkephalin precursor. However, quantification of
this observation must await appropriate analysis using immunochemical techniques.

Regardless of what event triggers the increase in ENK immunoreactivity, the rapid increase of ENK immunoreactive staining
implies a dramatic increase in the synthesis of enkephalin. This
increase could be mediated by a specific enkephalinase which
cleaves leu^5- and/or met^5-enkephalin from a larger enkephalin
peptide. If this is the case, ENK immunoreactivity observed before
hatching may be in part due to cross reactivity between the enkephalin antiserum and a larger enkephalin precursor molecule. Other
studies suggest such a sequence is plausible in view of the

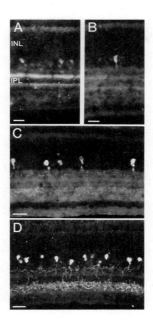

Figure 15. ENK immunoreactivity in the developing chick retina.
ENK immunoreactivity is first observed in somata about embryonic
day 13 or 14. ENK-containing somata are clearly present at embryonic
days 18 and 19 (A, B). ENK-containing somata and processes are
apparent after hatching on post-hatching day 1 (C). Intensely
labeled somata and processes are seen several days after hatching
as illustrated at posthatching day 3 (D). Calibration bars, 25 µm.

appearance of neurophysin-like immunoreactivity several days before
vasopressin-like immunoreactivity in the mammalian hypothalamus
(Sachs et al., 1975; Silverman, 1975; Choy and Watkins, 1979).

Glucagon-like Immunoreactivity in the Avian Retina

    GLU immunoreactivity is present in retinal cells located in
the INL and in processes which are most prominent in lamina 1 of
the IPL and in the ora serrata (Brecha et al., 1982, 1983; Kuwayama
et al., 1982; Cilluffo et al., 1983)(Figure 16). In central retina,
the majority of GLU immunoreactive cells have a round shape and
give rise to one or more medium caliber primary processes which
arborize in lamina 1. These processes in turn give rise to

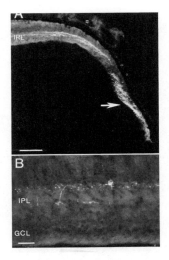

Figure 16. GLU immunoreactivity in the adult avian retina. A
dense GLU immunoreactive plexus is present near the ora serrata
(arrow)(A). GLU is observed in at least 3 cell types; the smallest
are distributed in all retinal regions (B). Calibration bars, A,
100 μm; B, 25 μm.

secondary processes which descend to and arborize within a thin
band in lamina 3 of the IPL (Figure 16B). A second GLU immunoreactive retinal cell population is present most prominently in a broad
band spanning the ventral retina. These medium to large cells have
a round soma and are characterized by a thick primary process which
courses tangential to the vitreal surface in lamina 1 of the IPL
for a short distance before ramifying into many fine processes
which are distributed to laminae 1, 3 and 5 of the IPL. One of
these fine processes courses in lamina 1 directly to the edge of
the retina where it joins a fascicle of GLU immunoreactive
processes within the ora serrata. A third population of GLU immunoreactive cells are present in peripheral retinal regions. These
cells have a medium size, round somata and two or three primary
processes which ramify in laminae 1 and perhaps deeper laminae of
the IPL. Some of these processes also join the fascicle of GLU-
containing processes which appear to course through the ora serrata
to en circle the retina (Figure 16A). These observations suggest
at least 3 types of GLU-containing cells: The majority of cells
present in central and peripheral retinal regions appear to be uni-

and/or bistratified amacrine cells. Medium to large diameter bi-
and/or tristratified immunoreactive cells are located in ventral
and peripheral retinal regions.

Ontogeny of Glucagon-like Immunoreactivity in Retinal Cells

GLU immunoreactivity in chick retina is first detected by
radioimmunoassay a day or two prior to the appearance of GLU
immunoreactive somata. Assayed GLU immunoreactivity increases
gradually from embryonic day 11 up to a peak at or near hatching
(Figure 17). GLU immunoreactive content then decreases until post-
hatching day 5, at which point stable adult values are attained.

GLU-containing somata, but not processes, are first observed
about embryonic day 13 or 14 in central retinal regions (Table 3
and Figure 18). These immunoreactive cells have an uneven, rough
appearing somata and are usually located in the second or third
cell tier from the border of the INL and IPL. They are likely to
be immature amacrine cells which have not given rise to their
processes. At embryonic days 15 and 16, a mixture of both immature
and mature appearing somata are observed. At these ages, GLU
immunoreactive processes are apparent in the IPL but their density
seems to be less than that observed in older embryonic and adult
retinas. At these ages, some of the large and/or medium sized GLU
immunoreactive cells are likely to be well developed since a well
defined plexus of processes within the ora serrata is evident. By
embryonic days 18 or 19, a day or two before hatching, GLU-containing cells appear to be similar if not identical in their numbers
and morphologies to GLU-containing amacrine cells present in the
adult retina. Furthermore, at this age, the density of processes
in the IPL and ora serrata appears similar to that observed in
adult retinas. GLU-containing cells thus appear to develop their
full immunoreactive staining pattern prior to hatching. As
mentioned above, GLU concentration continues to rise until just
after hatching, at which time it decreases to adult values
(Cilluffo et al., 1983).

Comparison of the Ontogeny of Peptide Immunoreactivity in Retinal Cells

The ontogeny of ENK, SRIF and GLU immunoreactivities in the
chick retina has been examined (Brecha et al., 1980; Morgan et al.,
1981; Cilluffo et al., 1983). In chick retina, a similar sequence
is observed for the development of SRIF and GLU immunoreactivity.
That is, there is a gradual increase in peptide-like content during
early embryonic ages, a more rapid increase during later ages
through hatching and, at least for GLU immunoreactive content, a
slight decrease to adult values soon after hatching. These changes
are likely to reflect the morphological maturation of these two
retinal cell types. That is, for GLU-containing cells there is a

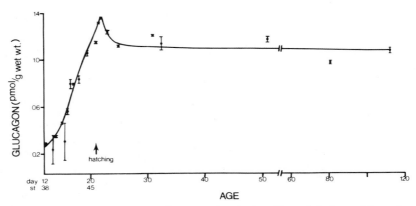

Figure 17.   GLU immunoreactive content in the chick retina increases gradually during development, peaks at or just after hatching and decreases slightly to adult values.

concomitant increase in 1) the number of mature appearing somata as well as density of processes within the IPL and 2) the concentration of GLU immunoreactivity during development (Table 3 and Figure 18). There are some marked differences in the temporal appearance, by immunohistochemistry, of peptide-like immunoreactivity. In some cases, such as for GLU-containing cells, GLU immunoreactivity first appears in immature apeparing cells and is thus likely to be present in these cells as they elaborate their processes. The GLU cells appear nearly identical to those observed in the adult a day or two before hatching. In contrast, ENK-containing cells show poor immunohistochemical staining before hatching and do not show adult staining patterns until at or just after hatching. The ENK-containing population of amacrine cells are thus delayed in the appearance of their immunoreactivity when compared to the GLU-containing retinal populations. This same observation was made in developing goldfish retina where SP immunoreactive amacrine cells and their processes are not observed in retinal regions still undergoing histogenesis and morphogenesis (Brecha et al., 1981B). That is, SP immunoreactivity in the goldfish appears abruptly throughout the somata and processes of amacrine cells which ramify in laminae 3 of the IPL. These cells are first characterized by a granular distribution of SP immunoreactivity within their soma and their processes are localized to the appropriate lamina of the IPL. At slightly older ages these immunoreactive cells appear to be mature in that they are similar in appearance to adult SP immunoreactive amacrine cells. Interestingly, in neither goldfish nor chick were SP-, ENK- or GLU-containing cells detected in distal retinal regions. Immunoreactive somata were only observed in the proximal retina, near to or at their final adult position.

Table 3

Observations of GLU immunoreactivity in the developing chick retina

Age	Stage	Location of glucagon		
		INL (somata appearance)	IPL	ora serrata
el3	39	immature		
el4	40	immature	1	±
el6	42	immature & mature	1	+
el7	43	mature	1,3	+
el8	44	mature	1,3	+
el9.5	45	mature	1,3,5	+

Immunohistochemical studies thus suggest that for some peptide-like substances (i.e. GLU and SRIF) the earliest stage they can be detected in retinal cells is at or just before these cells begin to give rise to their processes within the IPL; these cells are likely to be immature due to their rough uneven appearance and lack of processes. In other cases (i.e. ENK and SP) these peptides are seemingly not distributed in the cell until after it has elaborated its processes. Reasons for these different developmental profiles is unknown. Finally, an exact determination of the earliest age at which peptides are present in a particular cell population is difficult, if not impossible to determine using current immunohisto-chemical techniques. Indeed, the radioimmunoassay results suggest these peptides are present in the retina a day or two before they are detected by immunohistochemistry. But the current studies do clearly demonstrate that peptide-like substances (or precursors with similar immunoreactivity) are only present in those cells which are likely to contain that substance in the adult retina and not in a transient appearing cell population.

Some studies, including those above, also suggest the possibility that the retinal content of some peptides is dependent upon light stimulation. In rat retina, thyrotropin-releasing hormone-like (TRH) immunoreactivity is not detectable before the eyes open, is low at eye opening (day 8) and does not reach adult concentrations until after hatching and light exposure (Martino et al., 1980).

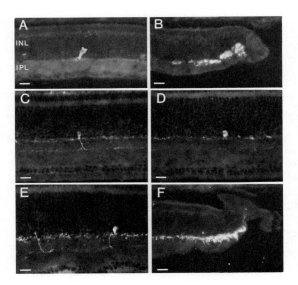

Figure 18. GLU immunoreactivity in the developing chick retina.
GLU is observed in somata and the ora serrate on embryonic day 16
(A, B). Many somata have an immature appearance as in A. The
immunoreactive pattern is similar if not identical to the adult a
day or two before hatching. C, D are at embryonic day 20 and E, F
are at posthatching day 1. Calibration bars, 25 μm.

Interestingly, the appearance of TRH immunoreactivity in the developing rat retina is prevented by maintaining the rat pups in the
dark. A second example implying that peptide content in retina is
dependent on light stimulation is the dramatic appearance of ENK
immunoreactivity in amacrine cells just after but not before
hatching. That is, ENK-containing amacrine cells are likely to
have elaborated their processes during mid to late embryonic stages
(Castro, 1966), and ENK immunoreactivity is only observed throughout their soma and processes after hatching, these two observations
suggest that the presence of "adult" levels of ENK immunoreactivity
is correlated with light stimulation at hatching.

Information concerning avian amacrine cell histogenesis and
morphogenesis is insufficient to fully evaluate the ontogeny of
peptide immunoreactivity in this context. The histogenesis of
amacrine cells occurs over several days and whether peptide immunoreactivity is associated with only those cell populations arising
at a given time point or with cell populations arising during the
entire histogenetic period is unknown. Likewise the data available

on the morphogenesis of amacrine cells is not sufficiently extensive to determine whether each amacrine cell population elaborates its processes over a given time span or over the entire developmental period. As in the other neuronal systems discussed in this chapter, combined ^{3}H-thymidine autoradiographic and immunohistochemical studies, as well as a detailed developmental Golgi analysis are needed to answer these questions.

CONCLUSIONS

As one reviews the data on the ontogeny of neuropeptides in retina, visual cortex and hippocampus, a few similarities can be seen. In some instances, most notably ENK immunoreactivity in both retinal amacrine cells and hippocampal mossy fibers, this peptide appears abruptly, well after neurogenesis and initial morphogenesis. In contrast, in other cases such as retinal GLU, hippocampal DYN and cortical VIP immunoreactivity, there is a slow emergence of immunoreactivity in coordination with morphological elaboration. The parallel emergence of neurophysin-like immunoreactivity with the morphological elaboration of hypothalamic magnocellular neurons has also been described (Gash et al., 1980). However, despite these occasional similarities, a general set of principles concerning peptide development both within the same and across different neuronal systems don't really emerge. In fact, one is struck by both the heterogeneity seen in the development of the same peptide substance in different cellular systems (e.g. ENK immunoreactivity in the hippocampal mossy fibers and lateral entorhinal efferents) and the heterogeneity seen between peptides within the same cellular systems (i.e. ENK and GLU immunoreactivity in amacrine cells; ENK and DYN immunoreactivity in mossy fibers). Therefore, in response to those questions posed in the introduction to this chapter we can answer several times in the negative. No, a consistent relationship has not been observed between the appearance of peptide immunoreactivity and neurogenesis. No, an obvious correlation betwen the appearance of immunoreactivity and either the morphogenesis of the parent neuron or other elements in the parent neuron environment (such as afferent innervation) was not seen.

The above data argues that there must be a heterogeneity in the relationship of the various new peptides to physiological development. Unfortunately we have very little specific information on physiological development that can be used to interpret these changes in relationship to the emergence of neuropeptides. Two of the described systems however, are likely candidates for studies along this line. We know the hippocampal mossy fiber system is active and physiologically competent (i.e. can activate target neurons) as early as five days postnatal (Bliss et al., 1974) -- approximately one week prior to the appearance of ENK immunoreactivity. Similarly, in the avian retina both an electroretinogram and visual evoked responses can be recorded at least a day or two before hatching (Witkovsky, 1963; Rager, 1979) -- again prior to the appearance of terminal contained ENK immunoreactivity. Both systems are accessible to studies directed towards detecting changes in synaptic physiology that correspond with the developmental appearance of enkephalin.

In summary, from the data in hand we must conclude that knowledge of the ontogeny of peptide immunoreactivity in a particular neuronal system does not have predictive value as to the ontogeny of that same peptide within another neuronal system. It seems that the determination of the ontogeny of each peptide type in each neuronal system will have to be evaluated independently. Although the results of such ontogenetic studies cannot be extrapolated to apply to unstudied brain areas they can be of tremendous importance in directing physiological studies such as those suggested above. The conclusions drawn from a combined anatomical/physiological analysis of the ontogeny of neuropeptides in one area could then have very broad applicability indeed, in that it could be used to identify the physiological impact of the appearance of the particular neuropeptides during development. This may be tantamount to identifying the function of those peptides in the brain.

ACKNOWLEDGEMENTS

We thank M. Cilluffo for her careful reading and helpful comments, and A. Boesman and L. Hendricks for their assistance in the preparation of this chapter. Research in this chapter was supported by Grants EY 04067 to N.B., BNS 82-00319 and Sloan Research Fellowship to C.G., and AM 17328 to G. Sachs.

REFERENCES

Amaral, D. and Deut, J., 1981, Development of the mossy fibers of the dentate gyrus: A light and electron microscopic study of the mossy fibers and their expansions. J. Comp. Neurol., 195:51-86.
Aubert, M.L., Grumbach, M.M., Kaplan, S.L., 1977, The ontogenesis of human fetal hormones. IV. Somatostatin, luteinizing hormone releasing factor, and thyrotropin releasing factor in hypothalmus and cerebral cortex of human fetuses 10-22 weeks of age. J. Clinical Endocrinology and Metabolism, 44:1130-1141.
Barden, N., Merand, Y., Rouleau, D., Moore, S., Dockray, G.J. and Dupont, A., 1981, Regional distributions of somatostatin and cholecystokinin-like immunoreactivities in rat and bovine brain. Peptides, 2:299-302.

Bayer, S., 1980, Development of the hippocampal region in the rat.
    I. Neurogenesis examined with ^{3}H-thymidine autoradiography.
    J. Comp. Neurol., 190:87-114.

Beinfeld, M.C., 1980, An HPLC and RIA analysis of the cholecystokinin
    peptides in rat brain. Neuropeptides, 1:203-207.

Beinfeld, M.C., Meyer, D.K. and Brownstein, M.J., 1980, Cholecysto-
    kinin octapeptide in the rat hypothalamo-neuohypophysial system.
    Nature, 288:376-378.

Beinfeld, M.C. and Palkovits, M., 1981, Distribution of cholecysto-
    kinin (CCK) in the hypothalamus and limbic system of the rat.
    Neuropeptides, 2:123-129.

Beinfeld, M.C. and Palkovits, M., 1982, Distribution of cholecysto-
    kinin (CCK) in the rat lower brain stem nuclei. Brain
    Research, 238:260-265.

Bennett-Clarke, C., Romagnano, M.A. and Joseph, S.A., 1980, Distri-
    bution of somastatin in the rat brain: telencephalon and dien-
    cephalon. Brain Research, 188:473-486.

Besson, J., Rotsztejn, W., Laburthe, M., Epelbaum, J., Beaudet, A.,
    Kordon, C. and Rosselin, G., 1979, vasoactive intestinal
    peptide (VIP): brain distribution, subcellular localization
    and effect of deafferentiation of the hypothalamus in male
    rats. Brain Research, 165:79-85.

Bliss, T.V., Chung, S.H. and Sterling, R.V., 1974, Structural and
    functional development of the mossy fiber system in the hippo-
    campus of the postnatal rat. J. Physiol., 239:92-94.

Blue, M.E. and Parnavalas, J.G., 1982, The effect of neonatal 6-
    hydroxydopamine treatment on synaptogenesis in the visual
    cortex of the rat. J. Comp. Neurol., 205:199-205.

Boycott, B.B. and Dowling, J.E., 1969, Organization of the primate
    retina: Light microscopy. Phil. Trans. R. Soc. Lond. B,
    255:109-184.

Brecha, N., 1983, A review of retinal neurotransitters: Histochemical
    and biochemical studies. In: Chemical Neuroanatomy (edited
    by P.C. Emson), New York, Raven Press, pp. 85-129.

Brecha, N., Cilluffo, M., Yamada, T., 1982, Localization and
    characterization of glucagon-like immunoreactivity in the
    retina. Soc. Neurosci. Abs, 8:46.

Brecha, N., Eldred, W., Kuljis, R.P. and H.J. Karten, 1983, Identi-
    fication and localization of biologically active peptides in
    the vertebrate retina. In: Progress in Retinal Research
    (edited by N. Osborne and G. Chader), New York, Plenum Press,
    in press.

Brecha, N.C. and Karten, H.J., 1983, Identification and localization
    of neuropeptides in the vertebrate retina. In: Brain Peptides
    (edited by D. Kreiger, M. Brownstein and J. Martin), New York,
    Academic Press, in press.

Brecha, N., Karten, H.J. and Davis, B., 1980, Localization of neuro-
    eptides, including vasoactive intestinal polypeptide and
    glucagon within the adult and developing retina. Soc. Neuro-
    sci. Abs., 6:346.

Brecha, N., Karten, H.J. and Laverack, C., 1979, Enkephalin-
    containing amacrine cells in the avian retina: Immunohisto-
    chemical localization. Proc. Natl. Acad. Sci. USA,
    76:3010-3014.
Brecha, N., Karten, H.J. and Schenker, C., 1981A, The localization
    of neurotensin-like and somatostatin-like immunoreactivity
    within amacrine cells of the retina. Neuroscience,
    6:1329-1340.
Brecha, N., Sharma, S.C. and Karten, H.J., 1981B, Localization of
    substance P-like immunoreactivity in the adult and developing
    goldfish retina. Neuroscience, 6:2736-2746.
Brownstein, M., Arimura, A., Sato, H., Schally, A.V., Kizer, J.S.,
    1975, The regional distribution of somatostatin in the rat
    brain. Endocrinology, 96:1456-1461.
Buckerfield, M., Oliver, J., Chubb, I.W., Morgan, I.G., (1981),
    Somatostatin-like immunoreactivity in amacrine cells of the
    chicken retina. Neuroscience, 6:689-695.
Cajal, S., Ramon y, 1893, La retine des vertebres. La Cellule,
    9:17-257.
Cajal, S., Ramon y, 1911, "Histologie du system Nerveux de l'homme
    et vertebres". Maloine, Paris.
Castro, G. de O, 1966, Branching pattern of amacrine cell processes.
    Nature, 212:832-833.
Choy, V.J. and Watkins, W.B., 1979, Maturation of the hypothalamo-
    neurohypophysial system. Cell Tiss. Res., 197:325-336.
Cilluffo, M., Yamada, T. and Brecha, N., 1983, Soc. Neurosci. Abs.,
    9, in press.
Coyle, J., Molliver, M., 1977, Major innervation of newborn rat
    cortex by monoaminergic neurons. Science, 196:444-447.
De Vries, G., Buij's, R. and Swaab, D., 1981, Ontogency of the vaso-
    pressinergic neurons of the suprachiasmatic nucleus and their
    extra hypothalamic projections in the rat brain-presence of a
    sex difference in the lateral septum. Brain Res., 218:67-78.
Dockray, G.H., 1980, Cholecystokinins in rat cerebral cortex: iden-
    tification, purification and characterization by
    immunochemical methods. Brain Res., 188:155-165.
Emson, P.C., 1979, Peptides as neurotransmitter candidates in the
    mammalian CNS. Progress in Neurobiology, 13:61-116.
Emson, P.C., Gilbert, R.F., Lorén, I., Fahrenkrug, J.F., Sundler, F.
    and Schaffalitzky De Muckadel, O., 1979, Development of vaso-
    active intestinal polypeptide (VIP) containing neurons in the
    rat brain. Brain Res., 177:437-444.
Emson, P.C., Hunt, S.P., Rehfeld, J.F., Golterman, N. and
    Fahrenkrug, J., 1980, Cholecystokinin and vasoactive intestinal
    polypeptide in the mammalian CNS: distribution and possible
    physiological roles. In: Neural Peptides and Neuronal Communi-
    cation (edited by E. Costa and M. Trabucchi), New York, Raven
    Press, pp. 63-74.

Emson, P.C., Rehfeld, J.F. and Rossor, M.N., 1982, Distribution of cholecystokinin-like peptides in the human brain. J. Neurochem., 38:1177-1179.

Fahrenkrug, J., 1979, Vasoactive intestinal polypeptide: measurement, distribution and putative neurotransmitter function. Digestion, 19:149-169.

Feldman, M.L. and Peters, A., 1978, The forms of non-pyramidal neurons in the visual cortex of the rat. J. Comp. Neurol., 179:761-794.

Feldman, S.C. and Lichtenstein, E., 1980, Morphology and distribution of somatostatin-containing neurons in the guinea pig neocortex. Anatomical Record, 196:55A.

Felten, D.L., Hallman, H. and Jonsson, G., 1982, Evidence for a neurotrophic role in noradrenaline neurons in the postnatal development of rat cerebral cortex. J. Neurocytol., 11:119-135.

Finley, J.C.W., Grossman, G.H., Dimeo, P. and Petrusz, P., 1978, Somatostatin-containing neurons in the rat brain: widespread distribution revealed by immunocytochemistry after pretreatment with pronase. Am. J. Anatomy, 153:483-488.

Fricke, R. and Cowan, W.M., 1977, An autoradiographic study of the development of the entorhinal and hippocampal afferents to the dentate gyrus of the rat. J. Comp. Neurol., 173:231-250.

Fuxe, K., Hokfelt, T., Said, S.I. and Mutt, V., 1977, Vasoactive intestinal polypeptide and the nervous system: immunohistochemical evidence of localization in central and peripheral neurons, particularly intracortical neurons of the cerebral cortex. Neurosci. Letters, 5:241-246.

Gall, C., Brecha, N., Chang, K.-J. and Karten, H.J., 1981, Localization of enkephalin-like immunoreactivity to identified axonal and neuronal populations of the rat hippocampus. J. Comp. Neurol., 198:335-350.

Gall, C., Brecha, N., Chang, K.-J. and Karten, H.J., 1983, Ontogeny of enkephalin-like immunoreactivity in the rat hippocampus. Neurosci., in press.

Gash, H., Sladek, C. and Scott, D., 1980, Cytodifferentiation of the supraoptic nucleus correlated with vasopressin synthesis in the rat. Brain Res., 181:345-355.

Goldstein, A., Tachibana, S., Lowney, L., Munkapiller, M. and Hood, L., 1979, Dynophin (1-13) an extraordinarily potent apioid peptide. Proc. Natl. Acad. Sci. USA, 76:6666-6670.

Greenwood, R.S., Godar, S.E., Reaves, T.A. and Harward, J.N., 1981, Cholecystokinin in hippocampal pathways. J. Comp. Neurol., 203:335-350.

Handelmann, G.E., Meyer, D.K., Beinfeld, M.C. and Oertel, W.H., 1981, CCK-containing terminals in the hippocampus are derived from intrinsic neurons: an immunohistochemical and radioimmunological study. Brain Research, 244:180-184.

Hjorth-Simonsen, A., 1972, Projections of the lateral part of the
    entorhinal area to the hippocampus and fascia dentata.
    J. Comp. Neurol., 146:219-232.
Hokfelt, T., Johansson, O., Ljungdahl, A., Lundberg, J.M. and
    Schultzberg, M., 1980, Peptidergic neurons. Nature,
    284:515-521.
Humbert, J., Pradelles, P., Gros, C. and Dray, F., 1979, Enkephalin-
    like products in an embryonic chicken retina. Neurosci.
    Letters, 12:259-263.
Ingaki, S., Sakanaka, M., Shiosaka, S., Sneba, E., Takatsuki, K.,
    Takagi, H., Kawai, Y., Minagawa, H. and Takyama, M., 1982,
    Ontogeny of substance P-containing neuron system in the rat:
    immunohistochemical analysis: I. Forebrain and upper brainstem.
    Neuroscience, 7:251-277.
Jones, E.G. and Hartman, B.K., 1978, Recent advances in neuroana-
    tomical methodology. Ann. Rev. Neurosci., 1:215-297.
Karten, H.J. and Brecha, N., 1980, Localization of substance P
    immunoreactivity in amacrine cells of the retina, Nature,
    283:87-88.
Khachaturian, H., Lewis, M.E., Hollt, V. and Watson, S.J., 1983,
    Telencephalic enkephalinergic systems in the rat brain,
    J. Neurosci., 3:844-855.
Kolb, H., Nelson, R. and Mariani, A., 1981, Amacrine cells, bipolar
    cells and ganglion cells of the cat retina: A Golgi study,
    21:1081-1114.
Krisch, B., 1980, Differing immunoreactivities of somatostatin in
    the cortex and the hypothalamus of the rat. Cell Tiss. Res.,
    212:457-264.
Kuwayama, Y., Ishimoto, I., Fukuda, M., Shimizu, Y., Shiosaka, S.,
    Inagaki, S., Senba, E., Sakanaka, M., Takagi, H., Takatsuki,
    K., Hara, Y., Kawai, Y. and Tohyama, M., 1982, Overall distri-
    bution of glucagon-like immunoreactivity in the chicken
    retina: an immunohistochemical study with flat-mounts.
    Invest. Ophthal. Vis. Sci., 22:681-686.
Laatsch, R.H. and Cowan, W.M., 1965, Electron microscopic studies
    of the dentate gyrus of the rat. I. Normal structure with
    special reference to synaptic organization. J. Comp. Neurol.,
    128:359-396.
Laemle, L.K., Feldman, S.C. and Lichtenstein, E., 1981, Somatostatin-
    like immunoreactivity in the rodent visual system. Soc.
    Neurosci. Abs., 7:761.
Lorén, I., Alumets, J., Hakanson, R. and Sundler, F., 1979, Immuno-
    reactive pancreatic polypeptide (PP) occurs in the central and
    peripheral nervous system: preliminary immunocytochemical
    observatiors. Cell Tiss. Res., 200:179-186.
Lorén, I., Emson, P.C., Fahrenkrug, J., Fjorklund, A., Alumets, J.,
    Hakanson, R. and Sundler, F., 1979, Distribution of vasoactive
    intestinal polypeptide in the rat and mouse brain.
    Neuroscience, 4:1953-1976.

Lorenté de Nó, R., 1934, Studies on the structure of the cerebral cortex. II. Continuation of the study of the ammonic system. J. Psychol. Neurol. (Leipzig), 46:113-177.

Loy, R., Lynch, G. and Cotman, C.W., 1977, Development of afferent lamination in the fascia dentata of the rat. Brain Res., 121:220-243.

McDonald, J.K., Parnavalas, J.G., Karamanlidis, A.N., Brecha, N. and Koenig, J., 1982a, The morphology and distribution of peptide containing neurons in the adult and developing visual cortex of the rat. I. Somatostatin. J. Neurocytol., 11:809-824.

McDonald, J.K., Parnavalas, J.G., Karamanlidis, A.N. and Brecha, N., 1982b, The morphology and distribution of peptide containing neurons in the adult and developing visual cortex of the rat. II. Vasoactive intestinal polypeptide. J. Neurocytol., 11:825-837.

McDonald, J.K., Parnavelas, J.G., Karamanlidis, A.N., Rosenquist, G. and Brecha, N., 1982c, The morphology and distribution of peptide-containing neurons in the adult and developing visual cortex of the rat. III. Cholecystokinin. J. Neurocytol., 11:881-895.

McDonald, J.K., Parnavelas, J.G., Karamanlidis, A.N. and Brecha, N., 1982d, The morphology and distribution of peptide-containing neurons in the adult and developing cortex of the rat. IV. Avian pancreatic polypeptide. J. Neurocytol., 11:985-995.

McGinty, J.F., Aguriksen, S.J., Goldstein, A., Terenius, L. and Bloom, F.E., 1983, Dynorphin is contained within hippocampal mossy fibers; immunochemical alterations after kianic acid administration and colchicine induced neurotoxicity. Proc. Natl. Acad. Sci. USA, 80:589-593.

McGregor, G.P., Woodhams, P.L., O'Shaughnessy, D.J., Ghatei, M.A., Polak, J.M. and Bloom, S.R., 1982, Developmental changes in bombesin, substance P, somatostatin and vasoactive intestinal polypeptide in the rat brain. Neurosci. Lett., 28:21-27.

Martino, E., Seo, H., Lernmark, A. and Refetoff, S., 1980, Ontogenetic patterns of thyrotropin-releasing hormone-like material in rat hypothalamus, pancreas and retina: selective effect of light deprivation. Proc. Natl. Acad. Sci. USA, 77:4345-4348.

Merchenthaler, I., Vigh, S., Petrusz, P. and Schally, A.V., 1982, Immunocytochemical localization of coritcoptropin-releasing factor (CRF) in the rat brain. Am. J. Anat., 165:385-396.

Morgan, I.G., Oliver, J. and Chubb, I.W., 1981, The identification and development of amacrine cells containing somatostatin-like immunoreactivity in chicken retina. Soc. Neurosci. Abs., 7:273.

Morrison, J.H., Magistretti, P.J., Benoit, R. and Bloom, F.E., 1981, The immunohistochemical characterization of somatostatin (SS) and vasoactive intestinal polypeptide (VIP) neurons within the cerebral cortex. Soc. Neurosci. Abs., 7:99.

Nishimura, Y., 1980, Determination of the developmental pattern of
    retinal ganglion cells in chick embryos by Golgi impregnation
    and other methods. Anat. Embryol., 158:329-347.
Osborne, N.N., Nicholas, D.A., Dockray, G.J. and Cuello, A.C.,
    1982, Cholecystokinin and substance P immunoreactivity in
    retinas of rats, frogs, lizards and chicks. Exp. Eye Res.,
    34:639-649.
Parnavelas, J.G., 1984, Physiological properties of identified
    neurons. In: The Cerebral Cortex (edited by E.G. Jones and
    A. Peters), New York, Plenum Press (in press).
Parnavelas, J.G., Bradford, R., Mounty, E.J. and Lieberman, A.R.,
    1978, The development of non-pyramidal neurons in the visual
    cortex of the rat. Anatomy and Embryology, 155:1-14.
Parnavelas, J.G. and McDonald, M.K., 1983, The cerebral cortex.
    In: Chemical Neuroanatomy (edited by P.C. Emson), New York,
    Raven Press, 505-549.
Peters, A. and Fairne, A., 1978, Smooth and sparsely-spined
    stellate cells in the visual cortex of the rat: A study using
    a combined Golgi-electron microscope technique. J. Comp.
    Neurol., 181:129-172.
Peters, A. and Kimerer, L.M., 1981, Bipolar neurons in rat visual
    cortex: a combined Golgi-electron microscope study.
    J. Neurocytol., 10:921-946.
Rager, G., 1979, The cellular origin of the b-Wave in the electro-
    retinogram - a developmental approach. J. Comp. Neurol.,
    188:225-244.
Sachs, H., Pearson, D. and Nureddin, A., 1975, Guinea pig neuro-
    physin: isolation, developmental aspects, biosynthesis in
    organ culture. Ann. N.Y. Acad. Sci., 248:36-45.
Shiosaka, S., Takatsuki, K., Sakanaka, M., Inagaki, S., Takagi, H.,
    Senba, E., Kawai, Y., Iida, H., Minagawa, H., Hara, V.,
    Matsuzaki, T. and Tohyama, M., 1982, Ontogeny of somatostatin
    containing neuron system of the rat: immunohistochemical
    analysis. II. Forebrain and diencephalon. J. Comp. Neurol.,
    204:211-224.
Silverman, A.J., 1975, The hypothalamic magnocellular neurosecretory
    system of the guinea pig. II. Immunohistochemical localization
    of neurophysin and vasopressin in the fetus. Am. J. Anat.,
    144:455-460.
Sims, K.B., Hoffman, D.L., Said, S.I. and Zimmerman, E.A., 1980,
    Vasoactive intestinal polypeptide (VIP) in mouse and rat
    brain: an immunocytochemical study. Brain Res., 106:165-183.
Steward, O., 1980, Topographic organization of the projections from
    the entorhinal area to the hippocampal formation of the rat.
    J. Comp. Neurol., 167:285-314.
Swanson, L.W., Sawchenko, P.E., River, J. and Vale, W.W., 1983,
    Organization of ovine corticotropin-releasing factor immuno-
    reactive cells and fibers in the rat brain: An immunohistochem-
    ical study. Neuroendocrinology, 36:165-186.

Sundler, F., Maghimzadeh, E., Hakausou, R., Ekeland, M. and Emson, P., 1983, Nerve fibers in the gut and pancreas of the rat displaying neuropeptide Y immunoreactivity. Intrinsic and extrinsic origin. Cell Tiss. Res., 230:487-493.

Takatsuki, K. Shiosaka, S., Sakanaka, M., Inagaki, S., Senba, E., Takagi, H. and Tohyama, M., 1981, Somatostatin in the auditory system of the rat. Brain Res., 213:211-216.

Tatemoto, K., 1982, Neuropeptide Y: Complete amino acid sequence of the brain peptide. Proc. Natl. Acad. Sci. USA, 79:5485-5489.

Tatemoto, K., Carlquist, M. and Mutt, V., 1982, Neuropeptide Y - a novel brain peptide with structural similarities to peptide YY and pancreatic polypeptide. Nature, 296:659-660.

Tornqvist, K., Lorén, I., Hakanson, R. and Sundler, F., 1981, Peptide-containing neurons in the chicken retina. Exp. Eye Res., 33:55-64.

Vincent, S.R., Skirboll, L., Hokfelt, T., Johansson, O., Lundberg, J.M., Elde, R.P., Terenius, L. and Kimmel, J., 1982, Coexistence of somatostatin and avian pancreatic polypeptide (APP)-like immunoreactivity in some forebrain neurons. Neuroscience, 7:439-466.

Walsh, J.H., 1981, Hormones and peptides in: Physiology of the Gastrointestinal Tract (edited by L.R. Johnson), New York, Raven Press, 59-144.

Watson, S., Khachaturian, H., Akil, H., Coy, D. and Goldstein, A., 1982, Comparison of the distribution of dynorphin systems and enkephalin systems in brain. Science, 218:1134-1136.

Witkovsky, P., 1963, An ontogenetic study of retinal function in the chick. Vision Res., 3:341-355.

THE EMBRYONIC DEVELOPMENT OF THE CEREBRAL CORTEX:

WHAT CAN WE LEARN FROM REPTILES?

A.M. Goffinet

Chargé de Recherches au F.N.R.S. (Belgium)
Unité de Neurologie du Développement
Faculté de Médecine UCL
Brussels, Belgium

INTRODUCTION

The development of the cerebral cortex has so far been primarily
examined in mammals, where a common sequence is constantly found
(cfr. Caviness and Rakic, 1978). Neuronal precursors proliferate
into germinative zones, lining the ventricles (ventricular zones:
VZ); post mitotic elements migrate outward, along radial glial
guides, and the majority of them settle into the telencephalic cortical plate (CP).

The cells in the CP are closely packed and radially oriented,
a property which appears to be under genetic control, for it is
affected by the reeler mutation in mice (Goffinet, 1979). This
radial presentation of cortical neurons is thought to be necessary
to the harmonious development of the cerebral cortex.

These widely accepted characteristics of cortical development
raise several questions, two of which will be more specifically addressed here. First, can this outline of cortical development be
generalized to include non-mammalian species and second, is the
radial presentation of cortical neurons a necessary feature of every
cerebral cortex in itself and finally what, if any, is its biological meaning?

In order to approach these questions, the development of the
cortical plate has been examined in reptiles, the vertebrates in
which the cortex is the most primitive. Embryos from turtles (Emys
orbicularis) and lizards (Lacerta agilis or virilis) have been

251

analyzed with morphological techniques, and compared with specimens
of Crocodilus niloticus and Sphenodon punctatus, available only as
embryological collections. These four species cover the four taxo-
nomic reptilian groups (see Fig. 4). Based on preliminary observations, two stages of development were selected: stage one is when
the cortical plate appears in the telencephalon; at stage two, the
cortical plate has acquired most of its cytoarchitectonic features.

OBSERVATIONS

Cell proliferation, migration, and synaptogenesis

      These general features of cortical development appear identical
in the two species, Emys and Lacerta, where they have been examined
in detail; they are presumably common to the development of all
reptiles.

      At the time of appearance of the cortical plate, the telenceph-
alic wall is composed of four concentric strata, namely an internal,
ventricular zone (VZ), a cell poor intermediate zone (IZ), the
cortical plate (CP) and an external, marginal zone (MZ); (Fig. 1).

      Mitosis is restricted to the ventricular zones, and occurs with
their spindles oriented parallel to the ventricular surface. Pro-
liferating elements have a neuroepithelial morphology; their ventricular surface is covered with ciliae, and they are joined together
on their lateral face by embryonic, primarily adhaerens junctions
(Fig. 2a,b). Cells in the VZ have a radial extension which spans
the whole thickness of the cerebral wall and ends against the basement membrane, forming characteristic end feet (Fig. 2c).

      In the intermediate zone, a few cells are seen, which are more
mature than neuroepithelial cells and correspond to post mitotic
neurons engaged in migration. The radial extensions from ventricular cells are often closely apposed to migrating elements and, by
analogy to mammals, these radial fibers probably serve as substrate
and guide during radial neuronal migration (Fig. 5). The IZ is rich
in fibers of various origin; the axons from neurons in the cortical
plate as well as afferent fibers arriving in the cortex run at this
level, as demonstrated by electron microscopy and Golgi impregnation.
In Lacerta and Emys, afferent fibers first form synapses at the level
of the marginal zone (MZ); these synapses have an asymmetrical morphology (Fig. 2d) and appear closely after the cortical plate begins
to differentiate. At later developmental stages, the number of
synapses increases dramatically in the VZ, and asymmetrical profiles
remain the most common. This situation is comparable to what occurs
in mammals, where synapses are also first encountered in the MZ:
however in mammals, synaptic profiles appear at the same time as
the cortical plate whereas in reptiles the CP appears first. This

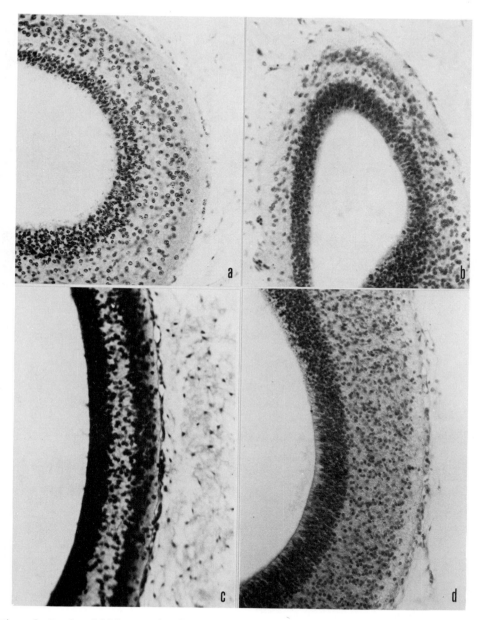

Fig. 1 Early differentiation of the cortical plate a) Emys orbicular-is stage one (X210),b) Lacerta agilis stage one (X225),c) Sphenodon punctatus stage one (X150),d) Crocodilus niloticus stage one (X170).

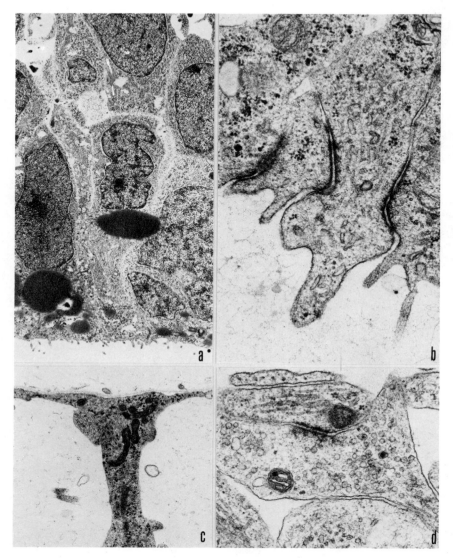

Fig. 2   a) Cells in the VZ (Lacerta), (X9000), b) junctions
between neuroepithelial cells (Lacerta), (X40000), c) radial glial
end foot (Lacerta), (X15000), d) synapse in the early MZ (Emys),
(X40000).

observation suggests that the afferent connections are not necessary
to the early histogenesis of the cortical plate.

The early development of the cortical plate

In contrast to other developmental events described above, the
histogenesis of the cortical plate is extremely different among the
reptilian groups examined, particularly regarding its cytoarchitectonic organization.

The CP reaches its best organization in lacertilians. From
the earliest stage of its differentiation, it appears as a condensation of cells at the level of the dorsal-external hemispheric
field (Fig. 1b). Three components become progressively individual-
ized, namely the medial or hippocampal cortex, the dorsal or general
pallium and the lateral or pyriform cortex; at stage two of development, the three components of the CP are clearly separated from
each other at the level of the superpositions of de Lange. Radial
orientation, and packing of the neurons into a plate, are more pronounced in the medial and dorsal cortex (Fig. 3b) than in the pyriform cortex. The radial organization of the lizard embryonic cortex
is also well appreciated on Golgi material, which displays the
harmonious dendritic arborization of neurons and the radial geometry
of the glial cells (Fig. 5b).

By contrast, the CP in Emys at all developmental stages appears
loose and poorly organized (Fig. 1a, 3a). The superpositions of
de Lange are not formed; the geometry of dendritic deployment is
more rudimentary and irregular, and the course of the radial glial
fibers more erratic than in Lacerta (Fig. 5a). In Sphenodon (Fig.
1c, 3c) the medial cortical plate is prominent and well defined,
quite reminiscent of its lizard counterpart, whereas the dorsal
cortex appears poorly organized, and the pyriform cortex is extremely small. In Crocodilus (Fig. 1d, 3d), all the cortical sectors
are well developed and densely populated but neurons never become
so closely packed and radially ordered as they are in lizards or in
the hippocampus of Sphenodon.

DISCUSSION

It has been suggested by Marin Padilla (1978) that the development of the mammalian cortex proceeds through a "reptilian stage",
called the primordial cortical organization. Our data shows that,
indeed, several steps of cortical development in reptiles are similar to early cortical histogenesis in mammals and that general principles of cortical development can probably be generalized to include
reptiles. However, they also stress important species differences
among the various reptilian taxons, particularly regarding the
histological organization of embryonic cortical neurons.

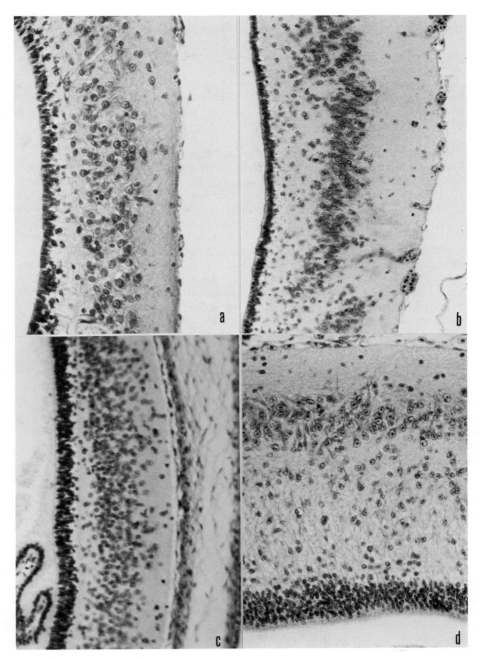

Fig. 3 The dorsal pallium at embryonic stage two. a) Emys orbicularis (X275), b) Lacerta agilis (X290), c) Sphenodon punctatus (X150), d) Crocodilus niloticus (X 260).

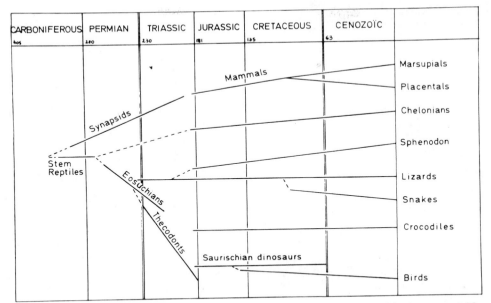

Fig. 4   Schema of evolutive filiations leading to living reptiles, mammals and birds (courtesy of Prof. C.B. Cox).

From the correlation between the distribution of the property of radial presentation (best expressed in lizards and rudimentary in turtles), and present views on paleontological filiations of reptiles (schematized on Fig. 4), it follows that this cytological characteristic of embryonic neurons in the CP has been acquired to various extents, at least twice, after phyletic divergence, in lacertilians and in mammalian ancestors. This provides an example of homoplasy or evolutive convergence in brain development and thus points to a similar and presumably beneficial way of solving a biological problem (Northcutt, 1981), namely the optimization of architectonic features.

This property of radial presentation of cortical neurons, discretely distributed, and differentially acquired during evolution, presumably responds to its own genetic determinism. In this respect it is interesting to note that a simple recessive defect, like the reeler mutation in mice, can electively perturb cortical architecture, while leaving cell differentiation and connections relatively unaffected (Caviness, 1977), so that in mammals the product of the

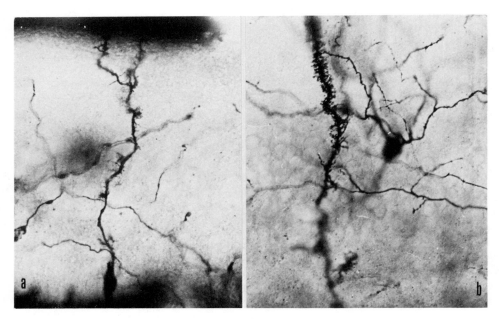

Fig. 5   a) Radial glial fiber with passing axons; dorsal cortex
of Emys stage two; Golgi stain (X 500), b) radial glial fiber with
neuron and passing neurites; dorsal cortex of Lacerta stage two;
Golgi stain (X 600).

wildtype allele at the reeler locus is necessary to the expression
of radial cortical organization.

    The morphological species differences observed at the level of
the developing cortical organization occur in parallel to differences
in the course and ramifications of the radial glial guides (Fig. 5).
This suggests that the radial guides, in addition to providing the
substrate for neuronal migration, could also act at the end of migration and influence the cytoarchitectonic differentiation. This hypothesis is in agreement with the theory of Rakic (1980) that radial
glial cells have a role in the areal differentiation of the CNS.
It receives some support from the work of Caviness (this volume) on
the abnormal cortical development in reeler mice, indicating that
the defect could reside at the level of the interaction between
radial glial guides and neuronal cells, at the end of their
migration.

SUMMARY AND CONCLUSIONS

The comparative study of cortical embryogenesis in reptiles reveals an invariant sequence regarding cell proliferation, migration, synaptogenesis. Important species differences exist in the developing cortical plate, particularly in the radial organization of the CP, best in lizards, rudimentary in turtles, intermediate in Sphenodon and Crocodiles.

When contrasted to paleontological filiation, this distribution is characteristic of an homoplastic character, an example of convergence in brain evolution (Northcutt, 1981). The species differences are reflected in the morphology of the radial glial guides, suggesting that the latter could play a key role in architectonic differentiation. Further work is in progress in order to get a better understanding of these phenomena.

ACKNOWLEDGEMENTS

I wish to thank Prof. C.B. Cox, Dr. Langerwerf, Dr. Pieau, Prof. A. Raynaud for their precious help and advice, and Mrs. J. Serneels for secretarial assistance. This work was supported by Credit au Chercheur F.N.R.S. No. 81/82-S2/5-FA-E14 and grant FRSM No. 3.4540.81.

REFERENCES

Caviness, V.S., 1977, Reeler mutant mouse: a genetic experiment in developing mammalian cortex, Neurosci. Symp., 27-46.
Caviness, V.S., and Rakic, P., 1978, Mechanisms of cortical development: a view from mutation in mice, Ann. Rev. Neurosci., 1:297-326.
Goffinet, A.M., 1979, An early developmental defect in the cerebral cortex of the reeler mutant mouse, Anat. Embryol., 157:205-216.
Marin Padilla, M., 1978, Dual origin of the mammalian neocortex and evolution of the cortical plate, Anat. Embryol., 152:109-126.
Northcutt, R.G ., 1981, Evolution of the telencephalon in non-mammals, Ann. Rev. Neurosci., 4:301-350.
Rakic, P., 1981, Developmental events leading to laminar and areal organization in the neocortex. In: The Cerebral Cortex, Schmitt, F.O., S.G. Dennis and F.G. Worden (eds.), MIT Press, pp. 7-28.

AN INVESTIGATION OF THE DEVELOPMENT OF OCULAR DOMINANCE AND

ORIENTATION COLUMNS IN CAT STRIATE CORTEX USING 2-DEOXYGLUCOSE

Ian Thompson, Margaret Kossut* and Colin Blakemore

The University Laboratory of Physiology
Parks Road, Oxford and
*The Department of Neurophysiology
The Nencki Institute of Experimental Biology
Warsaw, Poland

ABSTRACT

Neurophysiological studies on the striate cortex of immature cats have indicated that although oriented neurones occur they are broadly tuned and have a more imprecise columnar organization. Similarly transneuronal autoradiography reveals an initially incomplete segregation of the geniculo-cortical afferents. We have used 2-deoxyglucose autoradiography to examine the development of columnar metabolic label in the striate cortex of normal and binocularly deprived kittens following either monocular stimulation or stimulation with fixed orientations. In normal animals, both orientation and ocular dominance columns achieve an adult-like pattern at 5-6 weeks of age and indications of periodic labelling in both stimulus conditions are first apparent at 3 weeks. After stimulation with fixed orientations at 3 weeks, discrete foci of increased labelling are seen in layer IV; it is only in older animals that a full columnar pattern appears. At 3 weeks, ocular dominance columns extend through all cortical layers both ipsilateral and contralateral to the stimulated eye; the columns become more regular in older animals. Binocular deprivation appears to inhibit the formation of orientation columns as defined by deoxyglucose autoradiography; only in one 35 day old cat was there an indication of columnar labelling. Ocular dominance columns were less affected by binocular deprivation; at both 5 weeks and 3 months there was definite periodic label although the distribution in the younger animal was less regular than in a comparable normal animal.

261

A striking feature of striate cortex in adult cat and monkey is the columnar distribution of neurones displaying similar response characteristics. The electrophysiological experiments of Hubel and Wiesel (see Hubel, 1982) demonstrated that, in recordings made perpendicular to the cortical surface, neurones displayed similar orientation tuning and ocular dominance; while neurones recorded on tangential penetrations demonstrated gradual changes in response characteristics. This organization has been confirmed using other, autoradiographic, techniques. Transneuronal autoradiography demonstrates that geniculate input to layer IV of the striate cortex is periodic, forming an anatomical basis for ocular dominance columns, in both cat (Shatz, Lindstrom and Wiesel, 1977) and monkey (Wiesel, Hubel and Lam, 1974; LeVay, Hubel and Wiesel, 1980). The 2-deoxyglucose technique of Sokoloff (Sokoloff et al., 1977) also reveals columnar distributions of increased metabolism when the animal is stimulated either through one eye or binocularly with a single orientation (Kennedy et al., 1976; Hubel, Wiesel and Stryker, 1978; Albus, 1979; Singer, 1981; Schoppmann and Stryker, 1981).

While this columnar arrangement is precise and well ordered in the adult, it is less precise in the immature animal and is moreover malleable. In the cat, the adult periodicity of geniculate terminals in layer IV is not attained until about 6 weeks of age (LeVay, Stryker and Shatz, 1978). It does not develop in the absence of visual experience (Swindale, 1981) and can be altered by monocular deprivation (Shatz and Stryker, 1978). A similar pattern is observed in the monkey except that dark rearing fails to affect segregation (LeVay et al., 1980). Electrophysiological techniques indicate that orientation columns exist in visually inexperienced monkeys but the situation is less clear in the cat. While orientation tuned neurones do exist in immature cat striate cortex, many studies report that their tuning is broad and that they constitute a reduced proportion of the cortical population with rudimentary columnar organization (Blakemore and Van Sluyters, 1975; Fregnac and Imbert, 1978; Bonds, 1979) although Sherk and Stryker (1976) report that young visually deprived kittens display tuning characteristics which closely resemble those of the adult. As with ocular dominance, selective visual experience can alter the arrangement of orientation columns as determined by 2-deoxyglucose autoradiography: animals experiencing only one orientation demonstrate greatly expanded columnar labelling following stimulation with the rearing orientation (Singer, Freeman and Rauschecker, 1981).

We have used 2-deoxyglucose autoradiography to investigate the ontogeny of both ocular dominance columns and orientation columns in the cat. As the technique reveals activity in populations of neurones, it facilitates examination of any laminar variations in the development of these two columnar systems and, in the case of ocular dominance columns, how the development of periodic activity in cortical neurones correlates with the segregation of geniculo-

cortical afferents. The role of visual experience in determining
neuronal response characteristics in striate cortex is contentious
(see Swindale 1982a). This is particularly true for the cat in which
the neuronal properties are far less mature at eye-opening, compared
with those of the newborn monkey. We have also examined the development of periodic labelling in binocularly deprived animals to see
whether the patterns are disrupted or merely attenuated by comparison
with normal animals. It is also interesting to ask whether the
attenuation of pattern vision consequent on lid-suture has differential effects on the development of orientation and ocular
dominance columns since orientation tuning requires a more precise
spatial organization of the receptive fields.

Methods

     2-Deoxyglucose autoradiography was performed on 24 cats ranging
in age from 2 weeks to 3 months. Fourteen animals were binocularly
stimulated with gratings of fixed orientations and all but one of
these animals were paralyzed and anesthetized. To investigate ocular
dominance columns, 9 kittens were allowed to explore the normal laboratory environment, supplemented with patterned cards, with the
left eyelids sutured shut. The remaining animal explored with both
eyes open. Nine animals were binocularly deprived by bilateral eyelid suture prior to the time of normal eye-opening; they received a
maximum of 3 hours possible visual experience immediately prior to
the 2-deoxyglucose injection and this was minimized by occluding
the opened eyes with tape. All animals received 45 minutes of visual
stimulation after intravenous injection of 1.5 mCi/kg ^{3}H-2-
deoxylglucose (Amersham, 23 Ci/mmol; NEN, 8 Ci/mmol). The animals
were then anesthetized with pentobarbitone sodium and perfused with
the paraformaldehyde based fixative of McLean and Nakane (1974;
Durham, Woolsey and Kruger, 1981). After blocking the brain and
freezing it in isopentane at $-70\,^\circ$C, horizontal cryostat sections of
20 μm thickness were picked up on coverslips and snap-dried on a
hot-plate. The sections were exposed to LKB Ultrofilm for 4 weeks,
developed in Kodak D19 (5 min) and then printed at x6 magnification
on sheet film. Montages from three adjacent autoradiographs were
used to produce contact prints (Singer et al., 1981; Livingstone
and Hubel, 1981).

     The preparation of anesthetized, paralyzed animals for investi-
gation of orientation columns was as described in Thompson, Blakemore
and Kossut (1983). Briefly, after venous and tracheal cannulation
under althesin anesthesia, the animal was paralyzed with gallamine
triethiodide (10 mg/kg/hr) and artificially hyperventilated with a
75% N_2O:25% CO_2 anesthetic mixture; end-tidal pCO_2 was maintained
between 4.5 and 5%. The eyes were refracted and the areae centrales
or, in the youngest animals, the optic discs, aligned using a reversing ophthalmoscope. Visual stimulation commenced when althesin-
induced spikes had disappeared from the electroencephalogram and

the animal was judged to be in a steady state of light anesthesia.
Most animals were stimulated in the right visual hemifield with
vertical gratings, and with oblique gratings in the left hemifield.
The stimuli, generated by computer on a display screens subtending
a visual angle of about 25 deg, were drifting square waves with a
contrast of 0.75 (mean luminance, 250 cd/m^2). The spatial frequencies used were 0.05, 0.2 and 0.8 c/deg and the temporal frequencies
1 or 2 Hz, in either direction. The spatiotemporal characteristics
of the grating varied pseudorandomly, each combination was displayed
for 10 sec simultaneously on the vertical and oblique screens.
Preparation for monocular stimulation, with multiple orientations,
was simpler. Animals were induced with halothane (initially 5%) in
$95\%O_2:5\%CO_2$, the radial vein was cannulated and either the right
eyelids opened (BD animals) or the left eyelids sutured shut (normal animals). Local anesthetic was infused into all wounds. When
the animals had recovered from anesthesia and could walk freely,
the tape covering the right eye was removed and 5 minutes later the
2-deoxyglucose was given.

Results

Columnar development in normal kittens. Electrophysiological experiments indicate that the tuning characteristics and proportion of
orientation selective neurones reach adult values in the cat at 5-6
weeks of age (Blakemore and Van Sluyters, 1975; Fregnac and Imbert,
1978; Bonds, 1979; Derrington and Fuchs, 1981), coinciding with the
completion of terminal segregation in layer IV (LeVay et al., 1978).
2-Deoxyglucose autoradiographs at this age demonstrate clear columnar
label for both binocular stimulation with a single orientation and
simple monocular stimulation, as illustrated in Fig.7 1A-C. Figure
1A shows an autoradiograph of a horizontal brain section from a 35
day normal cat in which the right visual hemifield was stimulated
with vertical gratings and the left with oblique gratings. Both
visual cortices demonstrate distinct patterns of columnar label
within area 17. In any one column, increased label extends through
all cortical layers but it is densest in layer IV; the pattern resembles that described for the adult cat by Albus (1979) and
Schoppmann and Stryker (1981). There is some indication of continuous label within layer IV in Fig. 1A, presumably coinciding with
activity of geniculo-cortical terminals. In this animal the hemisphere stimulated with the vertical grating appeared to have a more
regular pattern of labelling, with a periodicity of about 1 mm, compared to the hemisphere stimulated with oblique gratings. Further
quantitative analysis will be necessary to confirm this impression.

Pronounced columnar label is also apparent in Figs. 1B and C
which show autoradiographs of horizontal sections from a 35 day and
a 43 day animal both of which viewed the laboratory environment monocularly for 45 minutes. In both animals, the hemisphere ipsilateral
to the stimulated eye has the more distinct periodicity, at about

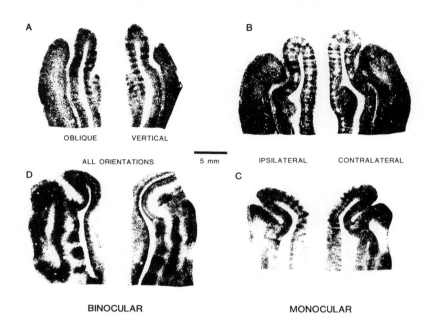

Figure 1. Orientation columns and ocular dominance columns in kittens 5 or 6 weeks old. All brains were cut horizontally and the sections exposed to KLB Ultrofilm for 4 weeks. Three adjacent autoradiographs were printed on sheet film at x6 magnification, superimposed and then used to make contact prints. A. Autoradiograph from a 5 week animal stimulated with oblique gratings in the left hemifield and vertical gratings in the right hemifield. Distinct columnar label can be observed in the striate cortex of both hemispheres, although it appears more regular in the left hemisphere. B and C. Autoradiographs from a 5 week (A) and a 6 week (B) animal both of which had explored the laboratory with the left eyelids sutured shut. In both animals the columnar pattern is stronger in the ipsilateral hemifield and, while evident in the 5 week animal, it is more apparent in the 6 week old kitten. D. This 5 week old animal was allowed to explore the laboratory with both eyes open. No regular columnar labelling patterns can be seen in striate cortex; anteriorly in the lateral bank periodicities are present. Their origin remains to be determined.

OCULAR DOMINANCE   ORIENTATION

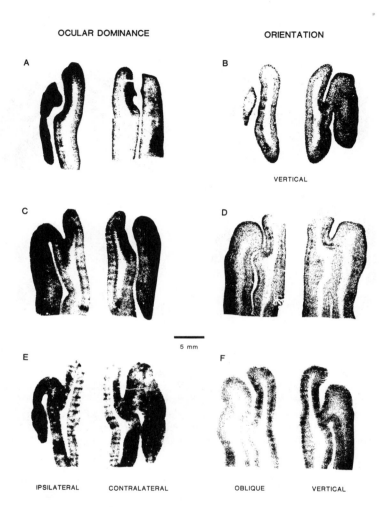

Figure 2. The development of ocular dominance and orientation columns as displayed in cats of 2 weeks (A,B), 3 weeks (C,D) and 4
weeks (E,F) of age. The three animals used to investigate ocular
dominance explored the laboratory with the left eyelids sutured.
The two oldest orientation animals (D,F) were paralyzed and anesthetized; the left hemifield was stimulated with oblique gratings and
the right hemifield with vertical gratings. The youngest animal
(B) was simply hand-held in front of the display screen for 45
minutes while vertical gratings drifted past; no columnar label was
seen in another, conventionally prepared 14 day old. While the
appearance of periodic label shows a similar time course for the

0.9 mm (Fig. 1B) and 1.2 mm (Fig. 1C). This agrees with results from transneuronal autoradiography (LeVay et al., 1978) which demonstrate a much clearer, and earlier, segregation of the ipsilateral geniculocortical terminals. The radial distribution of label in these two animals is rather different from that observed following stimulation with a single orientation. The focus of densest label does not always fall in layer IV, indeed there is a distinct band of relatively unlabelled cortex in deep layer IV possibly coinciding with the inner stripe of Baillarger. This pattern was reported for orientation columns in the 2-deoxyglucose study of Albus (1979) but this is not so apparent in the studies of Schoppmann and Stryker (1981) or Livingstone and Hubel (1981).

As the 2-deoxyglucose technique reveals local differences in metabolic activity, there is a possibility that intrinsic inhomogeneities in metabolism, independent of visual stimulation, generate the columnar pattern. Hendrickson and Wilson (1979) reported columnar labelling after binocular exposure to multiple orientations in a conscious monkey but no columns were observed in similar experiments on paralyzed, anesthetized cats (Schoppmann and Stryker, 1981; Tootell, Silverman and DeValois, 1981). We performed 2-deoxyglucose autoradiography on a 35 day kitten which was allowed to explore the laboratory with both eyes open. The majority of cortical sections revealed no columnar label within striate cortex, as illustrated in Fig. 1D. Occasional faint columns could be detected but the frequency of their occurrence was very much less than in animals stimulated through one eye or with a single orientation. This binocularly stimulated animal did show distinct columns in more lateral cortex (arrowed) which have a periodicity of about 2.3 mm. The origin of these columns remains to be determined.

If, at 5-6 weeks of age, the columnar pattern for both orientation and ocular dominance resembles the adult pattern, this is not the case for younger animals. Figure 2 illustrates the progression in labelling patterns in animals at 14, 21 and 28 days. In the youngest animals, at 14 days, neither monocular stimulation (Fig. 2A) nor binocular exposure to a single orientation (Fig. 2B) generates

two stimulus conditions, the extent of columnar labelling is greater in the monocularly stimulated animals. In animals presented with fixed orientations the main foci of periodic label are concentrated within layer IV in both the 3 and 4 week old animals. Another interesting feature of the autoradiographs is that extrastriate cortex is much more uniformly labelled in the orientation animals compared with the ocular dominance animals.

any obvious periodic label in area 17. The medial bank of the
lateral gyrus is uniformly labelled in both animals, although it is
possible that subsequent quantitative analysis might reveal intrinsic periodicities. Differential labelling can be observed in sections from these two animals, especially on the lateral bank of the
lateral gyrus which may coincide with area 18 although the cytoarchitectonic distinction between areas 17 and 18 is not very reliable
in these young animals. The existence of such patches indicates
that the immature cortex can demonstrate sufficient differential
responsiveness to generate significant discontinuities in 2-deoxy-
glucose uptake. If the same is true of striate cortex, it argues
that the absence of periodic label reveals the absence of specified
neurones rather than the absence of responsive neurones.

At 21 days, both the ocular dominance and orientation animals
display differential labelling patterns but with rather different
distributions. Monocular stimulation produces a faint columnar
pattern in the medial bank of striate cortex (Fig. 2C) which, interestingly, is more apparent in the contralateral hemisphere. Here
periodicities can be observed in most cortical laminae, both superficial and deep, with a repeat distance of about 1 mm. Both hemispheres also display a more intense and less regular pattern in the
postero-lateral bank of the lateral gyrus. A columnar pattern of
label is not obvious in the 21 day animal stimulated with fixed
orientations (Fig. 2D) but within a layer IV regular foci of label,
at 1 mm. intervals, appear in both hemispheres. By 28 days the
ocular dominance columns have become much more distinct (Fig. 2E)
especially in the ipsilateral cortex and the orientation columns
have extended into the superficial and deep laminae although not
invariably through the whole depth of the cortex. As in the 35 day
animal, it appears that the hemisphere stimulated with vertical
gratings has the more regular distribution of label down the medial
bank.

Columnar development in binocularly deprived kittens. The role of
visual experience in the specification of orientation tuning in cat
striate neurones is controversial. Long term binocular deprivation
greatly disrupts the specificity of neuronal responses (see Movshon
and Van Sluyters, 1981) but does this reflect a failure of normal
development of secondary atrophy of specified neurones? Some electrophysiological studies (Blakemore and Van Sluyters, 1975; Fregnac
and Imbert, 1978; Bonds, 1979) indicate that visual deprivation
arrests normal development whereas Sherk and Stryker (1976) found
that deprived cats of 3-4 weeks possessed neurones with orientation
tuning characteristics similar to those found in adult cats. We
examined the development of orientation columns in kittens visually
deprived by bilateral eyelid suture to ascertain whether periodic
labelling is present initially and subsequently disappears or whether

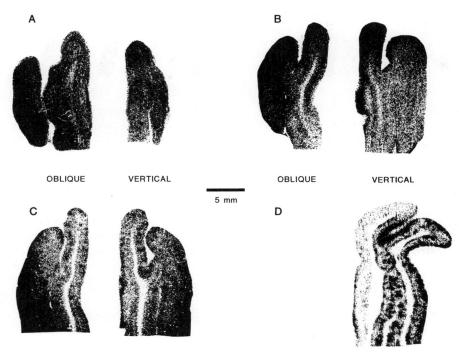

Figure 3. An examination of orientation columns in binocularly deprived cats, which underwent bilateral eyelid suture prior to the
time of normal eye-opening. The animals had their eyes opened at
various ages (3 weeks, A; 4 weeks, B; 5 weeks, C; and 8 weeks, D)
and, after a maximum interval of three hours, were stimulated with
gratings of a fixed orientation (oblique in the left hemifield and
vertical in the right hemifield). Compared with normal kittens
(Fig. 2B,D,F), there is little indication of columnar labelling in
striate cortex at any age. The 5 week animal (C) has some periodicities in the medial bank and the occasional column in postero-
lateral cortex. The 8 week animal (D) shows uniform label over
most of the striate cortex but there is differential label located
in the most superficial cortical layers. In more lateral cortex,
layer VI also appears to be differentially labelled. The right
hemisphere in this animal was cut parasagitally and displayed a
similar pattern.

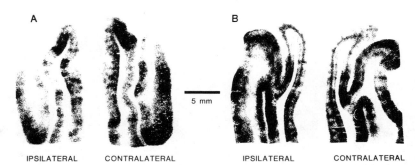

IPSILATERAL   CONTRALATERAL   IPSILATERAL   CONTRALATERAL

Figure 4. Monocular stimulation in binocularly deprived cats at 5 weeks (A) and 3 months (B) of age. The sutured eyelids over the right were opened one to two hours prior to stimulation, i.e. exploration of the laboratory. Differential label is clearly evident in the 5 week animal but is less regular than the pattern in the equivalent normal animal (Fig. 1B) although obviously more distinct than in the binocularly deprived animal stimulated with fixed orientations (Fig. 2C). Interestingly the pattern seems more regular in the 3 month deprived animal. Label is strongest, and apparently continuous, in layer IV but faint columns do extend throughout the depth of the cortex.

it ever develops. Representative sections from 4 kittens between 3 and 8 weeks of age, all binocularly deprived prior to normal eye-opening, are illustrated in Fig. 3. Each visual hemifield was stimulated with a single orientation and the autoradiographs reveal a very different pattern of 2-deoxyglucose uptake from that observed in normally reared animals (Figs. 1A and 2B, D, F). Only one animal (35 day, Fig. 3B) displays any periodic labelling within area 17. Patches of label somewhat denser than background are located in the posterior pole of the lateral gyrus but the label is much weaker and more diffuse than in the comparable normal kitten (Fig. 1A). The labelling pattern shown in Fig. 3B was the most distinct that we have observed in the seven binocularly deprived cats, including two at 28 days and two at 35 days, which we stimulated with fixed orientations. Surprisingly although no differential distributions of label within the bulk of area 17 are seen in the 8 week animal (Fig. 3D), there does appear to be an indication of periodic labelling in the superficial cortical laminae. Outside area 17 periodic label is much more obvious but whether this reflects the activity of orientation tuned neurones remains to be ascertained.

It could be argued that the immediate consequence of binocular deprivation is simply to reduce the responsivity of the neurones without altering their selectivity and so reduce the contrast of any differential label. If this is true, then one would expect to observe similar results for the development of ocular dominance columns in deprived kittens. Preliminary results suggest that this is not the case. Figure 4 illustrates autoradiographs from two binocularly deprived cats stimulated monocularly through the right eye. At 35 days of age, there are certainly discontinuities in striate labelling but, compared to a normal animals (Fig. 1B, C) the pattern is less regular (Fig. 4A, B). Columnar label in contralateral cortex is not particularly strong and ipsilaterally the distribution of the ocular dominance columns is uneven, not all columns extend through the whole depth of the cortex. However in an animal visually deprived until 3 months (Fig. 4C), the distribution of columnar label does not appear so disrupted. Regular columns are apparent outside layer IV but unlike normal, younger, animals there appears to be a strong continuous band of label located in layer IV. It is interesting that bilateral eyelid suture results in a similar failure of segregation of geniculocortical terminals (Swindale, 1982b) as in dark-reared kittens (Swindale, 1981) or after intra-ocular injections of tetrodotoxin (Stryker, 1981).

Discussion

The autoradiographs presented here reveal the development of the columnar pattern of increased metabolic activity in cat striate cortex which is associated either with monocular stimulation or else binocular stimulation with a fixed orientation. Interestingly, the two columnar systems appear to develop differently both in the laminar distribution of label within the columnar arrangement and in their susceptibility to the effects of visual deprivation. Consistent periodic labelling is first apparent in animals at 21 days of age. In animals stimulated with a single orientation, the pattern revealed is one of foci of label restricted to layer IV which, over the next fortnight, extend through all cortical layers. Electrophysiological studies on very young kittens do indicate that a small proportion of striate neurones are orientation specific and moreover that such neurones are preferentially located in layer IV (see Movshon and Van Sluyters, 1981), which is in agreement with the 2-deoxyglucose results presented here. LeVay et al. (1978), using transneuronal autoradiography, found that the distribution of geniculocortical afferents in striate cortex was uniform at 2 weeks of age but that fluctuations in the projection of the ipsilateral eye had appeared by 3 weeks coinciding with the first clear periodicities in the 2-deoxyglucose labelling following monocular stimulation. A similar temporal sequence for the development of ocular dominance columns has recently been reported by Silverman (1982). Although not well defined at this age, columnar label was present in both ipsilateral and contralateral cortex and could be observed in all cortical layers; it was not concentrated in layer IV.

The consequences of binocular deprivation on the appearance of orientation dependent periodicities in 2-deoxyglucose uptake is dramatic. The sequence observed in normal animals is totally disrupted and at no age does convincing columnar label appear. This result implies that visual deprivation results in a failure of the columns to develop rather than in secondary degeneration following an initial passive development. It could be argued that the deprivation has merely decreased neuronal responsivity to a level at which the deoxyglucose technique cannot resolve the columnar arrangement. However, the persistence of ocular dominance columns in BD animals argues that neurones are capable of responding adequately to a different stimulus. Neurones may demonstrate preferences for one or other eye and yet have poor orientation selectivities. It would be interesting to see whether 2-deoxyglucose autoradiography would reveal ocular dominance columns in dark-reared animals which receive no visual stimulation.

The advantage of 2-deoxyglucose technique is that it can reveal spatial inhomogeneities in the metabolic activity of populations of neurones but this characteristic also generates problems for interpretation. As the technique is essentially an averaging procedure, it may not reveal the existence of small numbers of neurones activated specifically by the stimulus amidst a background of nonspecifically activated neurones. Another problem is how 2-deoxyglucose uptake relates to neuronal activity generated by the stimulus. In the monkey, "hot-spots" of 2-deoxyglucose uptake exist which coincide with mitochondrian-rich, glutamic acid decarboxylase positive (GAD+ve) patches in striate cortex (Hendrickson, Hunt and Wu, 1981; Horton and Hubel, 1981). In the adult cat, neither cytochrome oxidase nor GAD+ve spots have been observed (Wong-Riley, 1979; Horton and Hubel, 1981; Hunt, 1982) nor is columnar label apparent following binocular stimulation with multiple orientations (Schoppmann and Stryker, 1981; Tootell et al., 1981; Fig. 1). Schoppmann and Stryker also demonstrated that the pattern of 2-deoxyglucose uptake in cat striate cortex following stimulation with a single orientation correlates with the orientation selectivity of neurones determined electrophysiologically. It would appear, for the adult cat visual cortex, that the 2-deoxyglucose technique does reveal the distribution of neuronal activity, certainly for oriented stimuli. The differences in the laminar distribution of label in the two developing columnar systems described above also suggest that the technique is not revealing intrinsic metabolic periodicities, rather periodicities which are dependent on the nature of the stimulus.

The exact nature of the influence of visual experience on the normal development of visual cortex remains to be defined and may well vary with species. Certainly in the cat, manipulations of

visual experience can affect the normal developmental mechanisms
to alter the distributions of both ocular dominance and orientation
tuning (see Movshon and Van Sluyters, 1981). But does this influence
of visual experience represent a separate developmental mechanism
or an integral component of the normal developmental processes?
Thus the results of binocular deprivation can be interpreted as
resulting either from a failure to provide necessary developmental
instructions or from a non-specific degenerative process. Data
from the monkey argue against visual experience being essential for
the establishment of orientation tuning. Orientated neurones are
present in the newborn animal and are not greatly disrupted by
short term binocular deprivation. Similarly, segregation of geniculocortical terminals is not affected by binocular deprivation
(LeVay et al., 1980) and the segregation of the retinogeniculate
afferents occurs well before birth in both monkey and cat (Rakic,
1976; Shatz and Kliot, 1982). Whether spontaneous neuronal activity
plays a role in these processes remains an intriguing question.
Certainly, functional retinogeniculate synapses are found in the cat
prior to terminal segregation (Shatz, Kirkwood and Siegel, 1982)
and the involvement of spontaneous activity has been postulated in
models of orientation column formation (Von der Malsburg and Cowan,
1982; and see Swindale, 1982c). If this is the case, then obviously
the effects of visual experience reflect mechanisms operating earlier
in development.

REFERENCES

Albus, K., 1979, ^{14}C-Deoxyglucose mapping of orientation subunits
    in the cats visual cortical areas, Exp. Brain Res.,
    37:609-613.
Blakemore, C. and R.C. Van Sluyters, 1975, Innate and environmental
    factors in the development of the kitten's visual cortex,
    J. Physiol., 248:663-716.
Bonds, A.B., 1979, Development of orientation tuning in the visual
    cortex of kittens. In Freeman, R.D., ed. "Developmental neuro-
    biology of vision", pp. 31-49 (Plenum, New York).
Derrington, A.M. and A.F. Fuchs, 1981, The development of spatial
    frequency selectivity in kitten striate cortex, J. Physiol.,
    316:1-10.
Durham, D., T.A. Woolsey and L. Kruger, 1981, Cellular localization
    of 2-[^{3}H]deoxy-d-glucose from paraffin-embedded brains,
    J. Neurosci.,1:519-526.
Fregnac, Y. and M. Imbert, 1978, Early development of visual
    cortical cells in normal and dark-reared kittens: relationship
    between orientation selectivity and ocular dominance,
    J. Physiol., 278:27-44.
Hendrickson, A.E. and J.R. Wilson, 1979, A difference in [^{14}]deoxy-
    glucose autoradiographic patterns in striate cortex between
    Macaca and Saimiri monkeys following monocular stimulation,
    Brain Res., 170:353-358.

Hendrickseon, A.E., S.P. Hunt, and J-Y. Wu, 1981, Immunocytochemical localization of glutamic acid decarboxylase in monkey striate cortex, Nature, 292:605-607.

Horton, J.C. and D.H. Hubel, 1981, Regular patchy distribution of cytochrome oxidase staining in primary visual cortex of macaque monkey, Nature, 292:762-764.

Hubel, D.H., 1982, Exploration of the primary visual cortex, 1955-1978, Nature, 299:515-524.

Hubel, D.H., T.N. Wiesel and M.P. Stryker, 1978, Anatomical demonstration of orientation columns in macaque monkey, J. Comp. Neurol., 177:361-380.

Hunt, S.P., 1982, GABA produces excitement in the visual cortex, Trends in Neurosci., 5:101-102.

Kennedy, C., M.H. Des Rosiers, O. Sakurada, M. Shinohara, M. Reivich, H.W. Jehle and L. Sokoloff, 1976, Metabolic mapping of the primary visual system of the monkey by means of the autoradiographic [14]-deoxyglucose technique, Proc. Natl. Acad. Sci USA, 73:4230-4234.

LeVay, S., M.P. Stryker and C.J. Shatz, 1978, Ocular dominance column and their development in layer IV of the cat's visual cortex:a quantitative study, J. Comp. Neurol., 179:223-244.

LeVay, S., T.N. Wiesel and D.H. Hubel, 1980, The development of ocular dominance columns in normal and visually deprived monkeys, J. Comp. Neurol., 191:1-51.

Livingstone, M.S. and D.H. Hubel, 1981, Effects of sleep and arousal on the processing of visual information in the cat, Nature, 291:554-561.

McLean, I.W. and P.K. Nakane, 1974, Periodate-lysine-paraformaldehyde fixative: a new fixative for immunoelectron microscopy, J. Histochem. Cytochem., 22:1077-1083.

Movshon, J.A. and R.C. Van Sluyters, 1981, Visual neural development, Ann. Rev. Psychol., 32:477-522.

Rakic, P, 1976, Prenatal genesis of connections subserving ocular dominance in the rhesus monkey, Nature, 261:467-471.

Schoppmann, A. and M.P. Stryker, 1981, Physiological evidence that the 2-deoxyglucose method reveals orientation columns in cat visual cortex, Nature, 292:574-576.

Shatz, C.J. and M. Kliot, 1982, Prenatal misrouting of the retinogeniculate pathway in Siamese cats, Nature, 300:525-529.

Shatz, C.J. and M.P. Stryker, 1978, Ocular dominance columns in layer IV of the cat's visual cortex and the effects of monocular deprivation, J. Physiol., 281:267-283.

Shatz, C.J., S.H. Lindstrom and T.N. Wiesel, 1977, The distribution of afferents representing the right and left eyes in the cat's visual cortex, Brain Res., 131:103-116.

Shatz, C.J., P.A. Kirkwood and M.W. Siegel, 1982, Functional retinogeniculate synapses in fetal cats, Soc. Neurosci. Symp., 12:815.

Sherk, H. and M.P. Stryker, 1976, Quantitative study of cortical orientation selectivity in visually inexperienced kitten, J. Neurophysiol., 39:63-70.

Silverman, M.S., 1982, The developmental topography of ocular dominance columns in the cat striate cortex, Soc. Neurosci. Abs., 8:3.

Singer, W., 1981, Topographic organization of orientation columns in the cat visual cortex: a deoxyglucose study, Exp. Brain Res., 44:431-436.

Singer, W., B. Freeman and J. Rauschecker, 1981, Restriction of visual experience to a single orientation affects the organization of orientation columns in cat visual cortex: a study with deoxyglu-cose, Exp. Brain Res., 41:199-215.

Sokoloff, L., M. Reivich, C. Kennedy, M.H. Des Rosiers, C.S. Patlak, K.D. Pettigrew, O. Sakurada and M. Shinohara, 1977, The [14]deoxyglucose method for the measurement of local cerebral glucose utilization: theory, procedure, and normal values in the conscious and anesthetized albino rat, J. Neurochem., 28:897-916.

Stryker, M.P., 1981, Late segregation of geniculate afferents to the cat's visual cortex after recovery from binocular impulse blockade, Soc. Neurosci. Abs., 7:842.

Swindale, N.V., 1981, Absence of ocular dominance patches in dark-reared cats, Nature, 290:332-333.

Swindale, N.V., 1982, The development of columnar systems in the mammalian visual cortex: the role of innate and environmental factors, Trends in Neurosci., 5:235-240.

Swindale, N.V., 1982, The effects of restricted visual experience on the development of ocular dominance patches in the cat, Soc. Neurosci. Abs., 8:296.

Swindale, N.V., 1982, A model for the formation of orentation columns, Proc. Roy. Soc. B., 215:211-230.

Thompson, I.D., M. Kossut and C. Blakemore, 1983, The development of orientation columns in cat striate cortex revealed by 2-deoxyglucose autoradiography, Nature, in press.

Tootell, R.B., M.S. Silverman and R.L. DeValois, 1981, Spatial frequency columns in primary visual cortex, Science, 214:813-815.

Von der Malsburg, C. and J.D. Cowan, 1982, Outline of a theory for the ontogenesis of iso-orientation domains in visual cortex, Biol. Cybern., 45:49-56.

Wiesel, T.N., D.H. Hubel and D.N.K. Lam, 1974, Autoradiographic demonstration of ocular-dominance columns in the monkey striate cortex by means of transneuronal transport, Brain Res., 79:273-279.

Wong-Riley, M., 1979, Changes in the visual system of monocularly sutured or enucleated cats demonstrable with cytochrome oxidase histochemistry, Brain Res., 171:11-28.

MUTATION-INDUCED DISORDERS OF MAMMALIAN FOREBRAIN DEVELOPMENT

Verne S. Caviness, Jr.* and
Alan L. Pearlman

*Director, Southard Laboratory
Eunice Kennedy Shriver Center for Mental
    Retardation, Inc.
Waltham, Massachusetts

+Departments of Neurology and Physiology
Washington University School of Medicine
St. Louis, Missouri

INTRODUCTION

Mutations at more than one hundred single gene loci modify unfavorably the development of the mammalian central nervous system (Sidman, Green and Appel, 1965; Caviness and Rakic, 1978). A few of these appear to involve a relatively small number of cellular events of development. The effect of the mutation may appear to be restricted to a given region or even to a given neural system in some instances. The present review is concerned with three groups of mutations which have particular significance in this way for the development of the forebrain:

1. The reeler mutation, which causes a systematic disorder of neuron position in cortical structures.

2. The tottering mutation, which is associated with an augmentation in cortical innervation derived from the locus ceruleus.

3. A variety of mutations that modify the trajectories of axon fascicles.

The reeler and tottering mutations also affect structures outside the forebrain, in particular the cerebellar cortex. These two

mutants have been observed only in mice. The effects of the third
group are limited to the forebrain or to forebrain and midbrain.
This group comprises a number of mutations affecting the development
of melanin as well as the acallosal mutation. Examples are widely
distributed among mammalian species, including man.

Developmental studies based upon this group of mutants offer
two compelling analytic advantages in comparison to studies based
upon experimental interventions. Firstly, certain critical events
of development altered by mutation are uniquely "dissected" out of
the overall developmental process (Benzer, 1973). With the exception of the acallosal mutant, such "dissections", or phenocopies,
have not been approximated by experimental means of intervention.
Secondly, the consequences of mutation, within a given strain of
animals, are highly characteristic from mutant animal to mutant
animal so that the effect of the mutation is usefully viewed as the
single variable altering the course of development. The effects of
experimental manipulations, by contrast, are in principle highly
variable and, often, difficult to determine. These analytic advantages of studies based upon mutant animals offset, to some extent,
the disadvantage that the molecular mechanism of mutant action is,
in no instance understood.

REELER - A MUTATION EFFECTING NEURON POSITION

Reeler is an autosomal recessive mutation which gives rise to a
generalized cytoarchitectonic anomaly of all cortical structures of
the forebrain (Caviness and Rakic, 1978). The cerebellar cortex is
also gravely malformed (Sotelo, this volume). Those cortical structures of the forebrain which are normally multilaminate, e.g., the
neocortex, piriform cortex and entorhinal cortex, are without laminar
differentiation in the mutant (Caviness and Sidman, 1972, 1973a;
Caviness, 1976a). The pyramidal cell layer of the hippocampal formation, normally uniform and compact, is dispersed and fragmented in
the reeler mutant (Caviness and Sidman, 1973a). The present discussion will consider the cellular events disrupted by the mutation
which lead to neuronal malposition. It will also consider the consequences of cell malposition upon the evolution of neuronal configuration on the one hand and the organization of neural systems on
the other.

NEURON MIGRATION

The neurons which occupy the adult neocortex are generated in a
pseudostratified epithelium (Sauer, 1935; Sauer and Walker, 1959)
which lines the ventricular cavity at the inner surface of the developing cerebrum (Sidman and Rakic, 1973). The majority of neurons
which constitute the cerebral cortex of the mouse are formed between
embryonic day 11 (E11 - here and in subsequent discussion, E0 is the
day of coitus) and embryonic day 17 (E17)(Angevine and Sidman, 1961;

Caviness and Sidman, 1973b; Caviness, 1982). At the completion of
their final divisions the young neurons migrate centrifugally toward
the surface of the cerebrum. The earliest formed cells complete
their migrations by E13 while the last continue their migrations a
day or so beyond the day of birth (PO).

As the earliest formed (E11) cells complete their migrations on
E13, they are distributed diffusely in a non-stratified pattern near
the surface of the cerebral wall. The pattern of cell distribution
at this time is indistinguishable in normal and reeler embryos
(Caviness, 1977, Caviness, Pinto-Lord and Evrard, 1981). Over the
next 24 hours, as the rate of cell arrival increases, the developing
neocortex of the normal animal acquires a trilaminate pattern. The
densely cellular cortical plate (CP) emerges between the plexiform
zone (PZ) above and the subplate (SB) below (Pinto-Lord and Caviness,
1979). During this same 24-hour period a strikingly different stratification plan emerges in the reeler cortex (Pinto-Lord and Caviness,
1979; Caviness, 1982). The superplate (SP), a zone which resembles
the subplate of the normal cortex in that the density of neuronal
somata is relatively low, occupies the most superficial cortical
plane. The cortical plate is immediately subjacent. The CP of the
mutant is relatively wide, extending centrally to the intermediate
zone (IZ), and is subdivided into upper and lower tiers by a plexiform zone (IPZ) which appears at an intermediate cortical level.

Migration and Disposition of Successive Neuronal Cohorts

Dramatic differences characterize the pattern of migration and
disposition of successively formed neuronal cohorts in normal and
reeler genotypes (Figure 1). With the appearance of the CP in the
normal animal, the initial (E11) cohort becomes subdivided into a
small contingent lying superficially within the developing PZ and
another somewhat larger group which becomes located in the SB
(Caviness, 1977, 1982). In reeler, by contrast, neurons of the E11
cohort remain together and retain their positions in the SP at the
most superficial plane of the cerebral wall. Subsequently arriving
cells contribute to the formation of the cortical plate subjacent
to the SP.

Cohorts of neurons generated thereafter, on E12 or later, enter
the CP of both normal and reeler cortex (Caviness, 1982). In the
normal animal, the neurons of successive cohorts bypass positions
held by their predecessors as they ascend all the way to the interface of CP and PZ. At this level migrating cells appear to encounter
an impediment to further outward movement, and their migrations are
halted. In reeler, by contrast, the young migratory neuron appears
to enjoy an unimpeded migratory ascent only while it crosses the intermediate zone. Soon after entering the cortical plate it appears
to encounter an obstruction to further ascent, and its migration is
halted at an anomalously deep position in the cortex (Caviness,1982).

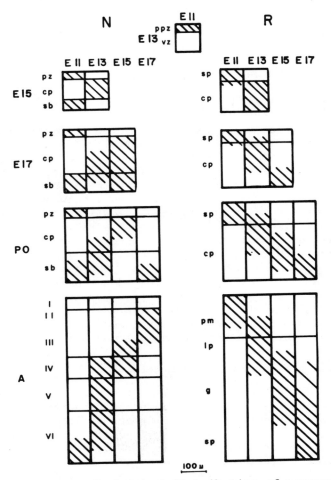

Figure 1. A summary of plots of distribution of neuronal cohorts at successive developmental stages (embryonic days E15, E17; the day of birth, PO) and in the adult (A), in normal (N) and reeler (R) animals. Cross-hatching indicates the zone occupied by the E11-E17 cohorts. Abbreviations: Normal - pz, plexiform zone; cp, cortical plate; sb, subplate; I-VI, cortical layers. Reeler - sp, super-plate; cp, cortical plate, pm, lp, g, sp, zones of polymorphic, large pyramidal, granule and small pyramidal cells. (From Caviness, 1982. Reprinted with permission).

In both normal and reeler cortex the post-migratory cell be-comes fixed in position at the termination of its migration, retaining indefinitely its position relative to other post-migratory

elements. Thus, successively generated cohorts are distributed to
and maintain complementary positions in the radial dimension of the
cortex (Caviness and Sidman, 1973b; Caviness, 1982). The differences
in the migratory path in the two genotypes thus leads in the normal
animal to an "inside-out" but in reeler an "outside-in" relationship between the sequence of migration and the radial order of
intracortical position.

Neuronal Migration and the Radial Glial Fiber

The young, post-migratory neuron is not attached to either the
ventricular or pial surface during its migratory ascent. In relation to its size, the distance of migration across the complex
terrain of the cerebral wall is great and becomes increasingly so
toward the latter days of the migratory epoch (Sidman and Rakic,
1973). The young neuron appears to be critically dependent for
guidance in this journey upon the assistance of a non-neuronal cell
class, the "radial glial cell" (Rakic, 1971, 1972). The somata of
the radial glial cells are located in or adjacent to the ventricular
zone. An elongated process, the radial glial fiber(RGF), ascends
from the soma to the outersurface of the cerebrum where its distal
expansions contribute to the glial limiting membrane.

The young, post-mitotic neuron assumes a fusiform configuration
with a radially extended leading process closely applied to the surface of the radial fiber (Rakic et al., 1974). In the normal animal,
the migrating cell is able to interpose its leading process between
the surface of the fiber and all post-migratory elements which it
encounters (Figure 2). It maintains close apposition to the fiber
throughout its ascent to the outermost level of the CP. Only in the
terminal segment of its ascent and in the subsequent phase of rapid
dendritic growth and cell differentiation as a post-migratory cell
does it surrender all but minimal contact with its guiding radial
fiber (Pinto-Lord, Evrard and Caviness, 1982).

In reeler the relationship of migrating cell and radial glial
fiber is normal as the cell crosses the intermediate zone. Upon
entry into the lower level of the cortical plate, however, the cell
appears unable to interpose its leading process between the surface
of the fiber and post-migratory elements (Figure 3; Pinto-Lord,
Evrard and Caviness, 1982). The leading process becomes blunted
and branched. Multiple neurites then sprout from the soma of the
cell and insinuate themselves into the interstices between
neighboring postmigratory neurons.

Thus arrested in its migration, the young neuron retains an
extensive contact with the surface of the radial glial fiber in the
mutant. This stands in contrast to the minimal contact retained
between the post-migratory cell and the surface of the fiber in the
normal animal. Subsequently arriving cells, in turn, are unable to

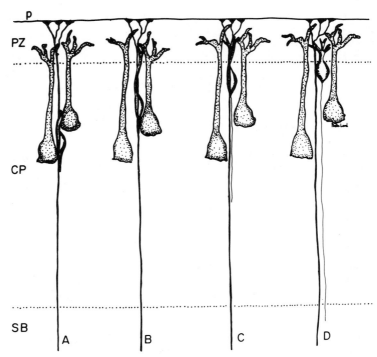

Figure 2. Schematic representation of the terminal phases of migration (A-D) of a young neuron (darkly shaded) in the normal cortex.
Postmigratory neurons (stippled) have minimal contact with the radial
glial fiber (RGF) and are readily displaced from its surface by the
leading process of the migrating cell. After the leading process
enters the plexiform zone (PZ) and begins to branch (B,C), the young
neuron also becomes largely disengaged from the RGF. At or near the
termination of migration an axon is observed to descend from the
inferior pole of the young neuron (C,D). Abbreviations: pz, plexiform zone; cp, cortical plate; sb, subplate. (From Pinto-Lord,
Evrard and Caviness, 1982. Reprinted with permission.)

displace the young neuron from the fiber and are similarly obstructed
from further upward migration. This set of observations, assembled
from combined Golgi-EM analyses (Pinto-Lord, Evrard and Caviness,
1982), suggests that the normal pattern of migration depends critically upon a change in adhesive affinity between the surface of the
radial glial fiber and that of the young neuron as the latter
switches from a migrating to a post-migratory state. In the normal
animal there is, apparently, a dramatic decrease in this affinity
which fails to occur in the mutant animal.

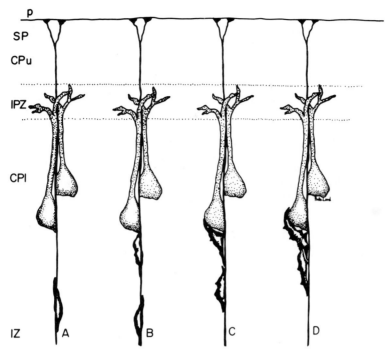

Figure 3.   Schematic representation of the terminal phases of migration (A-D) in the neocortex of reeler. The migrating neuron (dark
shading) ascends the radial glial fiber (RGF) normally until it encounters postmigratory cells (stippled) in CPl. The postmigratory
neurons have an abnormally extensive contact with the RGF. The
leading process of the migrating neuron becomes deflected away from
the RGF (B,C). A young neuron, fixed in position, gives rise to
multiple somatic sprouts (D). A second neuron ascending the same
RGF similarly becomes impacted against its predecessor (B-D).
Abbreviations: sp, superplate; cpu and cpl, upper and lower tiers
of the cortical plate; ipz, intermediate plexiform zone. (From
Pinto-Lord, Evrard and Caviness, 1982. Reprinted with permission).

CORTICAL DEVELOPMENT AND NEURON POSITION

     Neurons of the reeler neocortex are distributed to positions
with respect to their time of origin and migration which are systematically the inverse of those held by their normal counterparts.
Thus, as seen from the foregoing discussion, the neurons in the
mutant neocortex are "outside-in" while those of their normal
counterparts are "inside-out" with respect to time of origin. The
succeeding discussion will consider the consequences of this
systematic perturbation of cell position upon neuron configuration
and neural systems organization.

Cell Configuration

Neuron Form in the Adult Reeler

The normal and reeler neocortex contain the same broad morphological classes of neurons when considered from the perspective of
general cell stains (Caviness, 1976a, 1977). The relative positions
of corresponding classes is, however, systematically inverted in the
two genotypes (Figure 4). Polymorphic neurons, neurons varying
widely in shape and size, occupy the deepest neocortical layer (VI)
of the normal animal but the most superficial neuronal zone of the
mutant neocortex. A wide field of pyramidal cells extends superficially from the polymorphic cell zone to the external plexiform,
or molecular layer, of the normal animal and from the polymorphic
cell zone deeply to the central white matter of the mutant. In the
normal animal the largest of these are located deeply (layer V)
while medium and smaller pyramidal cells occupy successively more
superficial positions (layers III and II). In reeler, by contrast,
the largest of the pyramidal cells lies superficially just below
the polymorphic cell zone while the medium and small pyramids are
located in the depths of the cortex. In both genotypes, the granular
(stellate) cells are located at an intermediate cortical level inter-
calated between large and medium-sized pyramidal cells. In the
normal animal the stellate cells constitute the principal neuronal
population of layer IV.

The somatic size, configuration and staining properties of
these different neuronal classes appear essentially identical in the
two genotypes (Caviness, 1976b). If the details of cell configuration in the two genotypes are compared by Golgi impregnation, however, similarities and differences are apparent. In both normal and
reeler neocortex there is a similar spectrum of spine-bearing and
non spine-bearing forms. Among the former, pyramidal cells bear
characteristic apical as well as basal dendrites in the mutant.
Uncharacteristically, many are inverted in their polarity, and this
is particularly the case with respect to large pyramidal cells
located superficially and the medium-sized and small pyramidal
cells near the inferior margin of the cortex. Collaterals of the
apical dendrites as well as basal dendrites appear to be more than
normally abundant. Occasional pyramidal cells may be obliquely or
horizontally rather than radially aligned (Pinto-Lord and Caviness,
1979). Further, a substantial number of neurons with dendritic and
spine texture essentially the same as that of pyramidal cells are
more nearly bipolar or stellate than pyramidal in configuration.

As in the normal animal, axons of pyramidal neurons exit from
the cortical sector of origin in the mutant (Caviness, 1976b, 1977).
Some do this in reeler by descending radially from the cell body and
others by ascending to a fiber stratum just below the pial surface.

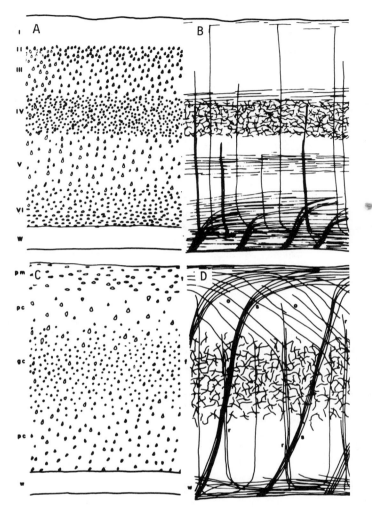

Figure 4. Schematic representation of cell and fiber patterns in the neocortex of normal (A and B) and reeler (C and D) mice. Roman numerals refer to the cortical laminae in the normal animal. The polymorphic cell zone (pm) lies superficially in the mutant cortex. Granule cells (gc) are concentrated at an intermediate level within the pyramidal cell zone (pc). (From Caviness, 1977. Reprinted with permission.)

The intracortical distribution of collaterals of these axons observes the same neuronal class affinities as those in the normal animal; collaterals of axons of medium-sized and small pyramidal cells ramify among the large pyramidal cells and may follow remarkable, anomalous

ascending trajectories to achieve this conjunction. Collaterals of
axons of large pyramidal cells ramify most richly at the level of
the cortex occupied by the cell body of origin of the axon. Spiny
stellate cells, typical of the dominant neuronal population of layer
IV of the normal neocortex, are also abundant at the mid-cortical
level of the mutant. As in the normal animal, the axonal arborization of this "interneuron" species is essentially confined to the
mid-cortical level.

Developmental Modulation of Pyramidal Cell Configuration

During the early phases of cortical development, dendrites
appear to grow only towards and within axon strata in both normal
and reeler neocortex (Pinto-Lord and Caviness, 1979). The different
positional relationships of postmigratory neurons with respect to
axon strata in normal and reeler neocortex are associated with dramatic differences in the configuration and the alignment of neurons
(Fig. 5). In the normal animal, for example, there is uniformity in
the positional relationships of the postmigratory pyramidal cell and
the principal early axonal strata of the molecular layer and the SB.
Thus, the pyramidal cell completes its migration with its leading
migratory process directed into the molecular layer. Its soma eventually comes to lie within the SB. The apical dendrite, realized by
transformation of the leading migratory process, ascends and develops
within the molecular layer while dendrites emerging from the cell
soma expand within the SB.

In reeler, by contrast, the apical dendrite may ascend or descend to the IPZ, depending upon the position of the cell soma with
respect to this fiber stratum (Fig. 5; Pinto-Lord and Caviness,
1979). On the other hand, if the cell soma is bracketed by the IPZ
and an ascending plexiform plane, the neuron may have two major polar
dendritic systems ascending and descending to thse respective axonal
strata. Finally, a cell fully confined within the IPZ appears to
achieve a stellate configuration with multiple dendrites radiating
in a spherically symmetric fashion from the soma into the surrounding axonal bed.

Connections

Despite the anomalies of cell positon in the cortical structures
of the forebrain of reeler, regional variations in the appearance of
neurons as well as their relative abundance and packing density are
closely parallel in normal and mutant cerebrum. A common cytoarchitectonic map may, therefore, be used for study of neural systems
organization in both genotypes. Comparative surveys of the principal
afferent and efferent connections of these forebrain cortical structures indicate that systems organization is essentially normal in
reeler (Devor, Caviness and Derer, 1975; Caviness and Yorke, 1976;
Caviness, Frost and Hayes, 1976; Stanfield, Caviness and Cowan,

1979; Caviness and Korde, 1981; Caviness and Frost, 1982). This generalization will be illustrated from the point of view of neocortical connections.

Efferent Projections of the Neocortex

Studies based upon retrograde transport of HRP indicate that homologous neurons in normal and reeler neocortex give rise to corresponding neocortical projections (Caviness, 1977; Simmons, Lemmon and Pearlman, 1982; Ivy, Caviness and Killacky, unpublished). Thus, in both genotypes polymorphic neurons are the source of the corticothalamic while large pyramidal cells give rise to subdiencephalic projections. Callosal connections of both normal and reeler neocortex arise principally from medium-sized and small pyramidal cells though the system also receives small contributions from polymorphic and large pyramidal cells.

Not only do corresponding systems arise from homologous cell classes, but the distribution of efferent neurons with respect to the neocortical cytoarchitectonic map are also normal in the mutant indicating that efferent systems organization is identical in the two genotypes (Fig. 6; Yorke and Caviness, 1975; Caviness and Yorke, 1976; Ivy, Caviness and Killackey, unpublished). Thus, in normal and reeler animals the callosal projection arises from a large area of the cortex but with a particularly heavy concentration of neurons of origin of this system at the 17-18a cytoarchitectonic border, corresponding to the vertical midline of the visual representations, and along the 1-3 border, corresponding to the trunk and proximal extremity of the SI representations. The spinal projection arises from respective regions of the SI, SII and MI cortical representations. Cortico-cortical connections within the same hemisphere are formed in reciprocal fashion between striate cortex (area 17) and the several representations of the visual field in extrastriate cortex (areas 18a and 18b). In both normal and reeler these interconnections are made with great precision; cortical zones representing particular points in the visual field are connected to zones in other visual areas that represent the same part of the visual field (Simmons, Lemmon and Pearlman, 1982). The cortico-tectal outflow receives contributions from the majority of fields. Only a few fields at the margin of the neocortex do not project to the tectum, and these are the same in both genotypes.

Neocortical Afferent Projections

The principal neocortical afferents of extrinsic origin arise in the thalamus and the opposite hemisphere. Axons of the reeler callosal projection descend radially from neurons of origin to the central white matter to decussate normally in the corpus callosum (Caviness and Yorke, 1976). As in the normal animal the distribution of axons in the contralateral hemisphere of reeler is homotopic with

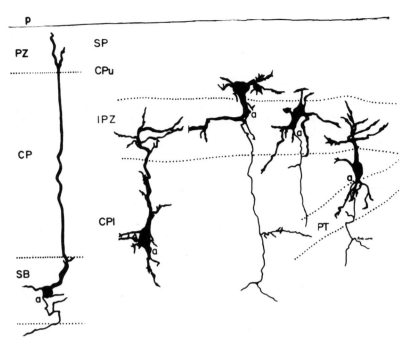

Figure 5.   Dendritic arborization with respect to axonal strata in
the developing normal (A) and reeler (B) neocortex.   In the normal
animal, the relationship of postmigratory cell to axonal strata is
uniform.   The apical dendrite ascends to branch within the plexiform
zone (PZ); somatic dendrites sprout into the subplate (SB).   The
relationship of postmigratory cell to axonal strata is varied in the
mutant.   Polar dendritic systems may ascend (1) or descend (2) to
the intermediate plexiform zone (IPZ).   Where the cell is bracketed
between two plexiform zones (4) it may direct a polar dendritic
system to each.   Where the cell lies within a plexiform zone (3),
dendrites issue radially from the cell soma.   In both genotypes,
axons (a) descend.   (From Caviness, Pinto-Lord and Evrard, 1981
Reprinted with permission.)

the distribution of cells forming the efferent system (Yorke and
Caviness, 1975; Caviness and Yorke, 1976).   In both genotypes axons
ascend radially into target cortical zones.   They terminate most
densely with respect to medium-sized and small pyramidal cells,
located in layers II and III of the normal but in the depths of the
mutant cortex.   A substantially weaker projection is distributed
among homologous cell populations of the infragranular zone of the
normal and the supragranular zone of mutant cortex.

The thalamocortical axons ascend as components of large fiber fascicles which extend between cortex and subcortical structures in both genotypes (Caviness, Frost and Hayes, 1976; Caviness and Frost, 1982). In the normal animal these axons enter and course through a fiber stratum which traverses the zone of polymorphic cells in the depths of the cortex. In the mutant, by contrast, the thalamocortical axons follow an anomalous course as components of sigmoid shaped fascicles which cross the full width of the cortex. As in the normal animal the axons of the reeler thalamocortical projection then course through a fiber stratum located within the polymorphic cell zone until they reach their target fields.

On the basis of differential degrees of divergence as well as different intracortical patterns of distribution, the thalamocortical projection of reeler, like that of normal animal, appears to be formed of two broad axonal classes (Frost and Caviness, 1980; Caviness and Frost, 1982). Terminals of the less divergent class I system are concentrated in tiers which overlap, in part, zones occupied by stellate, medium-sized pyramidal and polymorphic cells in both genotypes. The more divergent class II system has a diffuse intracortical distribution within the cortex. In the normal animal, depending upon the thalamic nucleus of origin, there may be a concentration of class II terminals in the molecular layer or in layer VI. The class I projection arising from a given thalamic nucleus is distributed to one or more complete cytoarchitectonic fields. Despite the anomaly of axon trajectory and neuron position in reeler cortex, the thalamic nucleus to neocortical field relationships are identical in the two genotypes. In both normal and reeler animals the overall projection is made up of several projections arising continuously from multiple adjacent nuclei and distributed to multiple adjacent fields. These projections each constitute a first-order transformation, since adjacent points within or between these sets of nuclei project to adjacent points within their target fields (Caviness and Frost, 1980, 1982). The ensemble is linked together identically in mutant and normal forebrain as a single second order, non-topologic transformation since in some instances adjacent thalamic nuclei project to fields which are separated from each other (Caviness and Frost, 1980, 1982).

Physiologic Properties of Cortical Neurons

Neurons of the normal visual cortex have distinctive functional characteristics that are determined by the complex set of excitatory and inhibitory connections they receive from the thalamus, from other cortical regions and from neurons intrinsic to the cortex. These functional characteristics may be determined by recording from individual neurons while presenting visual stimuli such as bars of light that can be varied in size, orientation, speed of movement and direction. Each cell in the visual cortex responds to stimulation in a particular part of the visual field; that part of the field is

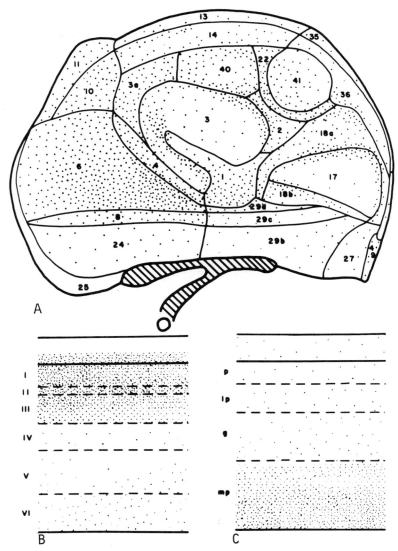

Figure 6.   The distribution of terminals of acallosal axons
(stippling) is projected upon the cytoarchitectonic map of the neocortex of normal and reeler mice (A).   In most cytoarchitectonic
fields of the normal cortex, terminals are most densely concentrated
at the level of the somata of small and medium-sized pyramidal cells
of layers II and III (B).   In the reeler (C), also, they are most
densely concentrated at the level of small and medium-sized pyramidal
cells (mp), but these lie in the depths of the mutant cortex.   (From
Caviness, 1977. Reprinted with permission.)

called the receptive field of the cell, and the stimulus features
that produce a response make up the receptive field properties of
the neuron.

The receptive field properties of individual neurons in area 17
of the normal and reeler mouse have been examined to determine
whether the connections that underlie these properties are established in the mutant despite the abnormality in cell position
(Drager, 1981; Lemmon and Pearlman, 1981; Simmons and Pearlman,
1982). Two sets of cortical neurons have been examined in detail.
In the normal mouse, many of the large pyramidal neurons of layer V
project to the superior colliculus. In reeler, this corticotectal
projection arises from large pyramidal cells that are concentrated
in the outer half of the cortex, although some neurons of this
class are scattered more deeply in the lower half of the cortex.
Corticotectal neurons in area 17 can be identified during physiological recording sessions in both normal and reeler mice by stimulating their axon terminals in the superior colliculus. In the
normal mouse corticotectal neurons have characteristic, large
receptive fields. They respond best to rapidly moving, relatively
small stimuli with very little enhancement of the response as the
stimulus is enlarged. They do not demonstrate either orientation
specificity or direction selectivity (Mangini and Pearlman, 1980;
Lemmon and Pearlman, 1981). The receptive fields of corticotectal
cells in the reeler mouse are indistinguishable from those in the
normal mouse. They have nonoriented, nondirectional receptive
fields with minimal areal summation. They do not differ significantly from normal in their average receptive field size, their
level of spontaneous activity, or their peak velocity sensitivity
(Fig. 7; Lemmon and Pearlman, 1981).

The neurons of area 17 that project to the opposite hemisphere,
although not restricted to a single cortical lamina like the corticotectal cells, can also be identified in both genotypes by
electrical stimulation of their terminals. Many of these neurons
have receptive fields that are tuned for the orientation of the
stimulus and demonstrate directional selectivity. Even these relatively complex and specific receptive field characteristics are not
significantly different in normal and reeler mice (Simmons and
Pearlman, 1982).

TOTTERING - A MUTATION AFFECTING INNERVATION DENSITY

Tottering (tg/tg) is an autosomal recessive mutation associated
with a wide-based ataxic gait and intermittent, focal motor seizures
beginning in the third to fourth week of postnatal life (Sidman,
Green, Appel, 1965; Levitt and Noebels, 1981). The density of locus
ceruleus derived, noradrenergic innervation of the cerebral, hippocampal and cerebellar cortices, the cochlear nuclei and the anterior
hypothalamus is increased by 2-3 times as determined by fluorescing

fiber density and quantitative recovery of norepinephrine (Levitt
and Noebels, 1981). By contrast the noradrenergic innervation
derived from non-locus ceruleus brainstem sources to the posterior
hypothalamus, basal forebrain and brainstem is normal. The increased
innervation density associated with the tottering mutation is
observed in target structures of normal volume (Levitt and Noebels,
1981). The apparent augmentation of axonal arborization in the
mutant is provided by a numerically normal complement of neurons in
the locus ceruleus, and the somatic size of these neurons appears to
be normal (Levitt and Noebels, 1981).

MUTATIONS AFFECTING AXON TRAJECTORY

    The formation of two axon pathways - the callosal decussation
connecting the cerebral hemispheres and the projection of the retina
upon the diencephalon and midbrain - illustrate the vulnerability of
developing axon trajectories to genetic mutation.

The Corpus Callosum

    Decussation of fibers of the corpus callosum first becomes
apparent soon after fusion of the paired cerebral vesicles between
the apposed septal regions rostral to the lamina terminalis (Silver
et al., 1982). In the course of normal development, fusion is
coincident with the formation of a bridging, interhemispheric
structure formed by glial cells which migrate toward each other from
proximate portions of the medial ependymal zones (Silver et al.,
1982). In the mouse this "glial sling" becomes established between
E14-15; lead fibers of the corpus callosum begin to fasciculate
along the medial margins of the hemisphere below the developing neocortex by E15 and to cross in large numbers by E17. Throughout the
period of crossing, early formed fibers invariably are interposed
bewtween their predecessors and the glial surface. Within 24 hours,
however, the rostrocaudal extent of axonal crossing far exceeds the
rostrocaudal extent of the sling; beyond P3, the sling is no longer
present.

    The callosal commissure is defective in approximately 30% of
adult animals of the BALB/cCF strain (Silver et al., 1982). The
phenotype observed in these animals approximates closely an acallosal condition transmitted by autosomal recessive inheritance in a
variety of species including man. In the mutant mouse, it has been
observed that septal fusion is delayed at least as late as E15-16,
and the interhemispheric fissure appears to contain clumped or
"tumor-like" mesenchymal tissue and hematomas. A glial sling is
not established. Callosally directed axons do not cross. Instead,
they are routed into a large fiber fascicle (Probst's bundle) which
follows a rostro-caudal trajectory subjacent to the cingulate
bundle in all mutant acallosal animals including the mouse. If the
sling is disrupted by surgical incision in E15 mouse embryos, the

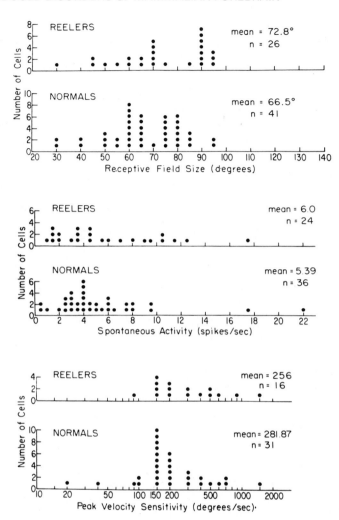

Figure 7. Histograms comparing the properties of identified cortico-tectal cells in the primary visual cortex (area 17) of the normal mouse with those from the reeler mutant. (From Lemmon and Pearlman, 1982. Reprinted with permission.)

acallosal condition, including Probst's bundle, is closely repro-duced in the resulting malformation.

The Retinal Projection

The eye develops as a vesicular evagination of the basal dien-cephalon (Silver and Sapiro, 1981; Silver and Robb, 1979; Silver and

Hughes, 1970). As the wall of the primary vesicle approximates the
ectoderm, the lens is induced in the latter. Subsequently, the
optic vesicle becomes ventrally invaginated to form the secondary,
or ocular, vesicle. Its ventral aspect is destined to become the
retina; subsequent, early stages of retinal development are induced
by reciprocal interaction with the developing lens. The dorsal
aspect of the vesicle is destined to become the pigment epithelium.
A sagitally aligned, ventral continuity of the ocular vesicle, the
ventral fissure, persists for a time in the optic stalk, but this
ultimately fuses.

From approximately E9.5-10.5 in mice and rats, pigment forms
rapidly in the dorsal aspect of the vesicle from where it spreads
centripetally along the dorsal aspect of the stalk for approximately
half of its length (Silver and Sapiro, 1981). The pigment formed in
the retinal primordium persists into adult life; the pigment formed
in the stalk, by contrast, is extruded or degenerates in the course
of prenatal development.

The dominant cellular population of the developing retinal
primordium is probably glial, in that many cells contain immunohisto-
chemically demonstrable glial fibrillary acidic protein (see
Atinitis, quoted in Silver and Robb, 1979). In the course of normal
retinal development, cell death is conspicuous in this cellular
population, in particular in the region of the ventral retinal primordium corresponding to the central retina and its continuity with
the optic stalk (Silver and Sidman, 1980). As cell death proceeds,
intercellular spaces, about 3 microns or greater in diameter, appear
between cells. As the spaces become more numerous, they appear to
become registered in the centripetal sense so as to form "channels"
which lead from the retina into the stalk.

Within 24 hours, at approximately E11.5, the earliest pioneer
fibers proceed centripetally, gathered in fascicles which course
through these channels. The earliest fibers, arising in the dorsal
central retina, proceed to the ventral midline of the stalk. Successively arising axons maintain their left and right positions in
the stalk relative to those in the center; more distally arising
late-comers pass between their predecessors and the glial limiting
membrane so that central to peripheral, tangential dimensions of the
retina are transformed to a central to peripheral relationship in
the radial dimension of the stalk. Upon reaching the diencephalon,
the majority of axons decussate. In the adult mouse, for example,
more than 80% of the projection to the lateral geniculate nucleus
and more than 90% of that to the superior colliculus is derived from
the contralateral retina (Drager and Olsen, 1980).

Two mutations recognized in mice are associated early in development with decreased cell death and little or no formation of
channels; both eventuate in aborted ocular development. The more

profoundly abnormal of the two, the anophthalmic mutation (strain
zrct, an) is associated with incomplete approximation of ectoderm
and primary vesicle which appears to be consequent to anomalous survival of interposed mesenchymal cells (Silver and Hughes, 1979).
Lens induction is incomplete or does not occur in the mutant.
Retinal development is aborted, and the eye degenerates by E16 in
the majority of mutant animals.

In the ocular retardation mutant (or^J) cell death proceeds
more slowly than normally in the posterior central retina, and the
formation of spaces and channels between the neuroepithelial cells
in this part of the retina is less conspicuous than in the course
of normal development (Silver and Robb, 1979). Axons emerging from
the retinal ganglion cells do, to some extent, become grouped in
fascicles. Rather than follow an orderly course through the channels into the stalk, many deviate chaotically in random directions,
some forming neuromas in the plane between retina and the primary
vesicle. The result is microphthalmia with rudimentary development
of the optic nerve, and this is associated with involution and
detachment of the retina.

Pigmentary Mutations

Mutations which give rise to abnormalities of retinal pigmenta-
tion are also associated with a reduced ipsilateral retinal projection. The phenomenon has proved general to multiple genetic loci
in a variety of mammalian species which affect melanin production
(LaVail, Nixon and Sidman, 1978). From a survey of 15 different
mutations in mice, involving multiple alleles at the albino locus,
the non-agouti locus and a third, heterogenous group of mutations
affecting the size or other aspects of the formation of retinal
melanosomes, it is apparent that the degree of reduction in the
ipsilateral retinal projection correlates with the total amount of
retinal pigment and tyrosinase activity (LaVail, Nixon and Sidman,
1978).

The albino mouse is an example of this class of mutation induced disorder (Drager and Olsen, 1980). Whereas the retinal zone
in which most ipsilateral projecting neurons are concentrated, a
crescent located inferotemporally, is decreased slightly in area in
the mutant, the number of such cells located outside this crescent
is greater than normal. The aggregate of ipsilaterally projecting
axons is, however, reduced approximately 30%, and the strength of
ipsilateral activation of binocularly driven neocortical neurons is
reduced in the albino animal.

The anomaly of decussation appears to be established from the
earliest phase of development of the retinal projection, as early as
the E11-12 interval in the rat, when "pioneer fibers" begin to enter
the optic stalk (Silver and Sapiro, 1981). At this time, the dorsal

sector of the optic stalk of the normal animal is still pigmented.
The pioneer axons entering the optic stalk are directed ventrally
and appear to avoid the zone occupied by melanin containing cells.
In the albino rat, the stalk is amelanotic (Silver and Sapiro,
1981).   The emergent axons invade the full circumference of the
distal stalk in anomalous fashion, establishing at the outset of
fascicle formation an aberrant topology of distribution of retinal
axons.   The behavior of centripetally growing axons at the chiasm
has not been clarified.   It is not known to what extent the early
misrouting described by Silver and Sapiro (1981) accounts for the
anomaly of decussation in the adult animal.

     Even though the mechanism by which the misrouting of fibers
from the temporal retina of albino animals at the optic chiasm takes
place has not been fully clarified, the misrouting provides an
opportunity to study how the resulting abnormal retinal projection
is handled at subsequent stages of organization of the visual system.
This aspect of the problem has been extensively studied with respect
to the projection of the retinal ganglion cells to the lateral geniculate nucleus in the thalamus (Guillery, 1969), in the projection
of the lateral geniculate to the visual cortex (Hubel and Wiesel,
1971; Guillery and Kaas, 1971) and in the interconnection of the
visual cortex of the two hemispheres (Shatz, 1979).   In each of
these detailed studies the Siamese cat, an example of this class
of pigment mutants, has been the subject of analysis.

     As a consequence of the inversion produced by the optics of
the eye, the nasal visual field projects to the temporal aspect of
the retina, and the temporal field projects to the nasal part of the
retina.   In the mammalian visual system, information from overlapping parts of the visual field of the two eyes is brought together
on one side of the brain.   For example, fibers from the left eye,
representing the temporal visual field (nasal retina), cross in
the optic chiasm and travel to the right lateral geniculate nucleus
(Fig. 8; Shatz and LeVay, 1979).   They are joined in the optic
chiasm by fibers from the right eye that represent the nasal field.
These fibers do not cross in the chiasm; instead they remain on the
same side and terminate in the right lateral geniculate.   The proportion of retinal fibers that remains on the same side is related
to the position of the eyes in the head.   Mammals with laterally
placed eyes, like mice and rats, have only a small overlap in the
visual field representation of two eyes, and thus only a small portion of retinal fibers terminating in the ipsilateral lateral geniculate.   Frontally placed eyes, like those of cats and monkeys,
result in a large overlap in the visual field representation of the
two eyes, and thus a large proportion of retinal fibers (nearly 50%
in monkey and man) that do not normally cross in the optic chiasm.

     Although fibers from the two eyes, representing the contralat-
eral visual field, terminate in the lateral geniculate, they remain

anatomically segregated. In carnivores and primates this segregation takes the form of separate layers for the fibers of each eye.
In the cat there are several such layers (Guillery, 1969), but we
shall be concerned here only with the two prominent dorsal layers,
A and Al. Layer A normally receives a representation of the contralateral visual field arising from the nasal retina of the contralateral eye, while Al receives a representation of the contralateral
field from the ipsilateral eye. These representations are in
register, one above the other, with the midline of the visual field
represented in the medial aspect of the geniculate laminae, and the
remainder of the field represented in precise retinotopic fashion in
each lamina.

The lateral geniculate nucleus of the Siamese cat receives an
abnormal representation from the contralateral eye: fibers from a
portion of temporal retina extending 15-20° from the midline cross
in the chiasm and thus terminate wrongly in the contralateral
lateral geniculate (Fig. 8). These aberrant fibers terminate in the
medial aspect of layer Al on the cells that should instead have
received input from a 15-20° sector of the ipsilateral retina (Fig.
8). The medial aspect of lamina Al thus contains a representation
of a part of the central aspect of the ipsilateral visual field that
is mirror-symmetric about the midline with respect to the representation of the contralateral field in layer A above with which it is
in register. The remainder of layer Al contains a normal, non-
crossed projection of the remaining temporal retina providing a
representation of the corresponding part of the contralateral
peripheral field (Guillery and Kaas, 1971).

The aberrant projection from retina to lateral geniculate is
thus handled in an orderly fashion that appears to take account of
retinal coordinates in matching afferent fibers with geniculate
neurons (Shatz, 1979). Cells in the medial aspect of layer Al
receive input from ganglion cells near the midline of the field,
even though they come from the wrong eye. How then is this abnormal
topographic representation handled in the projection of the lateral
geniculate onto the primary visual cortex, and what information does
the organization of this pathway in Siamese cats provide us for
understanding normal developmental mechanisms?

The primary visual cortex (area 17) of the cat normally receives
afferent fibers from radially registered points in layers A and Al.
The same pattern seems to be followed in the "Midwestern" variety
of Siamese cats (first discovered by Guillery in Madison, Wisconsin)
with the consequence that a given cortical point receives input from
two mirror-symmetric points in the visual field (Guillery and Kaas,
1971). The anomalous input misrouted from the contralateral temporal retina through the geniculate layer Al is apparently suppressed in some unknown manner, since it is not evident in physiological
recordings from single cortical neurons (Guillery and Kaas, 1971).

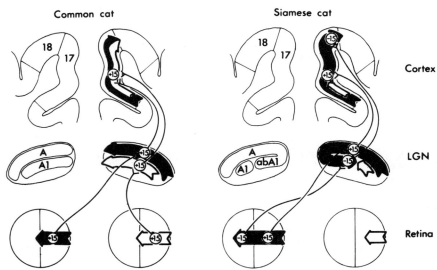

Figure 8.   Diagrammatic representation of the connections between
retina, lateral geniculate, and primary visual cortex (area 17) in
the common cat and the Boston Siamese cat. The contribution from
the left retina is shown by black arrows and from the right retina
by open arrows. Only the projections to the right hemisphere are
indicated. Each retinal representation is divided by a vertical
line that indicates the vertical midline of the visual field. The
locations of neurons with receptive fields 15° contralateral to the
vertical midline of the visual field are represented by the diagrammatic neuron labelled +15, while neurons with receptive fields in
the mirror image location in the ipsilateral field are labelled -15.
The medial aspect of lamina Al (abAl) in the Siamese cat receives
the aberrant, crossed projection representing the ipsilateral field;
the lateral aspect of Al receives the normal, uncrossed projection
representing the remainder of the normal contralateral field.
(From Shatz and LeVay, 1979.   Reprinted with permission.)

        Siamese cats studied in Boston by Hubel and Wiesel (1971) have
a different pattern of cortical organization. Instead of the suppression of the abnormal input that occurs in the Midwestern Siamese
cat, the Boston variety has a representation of the abnormal ipsilateral field crowded into area 17 in an orderly fashion adjacent to the
normal representation of the contralateral field (Hubel and Wiesel,
1971).   The   abnormal ipsilateral field representation in area   17
comes from the medial aspect of layer Al; it is continuous with the
representation   of   the   contralateral field coming from   layer   A
(Fig. 8).   Thus in the Boston Siamese cat some aspect of the retinal
coordinate system may in turn be controlling the   organization   of

the geniculo-cortical pathway, since the result is that adjacent parts of the retina are represented in the cortex in orderly fashion (Shatz, 1979).

In the Boston Siamese cat the abnormal visual field representation in the cortex also affects the interconnections of the visual cortical regions across the corpus callosum. In the normal cat the representation of the midline of the visual field lies along the border between cortical fields 17 and 18 and the 17/18 border is reciprocally interconnected across the corpus callosum. The remainder of fields 17 and 18, including more temporal regions of the visual field representations, by contrast, are sparsely interconnected by the callosal system (Hubel and Wiesel, 1965; Wilson, 1968; Fisken et al., 1975; Shatz, 1977). In the Boston Siamese cat the vertical midline of the visual field, including its system of callosal interconnections, is displaced away from the 17/18 border into a part of field 17 which is normally not interconnected by callosal axons. The callosal interconnections have also been reorganized so that the 17/18 border on one side is not connected with the 17/18 border on the other side but rather with regions well within areas 17 and 18. This reorganization leads to the interconnection of functionally appropriate regions, i.e. regions subserving the same part of the visual field (Shatz, 1977). Connecting the 17/18 border on the two sides would mean connecting points that were in mirror-symmetric parts of the visual field, a result that would seem to be functionally disastrous. The ability to form functionally appropriate connections is not foolproof, however. The 17/18 border apparently also forms connections with zones of area 17 and 18 that represent mirror-symmetric parts of the field (Shatz and LeVay, 1979).

COMMENT

Three morphogenetic events, critical to forebrain development, have been observed to be disrupted among the mutants under review: neuronal migration to the cerebral cortex, axonal decussation to form the corpus callosum and the orderly centripetal growth of axons from the retinal primordium to the basal diencephalon and mesencephalon. Analyses of these developmental events in normal animals identify constant relations between neuronal and glial elements: the migrating neuron with the radial glial fiber, the decussating callosal axons with a glial sling and the orderly course of exiting retinal axons through pre-existing channels within the population of neuro-epithelial cells. One might infer that these cellular associations observed in normal animals reflect critical morphogenetic cellular interactions.

The mutant studies provide complementary observations in support of this inference. In each instance where the developmental event is altered by mutation, there is an associated disruption of the neuron-glial relationship. In reeler the migrating neuron is unable to displace post-migratory cells from the surface of the radial glial fiber as it ascends through lower levels of the developing cortex. The glial sling does not form in the acallosal mutant. Channels do not form in the or^J mutant. The pigment containing "barrier" zone in the dorsal aspect of the distal optic stalk is defective in pigmentary mutants.

Whereas mutant studies and those in normal animals may identify cellular associations critical to morphogenetic events, as yet they provide no insight into the molecular mechanisms which mediate the cellular interactions. However, it is plausible that where these interactions are disrupted by single gene mutation the phenomena are mediated by specific diffusable trophic substances for which the allele in question is the structural gene. Equally plausible, how-ever, is the counter hypothesis that molecular mechanisms disrupted by mutation effect these cellular events in some less-specific way, related, for example, to the metabolic state of one or more critical cell populations or circulating systemic factors that might alter the metabolism of cells.

The cellular events leading to hyper-innervation by the locus ceruleus projection in the tottering mutant have not been identi-fied in developmental studies. The observations, as they stand, are consistent with the view that the terminal arbor of each cell of the locus ceruleus is increased several times without there being an increased size in the soma of the cell. Possibly, as suggested by Levitt and Noebels (1981), the phenomenon is secondary to an action of the mutant gene which directly modifies the cells of the locus ceruleus and is independent of modulating effects of tissue which is target to the projection. The thesis gains support from experiments where target tissues are destroyed either as a consequence of mutant gene action (Landis et al., 1970) or of teratogenic agents in genetically normal animals (Johnston, Grzanna and Coyle, 1979). Under these circumstances the ratio of terminal arbor of the locus ceruleus projection to volume of tissue is substantially increased, indicating that there are no modulating mechanisms providing for a constant ratio of terminal arbor to tissue volume. Obviously such observations do not exclude the existence of trophic factors which might modulate terminal deployment of this noradrenergic system. The seizure disorder in the tottering mutant, for example, also might be secondary to mutation induced anomalies of metabolism in the cells of the target tissue. Tottering is obviously a provoca-tive model for analysis of mechanisms which do control the deploy-ment of monaminergic systems. The model is particularly attractive in that this system is among the earliest yet identified system efferent to the neocortex.

A substantial spectrum of morphogenetic events are disrupted in the mutants under review. It is an arresting realization that other morphogenetic events, perhaps some which are closely related, are unmodified as a consequence of the mutant gene-induced perturbations. Presumably, the latter have a true independence of the former. The most informative relate to the following developmental issue.

Neuronal Lineage and Development

Neurons of the reeler neocortex migrate to and differentiate within positions which are drastically anomalous. Despite this handicap, general features of neuronal configuration as well as patterns of afferent and efferent projection differ little from those of neurons formed simultaneously in genetically normal litter-mates. The general implication of these observations is that attributes of neuronal classes of the neocortex are achieved independently of the milieu in which the cells develop. Conceivably these attributes of neuronal class are consequent to genetically determined events occurring with the terminal division of the cell even prior to cell migration.

Fine details of neuronal form, particularly with respect to the configuration of the dendritic arbor and local patterns of axonal deployment, by contrast, are apparently readily modified by influences exerted by ambient structures. This developmental variation, "noise" as seen from the point of view of genetic regulation, presumably is teleologically advantageous in that it would provide for optimum articulation of interacting elements.

Afferent Projections

In the pigmentary mutants where the ipsilateral to contralateral retinal projection ratios are disordered and in reeler where terminal axon trajectories follow a transcortical course, there is still an orderly topologic transformation of the projecting structure upon its target. Axon fasciculation is essentially normal. In the fore-going mutants as well as tottering, apparently, afferent systems also observe the appropriate boundary markers of their target fields. Within these boundaries they become distributed to the appropriate neuronal classes. In reeler, for example, the thalamo-cortical projection (Class I) of a nucleus not only finds its appropriate target cells in their anomalous positions within the appropriate cortex but is distributed appropriately in a tiered pattern.

Evidently fasciculated axons in these mutants maintain neighbor-hood relationships of their cells of origin, even where the milieu through which the fascicles course is anomalous. That a projection observes boundaries of its target has a dual implication. First there is probably high affinity of the axons of the system for the target neuronal population. Second there may be a capacity to exclude the entry of other systems through competitive mechanisms.

Finally the observations that afferent axons find their appropriate target cells in reeler indicates that axons and cells are
able to communicate with and attract each other through space and
that the mechanism of communication is independent of the milieu.
Whereas the entry of monoaminergic systems has been observed in
embryos, it is evident that this system, at least, enters and seeks
out the appropriate target structures directly and without error.
Whereas axon fasciculation or the registration of axonal systems
and target fields are phenomenon that might be mediated through
surface interactions, axon terminal to target cell conjunction
would seem more readily understood as a consequence of trophic
attractions mediated by diffusable substances.

In each of the mutants reviewed the morphogenetic events which
have proceeded independently of perturbations created by mutation
appear to involve interrelationships of neuronal elements. This may
be simply a matter of coincidence. Thus, the effect of mutations
which alter relationships between neurons may be pleitropic and/or
grave enough to be inconsistent with survival. Those affecting
neuron-glial relationships may be restricted, if specific, or may
act non-specifically because of low threshold vulnerabilities of
glial cells or of neuron-glial interactions. Thus, these studies,
as is generally the case with analyses involving mutants, pose but
have not yet provided tests of the principal organizing hypotheses
of the molecular biology of forebrain development.

REFERENCES

Angevine, J., Jr., and Sidman, R.L., 1961, Autoradiographic study
    of cell migration during histogenesis of cerebral cortex in
    the mouse, Nature, 192:766-768.
Benzer, S., 1973, Genetic dissection of behavior, Sci. Am.,
    229:24-37.
Caviness, V.S., Jr., 1976a, Patterns of cell and fiber distribution
    in the neocortex of the reeler mutant mouse, J. Comp Neurol.,
    170:435-448.
Caviness, V.S., Jr., 1976b, Reeler mutant mice and laminar distri-
    bution of afferents in the neocortex, Exp. Brain Res., Suppl.
    1:267-273.
Caviness, V.S., Jr., 1977, The reeler mutant mouse: a genetic exper-
    iment in developing mammalian cortex, Soc. Neurosci. Symp.,
    2:27-46.
Caviness, V.S., Jr., 1982, Neocortical histogenesis in normal and
    reeler mice: a developmental study based upon [^{3}H] thymidine
    autoradiography, Dev. Brain Res., 4:293-302.
Caviness, V.S., Jr., and Frost, D.O., 1980, Tangential organization
    of thalamic projections to the neocortex in mouse, J. Comp.
    Neurol., 194:335-367.
Caviness, V.S., Jr., and Frost, D.O., 1982, Thalamocortical projec-
    tions in the reeler mutant mouse, submitted for publication.

Caviness, V.S., Jr., Frost, D.O., and Hayes, N.L., 1976, Barrels in somatosensory cortex of normal and reeler mutant mice, Neurosci. Lett., 3:7-14.

Caviness, V.S., Jr., and Korde, M.G., 1981, Monoaminergic afferents to the neocortex: a developmental histofluorescence study in normal and reeler mouse embryos, Brain Res., 209:1-9.

Caviness, V.S., Jr., Pinto-Lord, M.C., and Evrard, P., 1981, The development of laminated pattern in the mammalian neocortex. In: Morphogenesis and Pattern Formation, pp. 103-126, L.L. Brinkley, B.M. Carlson and I.G. Connolly, eds, Raven Press, New York.

Caviness, V.S., Jr., and Rakic, P., 1978, Mechanisms of cortical development; a view from mutations in mice. In: Annual Review of Neuroscience, vol. 1, pp. 297-326, W.M. Cowan, Z.W. Hall, and E.R. Kandel, eds., Annual Reviews, Inc., Palo Alto.

Caviness, V.S., Jr., and Sidman, R.L., 1973a, Retrohippocampal, hippocampal and related structures of the forebrain in the reeler mutant mouse, J. Comp. Neurol., 147:235-254.

Caviness, V.S., Jr., and Sidman, R.L., 1973b, Time of origin of corresponding cell classes in the cerebral cortex of normal and reeler mutant mice: An autoradiographic analysis, J. Comp. Neurol., 148:141-152.

Caviness, V.S., Jr., and Yorke, C.H., Jr., 1976, Interhemispheric neocortical connections of the corpus callosum in the reeler mutant mouse: a study based on anterograde and retrograde methods, J. Comp. Neurol., 170:449-460.

Devor, M., Caviness, V.S., Jr. and Derer, P., 1975, A normally laminated afferent projection to an abnormally laminated cortex: some olfactory connections in the reeler mouse, J. Comp. Neurol., 164:471-482.

Drager, U.C., 1981, Observations on the organization of the visual cortex in the reeler mouse, J. Comp. Neurol., 201:555-570.

Drager, U.C., and Olsen, J.F., 1980, Origins of crossed and uncrossed retinal projections in pigmented and albino mice, J. Comp. Neurol., 191:383-412.

Fisken, R.A., Garey, L.J. and Powell, T.P.S., 1975, The intrinsic association and commissural connections of area 17 of the visual cortex, Philos. Trans. R. Soc. London Biol. Sci., 272:487-536.

Frost, D.O., and Caviness, V.S., Jr., 1980, Radial organization of thalamic projections to the neocortex in the mouse, J. Comp. Neurol., 194:369-393.

Guillery, R.W., 1969, An abnormal retinogeniculate projection in Siamese cats, Brain Res., 14:739-741.

Guillery, R.W., and Kaas, J.H., 1971, A study of normal and congenitally abnormal retinogeniculate projections in cats, J. Comp. Neurol., 143:73-100.

Hubel, D.H., AND Wiesel, T.N., 1965, Receptive fields and functional architecture in two non-striate visual areas (18+19) of the cat, J. Neurophysiol., 28:229-289.

Hubel, D.H., and Wiesel, T.N., 1971, Aberrant visual projection in
    the Siamese cat, J. Physiol. London, 218:33-62.
Johnston, M.V., Grzanna, R., and Coyle, J.T., 1979, Methylazoxymeth-
    anol treatment of feta rats results in abnormally dense nor-
    adrenergic innervation of neocortex, Science, 203:369-371.
Landis, S.C., Shoemaker, W.J., Schlumpf, M., and Bloom, F.E., 1975,
    Catechomalmines in mutant mouse cerebellum: Fluorescence micro-
    scopic and chemical studies, Brain Res., 93:253-266.
LeVail, J.H., Nixon, R.A., and Sidman, R.L., 1978, Genetic control
    of retinal ganglion cell projections, J. Comp. Neurol.,
    182:399-422.
Lemmon, V., and Pearlman, A.L., 1981, Does laminar position
    determine the receptive field properties of cortical neurons?
    A study of cortico-tectal cells in area 17 of the normal mouse
    and the reeler mutant, J. Neurosci., 1:83-93.
Levitt, P., and Noebels, J.L., 1981, Mutant mouse tottering:
    selective increase of locus ceruleus axons in a defined single-
    locus mutation, Proc. Natl. Acad. Sci., 78:4630-4634.
Mangini, N.J., and Pearlman, A.L., 1980, Laminar distribution of
    receptive field properties in the primary visual cortex of the
    mouse, J. Comp. Neurol., 193:203-222.
Pinto-Lord, M.C., and Caviness, V.S., Jr., 1979, Determinants of
    cell shape and orientation: A comparative Golgi analysis of
    cell-axon interrelationships in the developing neocortex of
    normal and reeler mice, J. Comp. Neurol., 187:49-70.
Pinto-Lord, M.C., Evrard, P., and Caviness, V.S., Jr., 1982,
    Obstructed neuronal migration along radial glial fibers in the
    neocortex of the reeler mouse: a Golgi-EM analysis, Dev. Brain
    Res., 4:379-393.
Rakic, P., 1971, Guidance of neurons migrating to the fetal monkey
    neocortex, Brain Res., 33:471-476.
Rakic, P., 1972, Mode of cell migration to the superficial layers of
    fetal monkey neocortex, J. Comp. Neurol., 45:61-84.
Rakic, P., Stensas, L.J., Sayre, E.P., Sidman, R.L., 1974, Computer-
    aided three-dimensional reconstruction and quantitative
    analysis of cells from serial electron microscopic montages of
    foetal monkey brain, Nature, 250:31-34.
Sauer, F.C., 1935, Mitosis in the neural tube, J. Comp. Neurol.,
    62:377-405.
Sauer, M.E., and Walker, V.E., 1959, Radioautographic study of
    interkinetic nuclear migration in the neural tube, Proc. Soc.
    Exp. Biol. Med., 101:557-560.
Shatz, C.J., 1977, Anatomy of interhemispheric connections in the
    visual system of Boston Siamese and ordinary cats, J. Comp.
    Neurol., 173:497-518.
Shatz, C.J., 1979, Abnormal connections in the visual system of
    cats, Soc. Neurosci. Symp., 4:121-141.
Shatz, C.J., and LeVay, S., 1979, Siamese cats: altered connections
    of visual cortex, Science, 204:328-330.

Sidman, R.L., Green, M.C., and Appel, S.H., 1965, Catalog of the
    Neurological Mutants of the Mouse, Harvard University Press,
    Cambridge, Mass.
Sidman, R.L., Rakic, P., 1973, Neuronal migration, with special
    reference to developing human brain: A review, Brain Res.,
    62:1-35.
Silver, J., and Hughes, J.F.W., 1979, The relationship between
    morphogenetic cell death and the development of congenital
    anopthalmia, J. Comp. Neurol., 157:281-302.
Silver, J., Lorenz, S.E., Wahlsten, D. and Coughlin, J., 1982,
    Axonal guidance during development of the great cerebral
    commissures: descriptive studies, in vivo, on the role of
    preformed glial pathways, J. Comp. Neurol., in press.
Silver, J., and Robb, R.M., 1979, Studies on the development of the
    eye cup and optic nerve in normal mice and in mutants with
    congenital optic nerve aplasia, Dev. Biol., 68:175-190.
Silver, J., and Sapiro, J., 1982, Axonal guidance during development
    of the optic nerve: The role of pigmented epithelia and other
    extrinsic factors, J. Comp. Neurol., 202:521-538.
Silver, J., and Sidman, R.L., 1980, A mechanism for the guidance
    and topographic patterning of retinal ganglion cell axons,
    J. Comp. Neurol., 189:101-111.
Simmons, P.A., Lemmon, V., and Pearlman, A.L., 1982, Afferent and
    efferent connections of the striate and extrastriate visual
    cortex of the normal and reeler mouse, J. Comp. Neurol.,
    in press.
Simmons, P.A., and Pearlman, A.L., 1982, Retinotopic organization
    of the striate cortex (ara 17) in the reeler mutant mouse,
    Dev. Brain Res., 4:124-126.
Stanfield, B.B., Caviness, V.S., Jr. and Cowan, W.M., 1979, The
    organization of certain afferents to the hippocampus and
    dentate gyrus in normal and reeler mice, J. Comp. Neurol.,
    185:461-484.
Wilson, M.E., 1968, Cortico-cortical connexions of the cat visual
    areas, J. Anat., 102:375-386.
Yorke, C.H., Jr., and Caviness, V.S., Jr., 1975, Interhemispheric
    neocortical connectons of the corpus callosum in the normal
    mouse: a study based on anterograde and retrograde methods,
    J. Comp. Neurol., 164:233-246.

THE GENERATION OF BINOCULAR MAPS IN THE HAMSTER SUPERIOR COLLICULUS:

NORMAL AND NEONATALLY ENUCLEATED ANIMALS

Ian Thompson

The University Laboratory of Physiology
Parks Road
Oxford, England

ABSTRACT

In the mammalian retinotectal projection, the existence of
direct binocular projections exhibiting congruent binocular receptive
fields requires that the nasotemporal axis of the retina displays
mapping rules of opposite polarity for the crossed and uncrossed
projections. The aberrant ipsilateral retinotectal projection
arising after neonatal removal of one eye has been mapped in the
hamster to investigate possible strategies for determining the normal
differences in mapping polarity. The ipsilateral retinotectal projection in enucleates displays a dual representation which is mirror-
symmetric about the representation of the temporal retinal margin.
In rostral tectum, temporal retina maps with a polarity appropriate
for an uncrossed projection whereas in caudal tectum both temporal
and nasal retina are mapped, with a polarity appropriate for a
crossed projection. Although two mapping polarities are present in
a single projection, neighbour relations are preserved insofar as
adjacent points on the tectum receive input from adjacent points on
the retina. Possible implications of this mapping will be discussed.

The formation of orderly retinotectal connections has occupied
an important place in developmental neurobiology concerned as it is
not only with mechanisms determining the gross trajectory of axons
but also with mechanisms which determine the self-ordering of projections (see chapters by Gaze, Schwarz in this volume). It combines
the problems of target recognition and of pattern formation. Most
experimentation has been done on non-mammalian species which either
have experimentally more amenable developmental stages or display

307

neuronal regeneration. More recently similar questions are being
asked about mammalian retinal projections and insights have been
made into the initial targetting of retinal axons (see chapter by
Rakic).

The mammalian superior colliculus receives direct input from
both contralateral and ipsilateral retinae, unlike the optic tectum
in most non-mammalian species (but see Prasada Rao and Sharma, 1982).
Moreover, a binocularly driven neurone in the superior colliculus
will have receptive fields in the two eyes which have the same
location in visual space. Direct binocular retinal projections raise
two basic problems for the generation of orderly retinal connections.
There is a problem in establishing the line of decussation; in the
rodent superior colliculus, the whole extent of the retina projects
contralaterally but, as the size of the binocular field is less than
the total visual field, only a restricted region of temporal retina
projects ipsilaterally in the adult (Cowey and Perry, 1979; Drager
and Olsen, 1980; Jeffery and Perry, 1982). The other problem
created by binocular vision is that the retinotectal mapping rule
for the nasotemporal retinal axis of the crossed and uncrossed projections must display opposite polarities on the tectum in order to
ensure binocular congruence. This follows because the brain and the
retinae display bilateral symmetry but the visual field does not
(see Thompson, 1979 and Scholes, 1981).

An elucidation of the developmental strategies which determine
these two different mapping rules may well give insight into the way
in which ordered connections are generated. It is interesting that
the problem of binocular representation does raise the possibility
that mapping rules can be dissociated into mechanisms which separately specify the neighbor relations within the map and the polarity of
the mapping: a distinction first made for retinotectal projections
by Hope, Hammond and Gaze (1976) and by Gaze and Hope (1976). Sperry
in his 1963 paper also recognized the problem posed by binocular
representation for the generation of two mappings from one eye. His
solution was to suggest a coordinate system which was symmetrical
about the retinal decussation line. Retinal loci were specified by
a radial coordinate and by a latitudinal (dorsoventral) coordinate
to generate a bilaterally symmetric labelling pattern. While this
coordinate scheme is applicable to retinal projections which demonstrate a sharp hemiretinal decussation pattern (e.g. the cat retinogeniculate projection) it cannot immediately account for a projection
in which the whole eye projects contralaterally and together with a
restricted region which also projects ipsilaterally (e.g. the rodent
and cat retinotectal projection).

A number of strategies can be invoked to produce binocular
mappings. One possibility is functionally dependent matching of the
two projections such that neighbor relations were preserved but in
terms of visual space rather than retinal location. This mechanism

appears to function in the establishment of binocular maps in
Xenopus tectum where the registration of the ipsilateral and
contralatral inputs can be altered by manipulating visual experience, for instance by eye rotations in the light but not in the dark
(see Keating, 1974; Udin and Keating, 1981). However, the ipsilateral retinal input to Xenopus is indirect and the direct ipsilateral
projection to the diencephalon which arises at metamorphosis behaves
in more hard-wired manner (Kennard, 1981). In the rodent, the
initial uncrossed retinotectal projection has a greater retinal extent than in the adult animal and acquires its adult morphology
before the eyes have opened (Land and Lund, 1979; Bunt, Lund and
Land, 1983; Frost, So and Schneider, 1979). However, the early extensive projection can be stabilized by neonatal, or prenatal,
unilateral eye removal (Lund, Cunningham and Lund, 1973; Land and
Lund, 1979). In this chapter, I present retinotopic maps from
adult hamsters which had one eye removed at birth. The expanded
ipsilateral retinotectal projection display a topography quite
different from that observed in the normal animal and may shed some
light on possible strategies employed in generating the normal map.

Retinotopic mapping in the retinotectal projection of normal and
neonatally enucleated hamsters

Adult hamsters were prepared for electrophysiological mapping
as described by Thompson (1979) and Tiao and Blakemore (1976b,c).
Briefly, after cannulation of the femoral vein and of the trachea,
the animals were paralyzed with gallamine triethiodide (35 mg/kg/hr)
and anesthetized with urethane (25 mg/kg/hr) alone or with additional
chloralose (0.16 mg/kg/hr). The corneas were protected with trans-
lucent contact lenses and the optic discs plotted regularly with a
reversing ophthalmoscope. Receptive fields were plotted on a hemispheric dome and the coordinates were translated by the amount
necessary to bring the optic discs to a standard location 54° from
the vertical meridian of the visual field and 25° above the horizontal meridian (Tiao and Blakemore, 1976a). Recordings were made in
the superior colliculus with tungsten-in-glass electrodes (Levick,
1972; Merrill and Ainsworth, 1972) and electrolytic lesions were
made at regular intervals to permit subsequent histological identification of the array of penetrations.

In the normal, pigmented hamster (Mesocricetus auratus) binocular responses are restricted to rostral tectum and the receptive
fields are located in both the ipsilateral and contralateral binocular visual hemifields. A map from a single pigmented hamster is
illustrated in Fig. 1A. The rostral region of the left superior colliculus was mapped carefully for binocular fields and the crossed
projection to the right colliculus was mapped more coarsely. A
comparison of the projection of the two eyes to the left superior
colliculus (the two visual field representations on the left) demonstrates the more extensive crossed input, with the uncrossed input

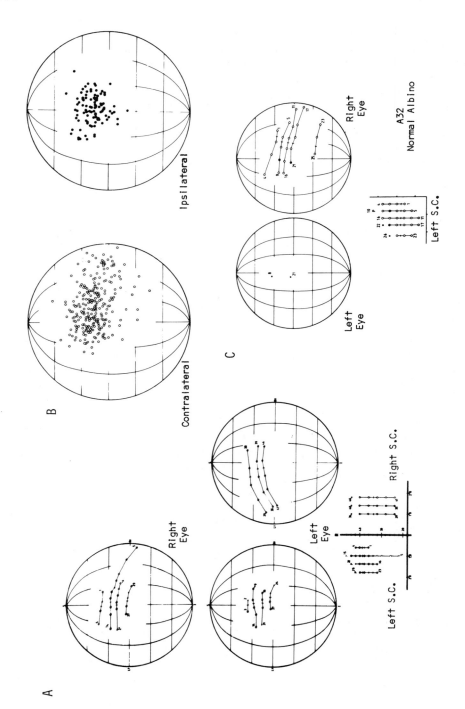

Figure 1. Retinotopic mappings and receptive field distributions in unoperated hamsters. In this figure, as in all the others, the visual field representation uses an axis-vertical coordinate system for the hemisphere whose anterior pole lies directly in front of the animal; the meridians and parallels are shown at 30° intervals. A. Retinal projections to both superior colliculi in a normal pigmented hamster. The projection of the left eye was mapped in both colliculi and the projection of the right eye was mapped in the left (contralateral colliculus). Receptive fields in both eyes recorded on penetrations into the binocular segment of left superior colliculus move together in visual space, thus preserving binocular congruence. Thus, for a rostrocaudal movement on the tectum, receptive fields in the left eye move in opposite directions in the crossed and uncrossed projections. The grid of penetrations is drawn with respect to the lambda, the distances are in millimeters. B. Pooled distribution of receptive fields recorded on 253 penetrations into the left superior colliculus of 12 normal, pigmented hamsters. Receptive fields recorded through the contralateral eye are shown on the left and the more restricted distribution of fields recorded through the ipsilateral eye (96 penetrations) is shown on the right. C. Retinotopic mapping of the left colliculus in an albino hamster; only two penetrations produced weak, binocular driving.

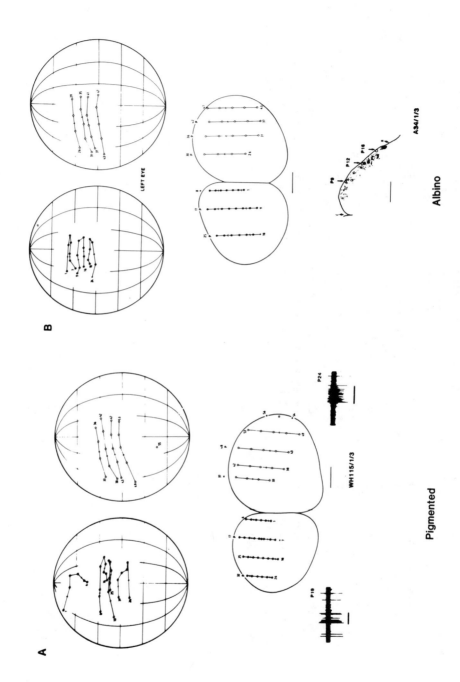

Figure 2. Individual retinotopic maps in the superior colliculi of two neonatally enucleated hamsters. The filled symbols indicate penetrations and corresponding receptive fields in the left, ipsilateral, colliculus and open circles those in the contralateral colliculus. The array of penetrations has been reconstructed from the location of lesions in sectioned material. A. Maps in a pigmented hamster enucleated on the day of birth. The remaining left eye displays an approximately normal map on the contralateral colliculus but ipsilaterally there is a duplicated map in which temporal retina is represented twice but separately. The two oscilloscope traces indicate visual responses recorded on penetrations P12 and P24 which produced receptive fields in similar locations, either side of the reversal. B. Retinotectal maps in an albino hamster which was enucleated on the day of birth. The mapping is essentially the same as that in the pigmented animal. The parasaggital section indicates the distribution of silver grains following injection of the eye with 3H-proline. The location of three lesions are illustrated to demonstrate that the point of reversal in the mapping is situated some distance from the rostral pole of the colliculus.

Tectal scale = 0.5 mm

being restricted to the representation of binocular visual field.
The fields in the two eyes are approximately in register and certainly move together in visual space as electrode location is
changed. This implies that, in nasotemporal retinal coordinates,
the mapping rules for the two eyes are opposite. This can be seen
more directly by comparing the left eye's projection to both the
left and right superior colliculi. As the location of the penetration moves more rostrally, the corresponding receptive field
locations in the left eye move in <u>opposite</u> directions in visual
space.

A cumulative plot of visual receptive locations in several
normal hamster illustrates the differences in visual field representation between the ipsilateral and contralateral projections (Fig.
1B). All recordings were made in the left superior colliculus and
consequently the bulk of the contralateral eye's responses are found
in the right visual hemifield although fields are found up to 35°
into the ipsilateral hemifield. In contrast, responses in the ipsilateral eye are restricted to the central 70° of visual space. It
is of course possible that some of these responses derive from indirect, across-the-midline projections rather than from the direct
uncrossed retinotectal projection. However, preliminary observations reveal that binocular responses persist after lesions of
either the overlying visual cortex or of the contralateral cortex
and superior colliculus. Further, recordings from a few normal
albino hamsters, which possess an anatomically reduced uncrossed
input, also indicated a reduced binocular representation (see
Fig. 1C).

After unilateral eye removal on the day of birth the uncrossed
retinotectal projection in both pigmented and albino hamsters is
greatly expanded (see Fig. 4C-F and Rhoades and Chalupa, 1980).
That this expanded projection maps in a very different way from the
normal projection is demonstrated in Fig. 2 which illustrates
mappings of both colliculi in a neonatally enucleated pigmented
(Fig. 2A) and an albino (Fig. 2B) animal. The maps in the two animals
are very similar which is quite different from the situation in
normal hamsters. The crossed projection to the right colliculus
(open symbols) is essentially normal: nasal retina projects to caudal
tectum and temporal retinal to rostral tectum. The ipsilateral projection is quite different due principally to a double representation
of temporal retina: in both animals the central 60° is represented
twice. The projection is continuous and has a point of reversal
corresponding to the temporal retinal margin, some 30° into the
contralateral visual hemifield. As the electrode is advanced from
caudal to rostral tectum, the corresponding receptive field
locations move first from just outside the binocular field (i.e.
more nasally on the retina) towards the extreme of the left eye's
visual field (i.e. the temporal retinal margin) and then back to
about 30° into ipsilateral visual hemifield (the limit of the ipsi-

lateral eye's representation in the superior colliculus of the
normal animal). The receptive field characteristics are similar in
the two limbs of the mapping except that responses are generally
weaker in caudal tectum. Thus one point in visual space can be
represented by two points on the tectum several hundred microns
apart. For instance, in the pigmented enucleate the receptive
fields recorded on penetrations P19 and P24 (whose neuronal responses are illustrated in Fig. 2A) were within 15° whereas the
tectal locations were separated by 600 µm; this distance corresponds
to a visual field separation of over 40° in the contralateral
superior colliculus. Histological reconstruction confirmed that the
point of reversal in the mapping was well inside the boundaries of
the superior colliculus. The parasagittal section in Fig. 2B indicates the location of three lesions (P12 corresponding to the point
of reversal) with respect to the rostral and caudal borders of the
colliculus. The location of terminal label was also determined in
this animal using axonal transport of ^{3}H-proline and is shown on the
section.

The existence of a reversal in the ipsilateral retinotectal projection was a constant feature of all animals enucleated on the day
of birth and recorded as adults. Since the representation displays
mirror symmetry about the temporal retinal margin, the mapping
polarities of the two components are equivalent to those normally
displayed by the crossed and uncrossed retinal projections. In the
caudal tectum of the enucleated animals, a caudal-to-rostral movement corresponds to a nasal-to-temporal movement on the retina which
is the polarity of the crossed retinotectal projection in a normal
animal, although here the actual tectal location of retinal points
is aberrant. Rostral to the point of reversal, the mapping polarity
is now appropriate for a normal uncrossed projection, and indeed the
positional correspondence is approximately that of the normal uncrossed projection. This mapping pattern, which was consistently
observed in 16 animals, is somewhat different from that reported, in
the enucleated hamster, by Finlay, Wilson and Schneider (1979) and
by Rhoades (1980). In Rhoades' study some animals displayed a
reversal in rostral tectum but most of the mapping was appropriate
for a crossed projection. Some rostrocaudal progressions in the
maps of Finlay et al. displayed two reversals; a pattern which was
observed in this study when the electrode entered pretectum. None
of the studies on the hamster have reported double receptive fields
like those described in the enucleated rat by Cunningham and Speas
(1975) suggesting two superimposed maps.

Some variability between animals was observed in the extent to
which nasal retina was represented in caudal tectum. In some enucleated animals responses could be recorded up to 90° ipsilateral
to the vertical midline, in others caudal responses were restricted
to the binocular visual field. Pooled receptive field locations in
the ipsilateral retinotectal projection of seven enucleated pigment-

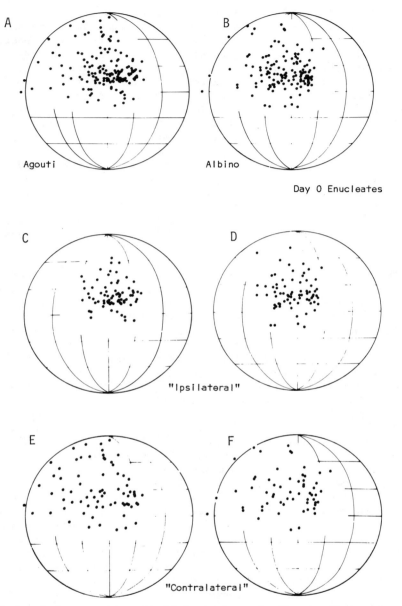

Figure 3. Pooled receptive field locations in the ipsilateral
superior colliculus of hamsters enucleated on the day of birth and
recorded as adults. Data for pigmented hamsters (147 fields in 7
animals) and for albino hamsters (128 fields in 8 animals) are shown
separately. A. and B.   Total distribution of receptive fields, independent of mapping rule in pigmented (A) and albino (B) animals.

ed hamsters and of eight enucleated albino hamsters are shown in
Fig. 3A and 3 respectively. As in Fig. 2, there is little difference between the albino and pigmented strains; receptive fields are
distributed over 120° of visual space, although there is a concentration of fields in what should correspond to binocular visual
field. In addition to the difference in mapping polarity of the two
components of the uncrossed map described above, there is also a
difference in the extent of visual field represented in the two
parts. This is documented in Fig. 3C-F in which receptive field
locations have been plotted separately according to whether they
occurred in that part of the map which mapped with a polarity appropriate for an ipsilateral projection (Fig. 3C,D, rostral tectum) or
with a polarity appropriate for a crossed projection (Fig. 3E,F,
caudal tectum). It is clear that the caudal, "contralaterally"
mapping component originates from a wider region of retina than the
"ipsilaterally" mapping component which is largely restricted to
central, binocular visual field. In fact, the difference between
the two distributions resembles the differences between the actual
crossed and uncrossed projections in the normal animal (Fig. 1B).

    As indicated above, the two limbs of the uncrossed retinotectal
projection occupy different tectal locations in any one animal, with
the retinally restricted "ipsilaterally" mapping rostral to the component which demonstrates a "contralateral" mapping polarity. In
order to examine the regularity of this division, the tectal locations of all electrode placements have been pooled and the result
is shown in Fig. 4A, B. A standard profile was constructed for the
ipsilateral superior colliculus of enucleated hamsters by averaging
the dimensions of several tecta and then scaling the actual locations
of the penetrations so that they occupied the same relative position
in the standard tectum. Figure 4A, B reveals that the tectum can be
divided into three areas. Most rostrally, there is a region in
which the mapping displays the polarity appropriate to an uncrossed
projection and which represents about 60° of retina away from the
temporal margin. In central tectum, the mappings display a "contralateral" polarity and correspond to about 120° of retina. Most
caudally there were very few penetrations, due to the overlying confluence of sinuses, but a higher proportion of penetrations failed
to elicit visual driving.

C. and D. Distribution of receptive fields in the two strains (C,
pigmented; D, albino) in the component of the mapping which demonstrates a mapping polarity appropriate for an uncrossed projection.
E. and F. Distribution of receptive fields in the component of
the mapping appropriate for a crossed projection (E, pigmented;
F, albino).

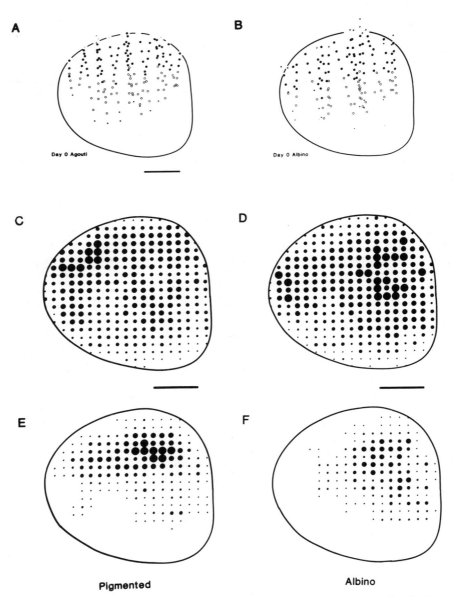

Pigmented   Albino

Figure 4. Tectal location of electrode penetrations and of the distribution of autoradiographic label in the ipsilateral superior colliculus of animals enucleated on the day of birth following injection of ^{3}H-proline into the remaining eye. The tectal profile is an averaged profile generated from several neonately enucleated animals and the location of penetrations or of label in individual

The pooled distributions imply a fairly sharp division between the two parts of the map and suggest that the rostral component of the ipsilateral projection is displaying not only an appropriate mapping polarity but also an approximately correct tectal location. In the normal hamster, the direct uncrossed retinal projection is characterized anatomically by clusters of terminals located deep to the crossed projection. In the enucleated animal the uncrossed projection now extends up to the tectal surface but closer analysis does reveal some deeper label especially in rostral tectum. The distribution of label following intraocular injections of ^{3}H-proline in the ipsilateral superior colliculus is displayed in a semi-quantitative way in Fig. 4C-F. The location and relative density (estimated by eye on a scale of 1-3) was transferred to the standard tectum and averaged across animals, the size of dot indicates the density of label. The uncrossed projection extends over virtually the whole of the ipsilateral colliculus when the superficial 100 μm of the stratum griseum superficiale (approximately the upper half) was examined (Fig. 4C, D). Label in the deeper half was confined to the rostral tectum, especially in the pigmented animal (Fig. 4E, F where it resembles the distribution of uncrossed label in a normal animal. The significance of this observation remains to be investigated. It could simply reflect a higher total density of terminals in rostral tectum so that some terminate in the deeper part of the stratum griseum superficiale. Certainly visual responses in rostral tectum were present in superficial as well as in deep layers and the receptive field location was essentially invariant with depth.

---

animals has been adjusted so that it occupies the same relative position in the standard tectum. A. and B. The location of penetrations in pigmented (A) and albino (B) animals. Filled circles indicate penetrations producing mappings with a polarity appropriate for an uncrossed projection and open circles those appropriate for a crossed projection. C. and D. The distribution of ipsilateral autoradiographic label in the superficial 100 μm of the stratum griseum superficiale averaged over 7 pigmented enucleates (C) and 5 albino enucleates (D). The size of spot correlates with the density of the label. E. and F. The distribution of label in the lower 100 μm of the stratum griseum superficiale in the same 7 pigmented (E) and 5 albino (F) animals.

Tectal scale = 0.5 mm.

Possible implications for binocular mappings in mammalian retinotectal projections

The ipsilateral retinotectal mappings of neonatally enucleated
hamsters presented here displayed a consistent form. The maps were
continuous and bilaterally symmetric about the nasotemporal retinal
axis thus displaying, within a single projection, mapping polarities
appropriate for both a crossed and an uncrossed projection. The
nature of the topography eliminates several possible strategies for
the generation of binocular mappings in the mammalian retinotectal
projection.

Point-to-point chemospecificity provides one such mapping mechanism in which the tectal locations of ipsilaterally and contralaterally projecting cells are separately specified, presumably
together with their laterality i.e. crossed or uncrossed. However
in the aberrant uncrossed projection of these enucleates, the double
representations of temporal retina are separate, not overlapping.
Thus retinal locations are terminating in tectal regions never observed in the normal animal and, as neither retina nor tectum has
been lesioned, tectal regulation is an unlikely possibility. The
existence of two mappings in one projection also eliminates an alternative strategy: that the laterality of the projection somehow
determines the mapping rule i.e. crossed projections always map in
one way and uncrossed projections in another. Neonatal excision of
one eye obviously removes the possibility of binocular vision, consequently it cannot be argued that visual experience is necessary
for the generation of the two mapping polarities evident in the
intact mammalian retinotectal projection. In normal binocular retinal projections, the uncrossed and crossed projections usually
display any laminar differences in their terminations; this is particularly clear in the lateral geniculate nucleus. If the different
laminae also displayed reversed mapping rules together with a label
specific for crossed or uncrossed projections, a binocular mapping
could be achieved. In the enucleates however, retinal fibers terminate outside their normal laminar location and do not display laminar
differences in retinotopicity. Thus in rostral tectum of the enucleated hamster, the location of the retinal projection from the
ipsilateral eye is the same in superifical and deep stratum griseum
superficiale. There does not appear to be any laminar segregation
of the mapping rules.

The observed mapping has two features: it contains two polarities in the representation and yet preserves a continuous mapping
insofar as neighboring tectal regions receive input from neighboring
parts of the retina, although the converse is not true. If the
retina contains two populations of ganglion cells programmed to map
with opposing polarities along the rostrocaudal axis of the tectum,
displaying only a weak positional specificity and a stronger tendency
to maintain neighbor relations, the outcome of inducing both these

populations to terminate on the same tectum may be the observed map. This hypothesis may also give insights into the albino abnormality. If, for some reason, the "ipsilateral" population of cells is mis-routed contralaterally it may behave as if it had gone ipsilaterally. It would project to the ipsilateral lamina of the terminal nucleus and map with the opposite polarity to the rest of the crossed pro-jection. Such an interpretation can be placed on the retinogenicu-late projections in the Siamese cat (Guillery and Kaas, 1971). For the albino hamster, the argument implies that neonatal removal of one eye "rescues" this "ipsilateral" population which in the intact albino would normally be eliminated, although the reason for its elimination remains to be determined.

As an explanation of the generation of binocular maps in the mammalian superior colliculus, the above postulation of two popula-tions of ganglion cells is obviously incomplete. It ignores the observation that the rostral ipsilateral tectum in enucleates contains an essentially normal map. If the expression of a double mapping could be demonstrated to be independent of tectal location, then the idea of two retinal populations differing in their mapping rules would be more attractive. Another problem not explicitly examined is why it is only temporal retina which contains cells displaying a mapping polarity appropriate for an uncrossed projec-tion. More generally, there are dangers in interpreting develop-mental rules from a consideration of the adult state alone. It is hoped that an examination of the development of retinotectal topo-graphy will give further insights into the rules governing the ordering of mammalian retinal projections.

REFERENCES

Bunt, S., R.D. Lund and P.W. Land, 1983, Prenatal development of
     the optic projection in albino and hooded rats. Dev. Brain
     Res., 6:149-168.
Cowey, A., and V.H. Perry, 1979, The projection of the temporal
     retina in rats, studied by retrograde transport of horseradish
     peroxidase, Exp. Brain Res., 35:457-464.
Cunningham, T.J., and G. Speas, 1975, Inversion of anomalous uncross-
     ed projections along the mediolateral axis of the superior
     colliculus: implications for retinocollicular specificity,
     Brain Res., 88:73-79.
Drager, U.C., and J.F. Olsen, 1980, Origins of crossed and uncrossed
     retinal projections in pigmented and albino mice, J. Comp.
     Neurol., 191:383-412.
Finlay, B.L., K.G. Wilson and G.E. Schneider, 1979, Anomalous ipsi-
     lateral retinotectal projections in Syrian hamsters with early
     lesions: topography and functional capacity, J. Comp. Neurol.,
     183:721-740.
Frost, D.O., K.-F. So and G.E. Schneider, 1979, Postnatal development
     of retinal projections in Syrian Hamsters: a study using auto-

radiographic and anterograde degeneration techniques,
    Neuroscience, 4:1649-1677.
Gaze, R.M., and R.A. Hope, 1976, The formation of continuously
    ordered mappings, Prog. Brain Res., 45:327-355.
Guillery, R.W., and J.H. Kaas, 1971, A study of normal and congeni-
    tally abnormal retinogeniculate projections in cats, J. Comp.
    Neurol., 143:73-100.
Hope, R.A., B.J. Hammond and R.M. Gaze, 1976, The arrow model:
    retinotectal specificity and map formation in the goldfish
    visual system, Proc. Roy. Soc. B, 194:447-466.
Jeffery, G., and V.H. Perry, 1982, Evidence for ganglion cell death
    during development of the ipsilateral retinal projection in the
    rat, Dev. Brain Res., 2:176-180.
Keating, M.J., 1974, The role of visual function in the patterning
    of binocular visual connections, Br. Med. Bull., 30:145-151.
Kennard, C., 1981, Factors involved in the development of ipsilateral
    retinothalamic projections in Xenopus laevis, J. Embryol.
    Exp. Morph., 65:199-217.
Land, P.W. and R.D. Lund, 1979, Development of the rat's uncrossed
    retinotectal pathway and its relation to plasticity studies,
    Science, 205:698-700.
Levick, W.R., 1972, Another tungsten micro-electrode, Med. Biol.
    Eng., 10:510-515.
Lund, R.D. and J.S. Lund, 1976, Plasticity in the developing visual
    system: the effects of retinal lesions made in young rats,
    J. Comp. Neurol., 169:133-145.
Lund, R.D., T.J. Cunningham and J.S. Lund, 1973, Modified optic pro-
    jections after unilateral eye removal in young rats, Brain
    Behav. Evol., 8:51-72.
Merrill, E.G. and A. Ainsworth, 1972, Glass-coated platinum-plated
    tungsten micro-electrodes, Med. Biol. Eng., 10:662-672.
Prasada Rao, P.D. and S.C. Sharma, 1982, Retinofugal pathways in
    juvenile and adult channel catfish, Ictalarus (Ameiurus)
    punctatus: an HRP and autoradiographic study, J. Comp. Neurol.,
    210:37-48.
Rhoades, R.W., 1980, Effects of neonatal enucleation on the func-
    tional organization of the superior colliculus in the golden
    hamster, J. Physiol., 301:383-399.
Rhoades, R.W. and L.M. Chalupa, 1980, Effects of neonatal enucleation
    on receptive-field properties of visual neurones in the superior
    colliculus of the golden hamster, J. Neurophysiol.,
    43:595-611.
Scholes, J.H., 1981, Retinal fiber projection patterns in the
    primary visual pathways to the brain. In Laverack, M.S. and
    D.J. Cosens, Eds. "Sense Organs", pp. 255-275 (Blackie, Glasgow
    and London).
Sperry, R.W., 1963, Chemoaffinity in the orderly growth of nerve
    fiber patterns and connections, Proc. Natl. Acad. Sci.,
    50:703-710.

Thompson, I.D., 1979, Changes in the uncrossed retinotectal projection after removal of the other eye at birth, Nature, 279:63-66.

Tiao, Y-C. and C. Blakemore, 1976, Regional specialization in the golden hamster's retina, J. Comp. Neurol., 168:439-458.

Tiao, Y-C. and C. Blakemore, 1976, Functional organization in the visual cortex of the golden hamster, J. Comp. Neurol., 168:459-482.

Tiao, Y-C. and C. Blakemore, 1976, Functional organization in the superior colliculus of the golden hamster, J. Comp. Neurol., 168:483-504.

Udin, S.B. and M.J. Keating, 1981, Plasticity in a central nervous pathway in Xenopus: anatomical changes in the isthmotectal projection after larval eye rotation, J. Comp. Neurol., 203:575-594.

DEVELOPMENT OF THE RETINOTECTAL PROJECTION IN CHICKS

Steven C. McLoon

Department of Anatomy
Medical University of South Carolina
Charleston, South Carolina

INTRODUCTION

Connections between neurons do not develop in a random fashion but rather in orderly predetermined patterns. This developmental phenomenon is commonly referred to as "neuronal specificity". There are many gradations of neuronal specificity which range from a population of neurons forming connections with another specific population of neurons to a single axonal branch synapsing with a specific region of a dendrite. The precision with which the connections between any two populations of neurons are predetermined and the mechanisms involved in the formation of these connections in an orderly manner are matters of considerable controversy and study.

The vertebrate visual system is a useful model for the study of neuronal specificity. In the visual system the retinal ganglion cells constitute the sole neuronal connections from the eye to the brain. The pattern of these retinofugal connections has been well characterized. The ganglion cell axons course from the eye to the chiasm, where in certain species some axons, which originate in specific retinal regions, enter the ipsilateral optic tract. The remaining axons decussate and enter the contalateral optic tract. Optic axons are then distributed only to certain nuclei within the brain. In these nuclei, for all cases thus far studied, the optic axons form connections in a retinotopic pattern.

Over the past hundred years a considerable amount of information has been acquired on the development of specific retinofugal connections primarily using morphological techniques. As studies begin

to focus more on the cellular mechanisms of neuronal specificity,
particularly using biochemical and tissue culture techniques, it is
essential that we constantly review those events and patterns of
development which shape the visual system to help evaluate the
importance of various molecular phenomena that are observed. The
chick retinotectal system is increasingly becoming the subject of
choice in molecular studies on the development of neuronal specificity. This is probably because large amounts of tissue are readily
and inexpensively available, and the system is not subject to the
regeneration or regulation inherent in the visual system of cold
blooded animals. With this in mind the following pages are aimed
at reviewing the more salient features of the developing chick
retinotectal system, concentrating primarily on those events which
have been described morphologically in vivo. Where possible, conclusions or hypotheses are drawn as to those mechanisms which may
act on the developing system. A large body of literature on visual
system development in other species was intentionally ignored,
keeping this primarily a review of studies done in the chick. The
studies presented are only offered as representative of the field
and by no means encompass everything known of the developing chick
visual system.

EARLY DEVELOPMENT OF RETINAL GANGLION CELLS

Ganglion cell genesis

     The pattern of retinal genesis and the early development of
ganglion cells have important implications for the formation of
proper retinotectal connections. Several laboratories have demonstrated that the neurons destined for the ganglion cell layer are
generated between embryonic day 3 (E3) and E12 (Fujita and Horii,
1963; Kahn, 1973, 1974). These results are based on incorporation
of tritiated thymidine by the dividing neuroblasts and then processing the retina at a later time for autoradiography to demonstrate
those cells with tritium label in their nucleus. This technique
has an interesting difference when used in chick embryos as
compared to developing mammals. Thymidine administered to mammals
is cleared from the system within a few hours after injection
(Nowakowski and Rakic, 1974). This results in pulse labelling of
only those cells which divide within that time. The yolk in the
avian egg is able to take up an injection of H^3-thymidine and then
release the exogenously-administered thymidine throughout the
remainder of development. In autoradiographs this results in all
cells being labelled which divided subsequent to the thymidine injection and cells which have already undergone their final division
remain unlabelled. Labelled thymidine injected into the egg on
E2.5 resulted in all the neurons in the ganglion cell layer being
labelled when the retina was processed on E16, and an injection on
E13 failed to label any of these cells. There is also a progressive genesis of ganglion cells from central to peripheral retina.

Kahn (1973, 1974) has shown that tritiated thymidine injected into the egg on E3 fails to label some of the cells in the ganglion cell layer of the central retina. Making thymidine injections later labels an annulus of cells around the central retina which is displaced more peripherally with later injections up to E12, where only a few cells around the most peripheral retina are labelled.

Axonal outgrowth

Immediately after withdrawing from the mitotic cycle the ganglion cell neuroblast migrates from its site of division at the outer limiting membrane (Fujita and Horii, 1963). Upon reaching the inner limiting membrane the ganglion cells puts out an axon and then breaks its attachment with this membrane (Nishimura, 1980). Using a silver stain, Goldberg and Coulombre (1972) have demonstrated that the earliest optic axons arise from cells in the central retina. There is a subsequent appearance of axons from ganglion cells situated more peripherally in the retina. It appears that the pattern of axonal outgrowth across the retina parallels the pattern of histogenesis, that is, central to peripheral. We have made a similar finding by injecting horseradish peroxidase (HRP) into the brain of embryos at various ages and observing the pattern of labelling in the retina. The first ganglion cells that could be retrogradely labelled in this manner were in central retina and found late on E6. Later injections added retrogradely labelled cells towards the retinal periphery. The importance of this pattern of cell genesis and axonal outgrowth will become clear in the discussion of development of retinotectal connections.

Development of different cell types

Up until recently the ganglion cell layer has been treated as homogeneous cell population in developmental studies. It is now clear that this layer is not only composed of numerous ganglion cell types but also at least one other neuronal type. Golgi studies were the first to reveal an amacrine-like cell in the ganglion cell layer (Galvez et al., 1977). A lesion of the optic tectum in an E3 chick embryo resulted, later in development, in the loss of 95% of the ganglion cells and appeared to leave this displaced amacrine cell population intact (Hughes and LaVelle, 1975; Hughes and McLoon, 1979). Furthermore, an early chick embryo eye explanted to the chorioallantoic membrane and thereby allowed to develop without making connections with the central visual nuclei loses its entire ganglion cell population but the displaced amacrine cell population remains (McLoon and Hughes, 1978a). We have used the tectal lesion paradigm coupled with tritiated thymidine labelling to show that genesis of the amacrine cells in the ganglion cell layer lags behind the wave of ganglion cell genesis. Past E10 the number, size and distribution of thymidine labelled cells in the ganglion cell layer contralateral to a tectal lesion exactly matches that

seen in the normal retina. We have concluded two things from
this; first, the last ganglion cells withdraw from the mitotic cycle
and begin differentiation by E10, and second, the genesis of amacrine
cells which are displaced to the ganglion cell layer accounts for
the thymidine labelled cells observed in this layer with injections
on E11 or E12. This also may explain why the peak number of axons
in the optic nerve is reached on E10 (Rager and Rager, 1978) rather
than E12 or 13 which would be expected if ganglion cell genesis
continued until E12.

When we move beyond differences in the genesis of displaced
amacrine cells and ganglion cells to differences in development of
different ganglion cell types, our knowledge is extremely limited.
This type of data may have significant implications for explaining
differences in the central projections of the different ganglion
cell types. It has been shown for the chick that there are at
least three different projection patterns of retinal ganglion
cells. Based on tectal lesion studies there seem to be small and
medium size ganglion cells in the ganglion cell layer which project
exclusively to the optic tectum (McLoon and Hughes, 1978b). Large
size ganglion cells in the ganglion cell layer, which survive tectal
lesions, appear to project to diencephalic visual centers (McLoon
and Hughes, 1978b), and other large size ganglion cells displaced
to the inner nuclear layer project to the ectomammillary nucleus
(Karten et al, 1977; Reiner et al., 1979). All these cell types
are found intermixed over the entire retina, and it is difficult to
imagine separate mechanical pathways for each of their axons to
follow to the appropriate termination site. Temporal differences
in genesis or maturation between the cell types could help determine
differences in the central projections. If each cell type in one
retinal area has a slightly different time of development, then
slight changes in other parameters of the system may direct the
axon of each succeeding ganglion cell type to different
terminal fields.

GUIDANCE OF GROWING OPTIC AXONS

Directing growth in the retina

Little is understood about the forces that guide the growing
optic axons. There is some evidence that pioneering optic axons
may course through preformed intercellular spaces. Just prior to
the outgrowth of optic axons there is a wave of cell death in the
inner portion of the chick retina which results in the formation of
intercellular spaces (Ulshafer and Clavert, 1979). Serial reconstruction of sections through the early retina revealed that these
spaces form channels oriented in a continuous fashion towards the
optic stalk (Krayanek and Goldberg, 1981). From studies in the
mouse retina it is known that in the absence of the early wave of

cell death the intercellular channels do not form, and optic axons fail to exit the eye (Silver and Robb, 1979). At the simplest level it could be suggested that the channels in the retina offer a path of least resistance for the growing axons to follow.

A physical channel could guide a growing axon purely by mechanical means but then one would expect axons to follow in either direction in these channels. However, studies on developing retina have failed to identify axons coursing in the improper direction (Goldberg and Coulombre, 1972). Since there is evidence for neighbor-to-neighbor relationships being maintained in the early retina (Bodick and Levinthal, 1980), it might be that an axon emerging from a cell follows the axon of the neighboring cell towards the optic fissure. This could explain the directed growth of later optic axons but can not explain the directed growth observed in the very first optic axons to emerge. Clearly factors other than mechanical guidance and neighbor-to-neighbor relationships are important in directing axonal growth in the retina.

An increasing amount of evidence suggests that an orientation cue must be present on the scleral surface of the inner limiting membrane. As axons emerge from the ganglion cells, they do not exhibit an oriented growth towards the optic stalk, but once the growth cones contact the inner limiting membrane their growth immediately becomes oriented towards the stalk (Suburo et al., 1979). Goldberg (1977) experimentally deflected the growth of optic fibers and found in general three types of results. Axons which were deflected outside the optic fiber layer exhibited random growth. Axons which remained within the optic fiber layer but grew along its scleral portion followed the oriented channels but in either direction through the channel. Finally, axons which grew in the inner portion of the optic fiber layer along the inner limiting membrane not only followed the channels but were always oriented towards the optic fissure. Furthermore, fixation of the early retina with hypertonic fixatives causes cell shrinkage and an exaggeration of the intercellular spaces; however, the growth cones of the optic fibers remain adherent to the inner limiting membrane (Krayanek and Goldberg, 1981). The basis of the association between optic axons and the inner limiting membrane or the polarity cue imparted by the membrane are the objects of current research (see Schwartz in this volume). One feature of the inner limiting membrane that needs to be kept in mind during future studies is that it undergoes constant change during development. The neuroepithelial cells undergoing mitotic division retract their processes from the inner membrane. After completion of division the cells reinsert a process into the membrane. Also, neuroblasts, having completed their final division and migrated to their ultimate position, retract their processes from the membrane and Muller cells mature and maintain a process in the membrane. It is is not impossible that one of these features is important in lending polarity cues to the inner limiting membrane.

It may also be that the the polarity cue in the developing retina
is present quite transiently.

Order in the optic pathway

The optic axons appear to be ordered in a retinotopic fashion
as they grow along the optic nerve and tract. Retinotopic order in
the nerve and tract has been clearly shown for the avian visual
system in the hatched chick. A discrete retinal lesion resulted in
a discrete patch of degeneration that could be traced throughout
the length of the optic nerve and tract (Bunt and Horder, 1983).
By reconstructing pathways from several animals with lesions it was
apparent that the nerve is organized in a retinotopic fashion.
Evidence that such an order is present in the early developing
chick system comes from several sources. A gradient from large to
small axons in the central to peripheral optic nerve exists in the
early embryo (Rager, 1980). Since the retina develops in a central
to peripheral fashion, it was suggested that these patterns in the
nerve represent retinotopic order in that the more mature axons
from central retina would be larger than the less mature axons from
peripheral retina. We have recently used HRP conjugated to wheat
germ agglutinin (HRP/WGA) injected in a small amount transsclerally
to label a few fascicles of axons in the retina. With post-injection
survival times as short as one hour, the optic axons immediately
around the injection site were labelled in their entirety without
affecting other axons. Within the optic nerve and tract a group of
labelled axons maintained close association with one another through
their entire course (figure 1). The only exceptions to this were
axons destined for the diencephalon (rather than the tectum) which
separated from the main group. Also an occasional fiber would
separate from the group in the retina and remain separated from the
group through the nerve and tract.

Several aspects of retinal development may serve to order the
optic axons in a retinotopic fashion as they form the optic nerve.
The first factor is that optic axons tend to associate in groups or
fascicles and maintain these groupings throughout their course.
Goldberg (1977) has shown that axons deflected outside the optic
fiber layer gather together in "well-defined thick fascicles". In
our own studies on the development of retinofugal projections it was
shown that small fascicles of axons enter the ipsilateral optic
tract at the chiasm in the early embryo. These axons remain as a
tight group up to the point where they enter their terminal nucleus
(McLoon and Lund, 1982). In the fish it has even been shown that
specific neighbor-to-neighbor relationships are maintained throughout the course of the optic axons (Bodick and Levinthal, 1980) but
such data does not yet exist for the chick. Thus, fasciculation
would tend to keep axons from the same retinal areas together. The
second important factor that may be responsible for establishing
the retinotopic order in the nerve is that growth cones of the op-

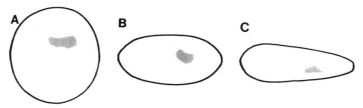

Figure 1. Reconstructions of A) the optic nerve about midcourse, B) the contralateral optic tract just after the chiasm, and C) the same optic tract just before reaching the tectum. The grey area represents the group of labelled axons resulting from a trans-scleral injection of HRP/WGA into the retina of the E9 chick followed by a one and a half-hour survival.

tic axons follow the scleral surface of the retinal inner limiting membrane (as discussed above). This results in young axons growing over their slightly older neighbors. Successive generations of ganglion cell axons would follow along the inner limiting membrane of the retina which is continuous with the inner limiting membrane of the nerve. Thus, fasciculation coupled with oriented channels delivers axons to the optic nerve with circumferencial order maintained and axons only growing along the inner limiting membrane would maintain age dependent or radial order.

Factors influencing the decussation of axons

Optic axons decussate completely at the chiasm and course to the contralateral side of the brain in the hatched chick. It has also been shown that unilateral enucleations performed during early embryonic development lead to a bilateral retinotectal projection (Ferreira-Berrutti, 1951; Raffin and Reperant, 1975; Mathers and Ostrach, 1979; O'Leary and Cowan, 1980). We examined the possibility of a transitory uncrossed pathway being present in early development which disappears unless the opposite eye is removed. Anterograde transport of horseradish peroxidase injected into one eye was used to visualize the central projections of that eye in chick embryos at different ages (McLoon and Lund, 1982). Besides the anticipated contralateral projection, a small projection was identified to primary visual nuclei on the side of the brain ipsilateral to the injected eye in embryos between E6 and E12. Whereas the optic fibers entered the contralateral tectum on E6, the ipsilateral projection did not arrive on the tectum until E8, suggesting that the time of development of the ipsilateral projection lags behind that of the contralateral projection. More surprisingly, a small projec-

jection was also identified from the injected eye into the contralateral optic nerve in a number of embryos.

In order to determine whether specific morphological features
of the developing chiasm influenced the decision of a growing optic
axon to decussate, we have studied the morphology of the developing
chiasm with electron microscopy and with serial 1 μm sections.
Several findings are of interest. First, we were unable to identify
oriented channels in the presumptive chiasm or optic tract which
might serve as a guide to the growing fibers. Oriented channels
are present along the ventral portion of the optic stalk. As the
optic stalk opens into the ventricle, the intercellular spaces
become less conspicuous in the neuroepithelium. Reconstruction of
serial 1 μm sections showed the spaces at this point lack regular
orientation or continuity. Second, the first fascicles of axons
from the two eyes remain separated from each other by numerous epithelial cells running between the ventricular surface and the limiting
membrane. This is true up until E6. On E6 the fascicles have increased in size to the point where there is some contact between
the fascicles from each eye. It is at this point in development
that we could first identify axons from an eye into the ipsilateral
tract and from one optic nerve into the contralateral nerve. There
are cellular partitions that remain between the fascicles from each
eye, but these partitions are discontinuous along the dorso-medial
extent. At this time the cells forming the partitions appear to
migrate from an area of cell proliferation into the ventro-lateral
chiasm. It is in the area of the chiasm most distant from these
regions of cell proliferation that the partitions are incomplete,
and it is in this area that fibers cross into fascicles of the
wrong eye. This has led us to suggest that the factors determining
whether or not an axon decussates at the chiasm, at least in the
chick, may be simple morphological constraints with no strict program within the growing axons. That is, an incomplete glial partition in portions of the chiasm seems to allow some axon fascicles
to pass through the partition and run with axons from the other
eye. For some reason in making this change the growing axons lose
the unidirectional constraints on their growth and can then grow in
either direction.

Another implication of these results is that the final ipsilat-
eral/contralateral distribution of axons in the mature system must
be determined by factors in the terminal field not at the chiasm.
In the case of the chick the total ipsilateral projection appears
to be eliminated. In the rat, however, where there is a substantial
ipsilateral projection at birth that arises from the entire retina,
only the ipsilateral projection from lower temporal retina is
retained (Land and Lund, 1979). It is still not clear what factors
exist in the terminal field which result in this elimination, but
it must involve competition between axonal populations since removal
of one eye early in development allows retention of these early

ipsilateral projections. It could be in the chick that the ipsilateral projection has a competitive disadvantage due to its late arrival in the terminal field relative to the contralateral axons.

EARLY INNERVATION OF THE OPTIC TECTUM

Evidence for changing connections

Previous studies using an autoradiographic technique have suggested that the first optic axons enter the tectum on E6 (Crossland et al., 1975). In the ensuing days the axons appeared to grow over the surface of the tectum, but they did not appear to penetrate the tectal layers below the stratum opticum until E10. This study suggested that the first fibers invaded the stratum griseum fibrosum superficiale on E10 in the center of the tectal surface. However, our laboratory reported a wave of cell death in the developing ganglion cell layer which proceeds from temporal to nasal retina. Based on the topographic pattern of connections between the retina and tectum, this would suggest that synaptogenic events in the tectum progress from rostral to caudal rather than central to peripheral (Hughes and McLoon, 1979). We have since re-examined the pattern of ingrowth and penetration of the retinal projections in the tectum using a newer more sensitive technique than that which was available previously (McLoon, 1982b). HRP or HRP/WGA was injected into the eye of chick embryos at various ages in order to anterogradely label the optic axons. The extent of the labeled optic axons in the tectum contralateral to the injected eye was reconstructed from serial sections using computergraphic techniques (Figure 2). As was shown previously, the first retinal fibers arrive on the tectum on E6, and these fibers enter at the rostral-ventral tectum. By later E6 the first evidence of penetration of label into the tectal layer below the stratum opticum is apparent. Penetration follows closely behind the advancing front of growing axons. During E7 and E8 the retinal projection grows dorsally to fill the most rostral extent of the tectum. From E9 through E12 the retinal axons grow caudally to cover the remaining tectum. During this entire period of growth the optic fibers penetrate the tectal layers in an area shortly after reaching that area. It is difficult to say why these results are so different from the results of Crossland et al. (1975). In the earlier study tritiated proline was injected into the eye, and the brain was processed for autoradiography. In young chick embryos there is a high propensity for the injected amino acids to be carried by the blood throughout the brain. This results in high background in autoradiographs which might obscure small projections.

Electron microscopic studies support a similar pattern of synaptogenesis in the tectum as that suggested by our HRP study (McGraw and McLaughlin, 1980). The first synaptic contacts were found in the rostral-ventral tectum on E6. A significant reduction in the number

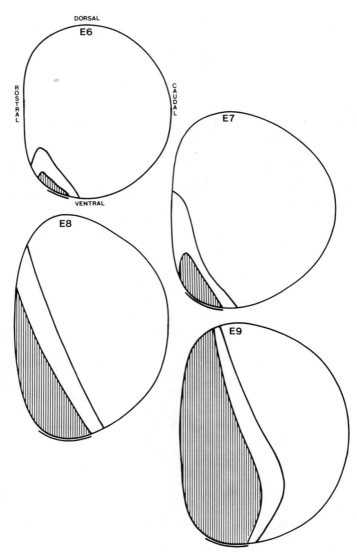

Figure 2. Reconstructions of the left tectum contralateral to an eye injected with HRP in embryos on successive days from E6 to E9. The crosshatched area represents the tectal area where the optic axons have penetrated below the stratum opticum. The unshaded area between between the crosshatching and the solid line represents the tectal area where optic axons are present in stratum opticum but have not penetrated deeper layers. The short line segment below each tectum represents that portion of the tectum which is continuous with the optic tract.

of these early synapses resulted from prior eye enucleations. HRP transport coupled with electron microscopy is needed to definitively show the optic origin of these early synapses and confirm this pattern of synaptogenesis.

These results suggest that the retinotectal projection in the chick develops in approximately a rostral-ventral to caudal-dorsal pattern. This is similar to the pattern of histogenesis and cellular maturation of the tectum as described by LaVail and Cowan (1971a, b) if their data is examined keeping in mind the rotation of the tectum which takes place during development (Goldberg, 1974). It is interesting that the pattern of tectal development imposes itself on the final maturation of the retina, as suggested by the temporal to nasal pattern of cell death in the ganglion cell layer.

The first optic axons arise from central retina, and the first optic connections are to rostral tectum. In the mature chick the central retina projects to central tectum. It must be concluded from these observations that the early optic axons slide their connections from rostral to central tectum. A similar sliding of connections has also been reported in developing Xenopus retinotectal connections (Gaze et al., 1974; Scott and Lazar, 1976). It is not clear what the incentive is for the terminals to shift during development. It is unlikely that competition for synaptic space has much of a role in the development of these connections. Partial retinal ablations have been made early in development such that the portion of the retina destined to innervate the rostral tectum is absent (Crossland et al., 1974). Even in this case, at the end of development the central retina is projecting to central tectum, and the rostral tectum is not innervated by the retina. This means that the retinal projection shifted from its early site of connection even in the absence of competition form the axons which would normally project to that region. Sliding connections have important implications for theories on neuronal specificity. Sperry (1943) postulated the existence of specific cytochemical markers on optic terminals and tectal neurons. A matching of the markers on the terminals with the appropriate tectal cell markers would result in the specific pattern of connections between the retina and the tectum. The studies of Crossland et al. (1974) have shown that the retinal neurons are specified very early in development. That is, a change in the relative position of the retinal neurons to one another by retinal lesions did not alter their ultimate site of termination in the tectum. The presence of sliding connections during development suggests that either the tectal neurons change their cellular markers during development or that specific cell markers do not exist.

Precision of the early projection

Theories have been proposed to account for the specificity in retinotectal connections which do not require precise cytochemical

markers. In one such theory, it was suggested that optic axons grow
from the eye in an orderly fashion and maintain this order into the
terminal field (Horder and Martin, 1979). As discussed above, it
appears that there is a high degree of retinotopic order in the optic
nerve and tract; however, it does not mean that this order is necessarily maintained into the terminal field. We have tried to assess
the degree of order between the optic axons as they grow over the
tectal surface (McLoon, 1982a). This was approached by making a
partial retinal ablation in embryos of various ages followed by an
injection of HRP into the eye with the lesion. It was expected that,
if the projection was tightly ordered, there would be no HRP label in
the portion of the tectum corresponding to the retinal lesion. What
was found, however, was a reduction in the amount of label in the
tectum corresponding to the retinal lesion but not a complete absence
of label (Figure 3). This was the case up through E12. Past E12 the
appropriate area of the tectum was completely lacking a projection.

     These results suggest that the early retinal projection to the
tectum lacks topographic precision and is refined during subsequent
development, leaving a tightly ordered retinotopic map on the tectum.
What is not clear is whether the initial retinal map on the tectum is
topographically organized but with large terminal arbors or if a considerable percentage of the cells project completely out of the proper pattern. Previous studies examined silver stained fibers on
the developing tectum and reported an apparent "meandering" of fibers
which then became progressively more organized as development proceeded (Goldberg, 1974). It is difficult to reconcile the apparent
diffuseness in the developing pathway with the theory that an orderly
ingrowth of optic axons to the tectum is the sole mechanism for generating the orderly projection. It is necessary to invoke mechanisms
which must involve either neighbor-to-neighbor or retina-to-tectum
recognition. It should be noted, however, that the bulk of the
retinal fibers on the tectum do appear to be properly positioned,
at least at a quadrantic level. This order might be accounted for
by mechanisms such as the orderly ingrowth of the optic axons onto
the tectum.

GANGLION CELL DEATH AND REFINEMENT OF THE EARLY PROJECTION

     During early development optic axons project broadly within the
confines of the visual system. Several aberrant projections, that
is, projections not incorporated into the adult visual system, present in early development of the chick visual system were described
in previous parts of this article. These include projections from
one retina into the contralateral nerve or ipsilateral optic tract
and projections not conforming to precise topographic order in the
tectum. The aberrant projections appear to be removed or corrected
during development. One possible method for removal of inappropriate projections is death of ganglion cells with an aberrantly
projecting axon. Substantial numbers of degenerating neurons have

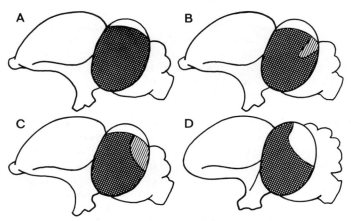

Figure 3.   Diagrams of the retinal innervation to tecta reconstructed from serial sections.   Double crosshatch represents normal
retinal input, single crosshatch represents a reduced retinal input
and white indicates no retinal projection.   A.   Shows the innervation in a normal embryo on E10.   B. Shows the reduced retinal input
to the caudal-inferior tectum in an E10 embryo resulting from a
superior-nasal retinal lesion induced on E8.   C.   Shows a similar
reduced input but resulting from a lesion induced on E3.   D.   Shows
the lack of retinal projection to the caudal-inferior tectum in an
E16 embryo resulting from a superior-nasal retinal lesion induced
on E3.

been observed in the retinal ganglion cell layer of the chick between E11 and E15 (Rager and Rager, 1978; Hughes and McLoon, (1979).
There is a concomitant loss of axons in the optic nerve during this
time.   By counting the number of axons in sample electron micrographs
of the optic nerve of embryos from E5 to E18 it was estimated that
40% of the ganglion cells degenerate during this period (Rager and
Rager, 1978).   This wave of cell death is unrelated to the cell
death that precedes initial axonal outgrowth as discussed previously.   The timing of the ganglion cell death corresponds to the timing
of the disappearance of certain aberrant projections.   The alterations in the topographic precision of the crossed retinotectal projection (McLoon, 1982a) and the complete disappearance of the
ipsilateral projection (McLoon and Lund, 1982) occurs between E12
and E15.   This correlation suggest that cell death may indeed be
involved in refining the early pattern of retinal projections.   It
also appears that axon retraction may play a role in remodeling the
early retinal projection pattern.   A small projection was identified

from one retina into the contralateral optic nerve in early chick
development. This projection disappears prior to E8, before the
major wave of ganglion cell death. Axon retraction not involving
cell death has previously been implicated in the remodeling of mammalian callosal projections (Innocenti, 1981; Ivy and Killackey,
1981; O'Leary et al., 1981). We can't as yet rule out the possibility that changes in topographic precision or laterality in the
developing chick visual system also involve retraction of axons or
axon collaterals and not strictly cell death.

The death of ganglion cells during this period of normal development may result from those cells which die being unable to form
sustaining connections in the brain. Destruction of the optic tectum
in an embryo prior to the arrival of optic axons results in a 70%
further loss of neurons in the ganglion cell layer (Hughes and
LaVelle, 1975). The temporal pattern of this increased cell loss
is the same as that for normal cell death (Hughes and McLoon,
1979). It also has been recently shown that survival of identified
ganglion cells in culture requires the presence of tectal cells or
tectum-conditioned media (Nurcombe and Bennett, 1981). Together
these results suggest that ganglion cells may require some trophic
substance and it is either delivered to the ganglion cell through
the synapse, or synapses may be required to maintain a sufficiently
large terminal arbor for uptake of an adequate quantity of the
trophic substance from the terminal environment. Thus, ganglion
cells not forming sufficient synapses in their target nucleus would
degenerate. In the case of optic axons not conforming to the proper
topographic pattern in the tectum during early development, they
may be prevented from forming or maintaining the critical minimum
number of synapses and hence, the cells would degenerate for lack
of trophic substance.

Further evidence for the importance of the tectum in ganglion
cell death comes from the pattern of cell death in the retina.
Counts from selected regions of retinal whole mounts revealed an
overall temporal to nasal progression of cell death (Hughes and
McLoon, 1979). This pattern corresponds in terms of the retinal
connections with the tectum to the pattern of tectal genesis and
maturation. That is, the first ganglion cell death is seen in the
temporal retina which connects to rostral tectum, the first part of
the tectum to develop. This suggests that the tectum may have to
reach a certain level of maturity before inappropriate projections
can be eliminated. Ganglion cell death commences at the same time
post-synaptic potentials can first be detected in the tectum
(Rager, 1980). An interesting possibility is that activity may play
a key role in eliminating inappropriate synapses in the developing
tectum. A mechanism has been proposed to account for such a phenomenon (Hebb, 1949; Stent, 1973). The basic idea is that synchroni-
zation between the activation of a synapse and the firing of the
post-synaptic cell would stabilize that synapse. Conversely if a

synapse was not activated in conjunction with the firing of a cell, it would be destabilized or even knocked off. There is some evidence for coupling of neighboring retinal ganglion cells during early development (Arees and DeLong, 1977). One could thus imagine neighboring retinal ganglion cells, that is, cells from a single retinal locus, firing synchronously and thus stabilizing their synapses onto a common group of tectal neurons. An aberrant axon, that is, from a cell in some other retinal locus, synapsing onto this same common group of tectal neurons would probably not fire synchronously, and its synapses would be eliminated. If this cell lacked synapses onto other properly located tectal neurons along with terminals from other cells in its same retinal locus, it might then be unable to acquire sufficient trophic substance and would degenerate. One important thing this model requires is that many of the retinal terminals be in proper topographic order on the early tectum. From experiments described above, we can suggest that this is true.

     In summary, the retina connects with the tectum in a specific pattern. The development of these specific connections appears to involve a combination of non-specific factors such as temporal gradients of maturation and mechanical guidance, more specific factors such as polarity gradients in the retina and tectum, and possibly even functional activity. Much more knowledge is needed particularly at the molecular and biochemical level before these processes can be completely understood.

REFERENCES

Arees, E.A. and DeLong, G.R., 1977, Temporary contacts formed between developing optic fibers in the chick, J. Embryol. Exp. Morphol., 37:211-216.
Bodick, N. and Levinthal, C., 1980, Growing optic nerve fibers follow neighbors during embyrogenesis, Proc. Natl. Acad. Sci. USA, 77:4374-4378.
Bunt, S.M. and Horder, T.J., 1983, Evidence for an orderly arrangement of optic axons within the optic nerves of the major non-mammalian vertebrate classes, J. Comp. Neurol., in press.
Crossland, W.J., Cowan, W.M., Rogers, L.A. and Kelly, J.P., 1974, Specification of the retino-tectal projection in the chick, J. Comp. Neurol., 155:127-164.
Crossland, W.J., Cowan, W.M., and Rogers, L.A., 1975, Studies on the development of the chick optic tectum. IV. An autoradiographic study of the development of retino-tectal connections, Brain Res.,91-23.
Ferreira-Berrutti, P., 1951, Experimental deflection of the course of the optic nerve in the chick embryo, Proc. Soc. Exp. Biol. Med., 76:302-303.
Fujita, S. and Horii, 1963, Analysis of cytogenesis in chick retina by tritiated thymidine autoradiography, Arch. Histol. Jap., 23(63):359-366.

Galvez, J.M.G., Puelles, L. and Prada, C., 1977, Inverted (dis-
    placed) retinal amacrine cells and their embryonic development
    in the chick, Exp. Neurol., 56:151-157.
Gaze, R.M., Keating, M.J. and Chung, S.H., 1974, The evolution of
    the retinotectal map during development in Xenopus, Proc. Roy.
    Soc. Lond. B, 185:301-330.
Goldberg, S., 1974, Studies on the mechanics of development of the
    visual pathways in the chick embryo, Devel. Biol., 36:24-43.
Goldberg, S., 1977, Unidirectional, bidirectional, and random growth
    of embryonic optic axons, Exp. Eye Res., 25:399-404.
Goldberg, S. and Coulombre, A.J., 1972, Topographical development
    of the ganglion cell fiber layer in the chick retina. A whole
    mount study, J. Comp. Neurol., 146:507-518.
Hebb, D.O., 1949, Organization of Behavior, Wiley and Sons, New York.
Horder, T.J. and Martin, K.A.C., 1979, Morphogenetics an an alter-
    native to chemospecificity in the formation of nerve connec-
    tions, Soc. Exp. Biol., 32:275-358.
Hughes, W.F. and LaVelle, A., 1975, The effects of early tectal
    lesions on development in the retinal ganglion cell layer of
    chick embryos, J. Comp. Neurol., 163(75):265-284.
Hughes, W.F. and McLoon, S.C., 1979, Ganglion cell death during
    normal retinal development in the chick: Comparisons with cell
    death induced by early target field destruction, Exp. Neurol.,
    66:587-601.
Innocenti, G.M., 1981, The development of interhemispheric connec-
    tions, Trends in NeuroSci., 4:142-144.
Ivy, G.O. and Killackey, H.P., 1981, The ontogeny of the distribu-
    tion of callosal projection neurons in the rat parietal cortex,
    J. Comp. Neurol., 195:367-389.
Kahn, A.J., 1973, Ganglion cell formation in the chick neural
    retina, Brain Res., 62:285-290.
Kahn, A.J. 1974, An autoradiographic analysis of the time of
    appearance of neurons in the developing chick neural retina,
    Devel. Biol., 38:38-40.
Karten, H.J., Fite, K.V. and Brecha, N., 1977, Specific projection
    of displaced retinal ganglion cells upon the accessory optic
    system in the pigeon. Proc. Natl. Acad. Sci., 74:1753-1756.
Krayanek, S. and Goldberg, S., 1981, Oriented extracellular channels
    and axonal guidance in the embryonic chick retina, Devel.
    Biol., 84:41-50.
Land, P.W. and Lund, R.D., 1979, Development of the rat's uncrossed
    retinotectal pathway and its relation to plasticity studies,
    Science, 205:698-700.
LaVail, J.H. and Cowan, W.M., 1971a, The development of the chick
    optic tectum. I. Normal morphology and cytoarchitectonic
    development, Brain Res., 28:391-419.
LaVail, J.H. and Cowan, W.M., 1971b, The development of the chick
    optic tectum. II. Autoradiographic studies, Brain Res.,
    28:421-441.

Mathers, L.H. and Ostrach, L.H., 1979, Mechanisms controlling axonal misrouting in the visual system of the chick embryo, Anat. Rec., 193:614.

McGraw, C.F. and McLaughlin, B.J., 1980, Fine structural studies of synaptogenesis in the superficial layers of the chick optic tectum, J. Neurocytol., 9:79-93.

McLoon, S.C., 1982a, Alterations in precision of the crossed retino-tectal projection during chick development, Science, 215:1418-1420.

McLoon, S.C., 1982b, Evidence for sliding connections in the development of the retinotectal projection in the chick, Soc. Neuro. Abs., 8, in press.

McLoon, S.C. and Hughes, W.F., 1978a, Ganglion cell death during retinal development in chick eyes explanted to the chorioallantoic membrane, Brain Res., 150:398-402.

McLoon, S.C. and Hughes, W.F., 1978b, Development and distribution of a ganglion cell subpopulation in the chick retina, Neurosci. Abs., 4:637.

McLoon, S.C. and Lund, R.D., 1982, Transient retinofugal pathways in the developing chick, Exp. Brain Res., 45:277-284.

Nishimura, Y., 1980, Determination of the developmental pattern of retinal ganglion cells in chick embryos by Golgi impregnation and other methods, Anat. Embryol., 158:329-347.

Nowakowski, R.S. and Rakic, P., 1974, Clearance rate of exogenous ^{3}H-thymidine from the plasma of Rhesus monkeys, Cell-Tiss. Kinet., 7:189-194.

Nurcombe, V. and Bennett, M.R., 1981, Embryonic chick retinal ganglion cells identified "in vitro". Their survival is dependent on a factor from the optic tectum, Exp. Brain Res., 44:249-258.

O'Leary, D.D.M. and Cowan, W.M., 1980, Observations on the effects of monocular and binocular eye removal on the development of the chick visual system, Soc. Neurosci. Abs., 6:297.

O'Leary, D.D.M., Stanfield, B.B. and Cowan, W.M., 1981, Evidence that the early postnatal restriction of the cells of origin of the callosal projection is due to the elimination of axonal colllaterals rather than to the death of neurons, Devel. Brain Res., 1:607-617.

Raffin, J.P. and Reperant, J., 1975, Etude experimentale de la specificite des projections visuelles d'embryons et de poussins de gallus domesticus L. microphtalmes et monophtalmes, Arch. Anat. Micro. Morph. Exp., 64:93-111.

Rager, G.H., 1980, Development of the Retinotectal Projection in the Chicken., Springer-Verlag, Berlin.

Rager, G. and Rager, U., 1978, Systems-matching by degeneration. I. A quantitative electron microscopic study of the generation and degeneration of retinal ganglion cells in the chicken, Exp. Brain Res., 33:65-78.

Reiner, A., Brecha, N. and Karten, H.J., 1979, A specific projection of retinal displaced ganglion cells to the nucleus of the

basal optic root in the chicken, Neurosci., 4:1679-1688.
Scott, T.M. and Lazar, G., 1976, An investigation into the
    hypothesis of shifting neuronal relationships during
    development, J. Anat., 121:485-496.
Silver, J. and Robb, R.M., 1979, Studies on the development of the
    eye cup and optic nerve in normal mice and in mutants with
    congenital optic nerve aplasia, Devel. Biol., 68:175-190.
Sperry, R.W., 1943, Effect of 180 degree rotation of the retinal
    field on visumotor coordination, J. Exp. Zool., 92:263-279.
Stent, G.S., 1973, A physiological mechanism for Hebb's postulate of
    learning, Proc. Natl. Acad. Sci. USA, 70:997-1001.
Suboro, A., Carri, N. and Adler, R., 1979, The environment of axonal
    migration in the developing chick retina: A scanning electron
    microscopic (SEM) study, J. Comp. Neurol., 184:519-536.
Ulshafer, R.J. and Clavert, A., 1979, Cell death and optic fiber
    penetration in the optic stalk of the chick, J. Morphol.,
    162:67-76.

INTERACTIONS OF AXONS WITH THEIR ENVIRONMENT:

THE CHICK RETINO-TECTAL SYSTEM AS A MODEL

Uli Schwarz and Willi Halfter

Max-Planck-Institut für Virusforschung
Biochemistry Department
Tübingen, Federal Republic of Germany

INTRODUCTION

In complex organisms, the different regions of the body and the various parts of the nervous system are interconnected via axons. These axons grow out from neural cell bodies in a timed and topologically defined manner resulting in the establishment of specific connectivity patterns during embryogenesis (for review see Cowan, 1978). Perhaps the best studied example of such a pattern is the projection of the retina onto the optic tectum.

Retino-Tectal Connections in the Chick as a System for Studying Nervous System Development

The retino-tectal system of the chick has several advantages as a model for both experimental and theoretical analysis of neuro-development. Firstly, all the neurons whose axons project out of the retina onto the optic tectum (i.e., the so-called ganglion cells) are arranged in a single two-dimensional layer. Secondly, the projection of these retinal axons onto the optic tectum is also analyzable in two dimensional terms and, more important, the pattern of axon endings on the tectum reflects in a topologically exact fashion the region of origin of the axons in the retina (Goldberg, 1974; Crossland and Cowan, 1975; Rager and van Oeynhausen, 1979). Thirdly, the system is accessible to experimental manipulation both in vivo and in vitro.

In the growth of axons from the retina to the tectum, three stages may be recognized:

1. Axonal growth within the retina to the appropriate exit point at the optic nerve-head
2. Axonal growth between the retina and tectum, this pathway forming the optic nerve, and
3. Axonal growth into the tectum, resulting in the selection of appropriate synaptic connections.

General Considerations on Axonal Guidance

The guidance of axons could be completely achieved by an intrinsic program without any interaction with the embryonic environment. This would be something like modern navigation systems in which all the parameters required for path finding such as times, coordinates, etc. are stored in a memory. This is not a very attractive solution for a biological system, as it is complicated and, above all, inflexible. It makes more sense to assume that constant interaction of axons with their environment takes place. In summary, five mechanisms, which are not mutually exclusive, have been proposed to explain the generation of correct axonal projections:

1. A timed order of the generation and outgrowth of fibers.
2. Mechanical guidance by the micromorphology of the environment.
3. An interaction of the fibers with each other.
4. Functional validation of the projections by activity of synapses.
5. An interaction of axons with the environment through chemical markers which are spatially distributed both in the tissue of axon origin (the retina) and in the axons's target tissue (in our case, the tectum).

None of these mechanisms acting alone may explain the development of neural maps such as the retino-tectal projection (for review see Gierer, 1982). However, many arguments point to the fifth of the above mentioned mechanisms as one essential cue used to generate neural maps. This assumption was introduced by Sperry (1963) as the chemoaffinity model. It was originally proposed that the surface of the axons could carry molecular markers specific for their region of origin, and that these would match position-specific markers on the target. This, however, would require a vast variety of different molecules as markers and very extensive random search of the axons on the target tissue for appropriate positions. There is so far no indication that such random search really takes place; in any case, nature may have found a more general solution to the problem of constructing neural connectivity maps. More recently, models which are more economical in molecular species have been proposed (Fraser, 1980; Gierer, 1982). These

models can explain not only the normal development of axonal pathways but also the results of artificial, surgical interferences
with development.

     Gierer's model, for example, proposes that substances on the
axonal growth cone, which are graded with respect to position of
origin on the retina, interact wth graded tectal components in producing guiding substances, in the simplest case one substance of
concentration p. Substance p, in turn, interacts with an intracellular pattern forming mechanism within the growing axon. In the tip
of the axon, a focus of activity in the direction of maximal slope
of the distribution of p would be initiated, resulting in oriented
growth. Growth would stop when the appropriate position of p is
reached. Many types of activating and inhibiting reaction based on
conventional kinetics are possible. According to the model, the
requirements for accurate projections are surprisingly simple, for
each dimension of the projecting and of the target area, one or two
graded compounds suffice and conventional enzyme kinetics are enough.
These properties make this model very attractive for a biochemist.
Chemo-affinity may be one essential mechanism underlying the development of highly specific projecitons and this speculation is the
basis of our experimental work. We posed the following questions:
Are individual retinal axons endowed with mechanisms to identify
their particular target cell or target area in the tectum? Similarly, how can the axons recognize the way to their target area?
Finally, we ask whether there is any hope to bridge the gap between
our descriptive understanding of the establishment of neural connections and the desired elucidation of the mechanisms underlying the
generation of neural networks in molecular terms.

THE RETINO-TECTAL SYSTEM OF BIRDS AS AN EXPERIMENTAL MODEL

Explant Cultures of Embryonic Retina

     Cultures from avian embryonic retina either as whole flat
mounts or as explants of sub-regions, are viable for about three
days. During this time, vigorous outgrowth of neurites is observed.
The timing of neurite outgrowth and the orientation of neurites
reflect quite exactly the generation of the axon pattern in the
retina of the developing animal.

     Various staining procedures (including silver impregnation)
reveal that a flat-mounted embryonic retina shows a centripetal
arrangement of axons. As schematically represented in Fig. 1, the
axon bundles intersect slightly ventral to the dorsal-most part of
the optic fissure where the axons merge to form the optic nerve.
When the retina of a 6-day-old chick embryo (E6), flattened out on
a membrane filter, is cut into strips which are transferred onto a
collagen substrate and cultured further, neurites grow out in abundance over the collagen surface. The neurites in all properties

tested behave like true axons: Horseradish peroxidase, taken up by
injured neurites in explant cultures labels large cell bodies indistinguishable from authentic ganglion cell bodies in size, shape,
and dendritic arborization. The labelled cell bodies in explants
all lie close to the inner limiting membrane on the vitreal side of
the retina (Halfter et al., 1982).

     The position and time of axon outgrowth in vitro closely cor-
responds to the normal changing pattern of withdrawal from the cell
cycle (Kahn, 1973) and axon extension (Goldberg and Coulombre,
1972) by retinal ganglion cells. The absolute rate of increase of
postmitotic ganglion cells reaches a maximum at E6 (Kahn, 1973).
Correspondingly, more axon outgrowth occurred from explants of E6
chick retina than from E4 and E5 retinae. In terms of retinal
regions, axons sprouted in cultures from E4 chick donors mainly
from the dorsal and central parts, as in the normal E4 retina
(Goldberg and Coulombre, 1972).

     On the other hand, there was a rapid decrease in axon produc-
tion from explants from chick embryos of E7 or older when few ganglion cells are born (Kahn, 1973) despite the presence at the time
of explantation, of axon-bearing ganglion cells born throughout
the E4 to E7 birth phase. Likewise, in terms of retinal regions,
axon outgrowth capacity ceased first in the dorso-temporal region
which is the developmentally oldest part of the retina (Hughes and
McLoon, 1979).

     Mitosis inhibitors Ara-C and FUdR do not affect outgrowth, indi-
cating that the culture system does not permit the transition from
mitotic ganglion cell precursors to post-mitotic, axon-bearing
neurons.

Axon Guidance within the Retina

     The orientation of axon growth during normal development -
leading to a centripetal orientation of fibers towards the optic
nerve head - is reproduced in tissue culture of retinal subregions.
In strips of retina, not only did most neurites emerge on the side
of an explant which originally was closest to the optic nerve-head
(Fig. 2), but also these neurites tended to grow in the direction
of the original position of the nerve-head. For example, neurites
from the nasal part of strips cut in a naso-temporal direction
tended to run slightly temporally while those from the temporal
part oriented slightly nasally (Fig. 2). The similarity between
the pattern in vivo and in vitro was also demonstrated in the
neurite outgrowth from naso-temporal strips cut directly through the
optic nerve-head (Fig. 2a). Here, neurites emerged as a thick central spray, with only a few neurites emerging laterally (Fig. 2b).
HRP-labelling confirmed that neurites from lateral zones ran within
these strips and turned abruptly to emerge centrally (Fig. 2c).

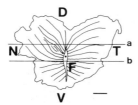

Figure 1. Camera lucida diagram of a flat mounted, embryonic (E6)
chick retina; silver staining shows the centripetal pattern of
axons. All axons converge on the optic fissure (F) and leave the
retina by the optic nerve-head (asterisks). (a) and (b) indicate
the positions of the explant strips represented in Fig. 3 and Fig.
4. D, V, N, T: Dorsal, Ventral, Nasal and Temporal. Bar: 1 mm.

    The striking maintenance of both orientation and direction of
axon sprouting does not depend on external factors such as the relative arrangement of retinal explants or even on the position of co-
cultured tectal tissue, nor on any apparent inherent orientation in
the collagen matrix on which the axons grew. A trivial explanation
for the polarization of axon outgrowth would be the notion that the
axons are already oriented in the piece of explant and simply maintain their given direction in the case of short axons not cut during
preparation, or that cut axons regenerate from severed stumps without
change of direction. This may be true for the very first axons leaving the explant. However, the maintenance of the axon pattern over
longer periods in culture depends on other parameters. This is
shown by experiments in which the vitreal surface, consisting of a
basal lamina plus the end- feet of Muller glia cells, is removed by
proteases. This treatment does not disarrange pre-existing axons
but newly outgrowing axons are dramatically disoriented (Figs. 3
and 4). This occurs not only in cultures of strips, but also in
protease-treated whole-mount retinal cultures. The orientation of
axonal out-growth does not depend on the basal lamina and the Muller
glial end-feet since preliminary experiments in which retinae were
cultured after non-enzymatic removal of these layers (W. Reckhaus,
personal communication) did not disorient axon growth. We are,
therefore, led to the conclusion that the local microenvironment of
the fiber layer in the retina plays a decisive role in the initial
choice of axon orientation and direction (Goldberg, 1977; Silver
and Sidmann, 1980; Krayanek and Goldberg, 1981). Once decided upon,
the orientation and direction of axonal growth tend to be maintained even without the absolute necessity of continued directional
information, because axons from strip cultures keep their orientation over randomly oriented col-substrates several millimeters
distant from the retinal tissue.

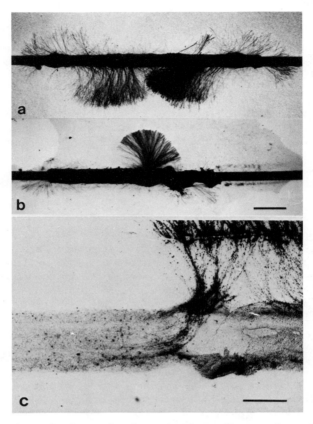

Figure 2. Sudan Black-stained retinal explants of an E5 quail embryo after 2 days of incubation (a and b). The original position of both explants is shown in Fig. 1. (c) Axons of an E6 chick retina explant after 2 days in vitro, showing the fiber pathway within the explanted tissue, after labelling with horseradish peroxidase. The explant is seen from the top; the filter strips appearing in (a) and (b) have been removed. This explant has the same retinal orgin as b. Bar (a) and (b): 1 mm. Bar (c): 250 μm.

In the explant system using retinal whole mounts, localized staining with rhodamine showed that most axons grew towards the optic nerve-head, that is, they initially chose both the correct orientation and direction. However, a very small percentage of axons had the correct orientation but the wrong direction and grew to the retinal periphery. On the other hand, many of the correctly

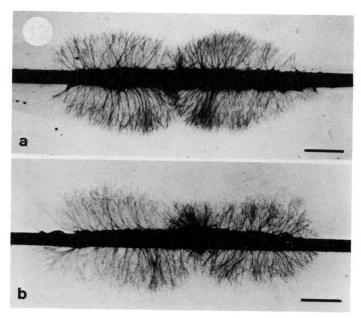

Figure 3. Chick retina explants (E6) after 2 days in vitro,
treated with trypsin and stained with Sudan Black. Before explantation, the whole retina had been treated with trypsin. Axons grow
on both sides of the strips in contrast to the orientation shown in
Fig. 2. The origin of the explants is shown in Fig. 1 and corresponds to that of the explants in Fig. 2 a and b. Bar: 1 mm.

oriented and directed axons, on reaching the site of the optic
nerve-head and being unable to exit from the retina as they would
in vivo, grew across to the opposite side of the retina, again in
the correct orientation but with the wrong direction; they could
even be mechanically forced to grow with wrong orientation (Fig.
5). This indicates that the choice of orientation and the choice
of direction may be separately controlled (Halfter, in preparation).

Recognition of Tectal Tissue by Retinal Axons

The interaction of axons with their environment may be important
not only for path-finding in the organism on the way to the target
tissue but also upon arrival there. The possible recognition of
target tissue by retinal axons was studied with our tissue culture
system described above. When a suspension of tectal cells, obtained

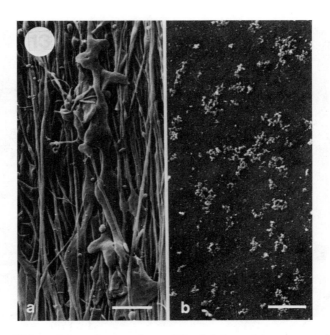

Figure 4.   Vitreal surface of an E6 chick retina seen in the scanning electron microscope. (a) The vitreal basement membrane and
glia end feet of the Muller cells have been removed by trypsin,
leaving the orientation of the optic axons untouched. (b) Untreated
control. Bar: 10 μm.

by mechanical dissociation of the tissue, was added to explants
after two days of culturing and incubated for another two hours, a
preferential adhesion of axons from the nasal part of the retina was
seen. Since, however, cells did not only adhere to axons but also
to each other and to the collagen matrix, the picture was not satis-
factorily clear. A very neat result was obtained with membrane
preferential adhesion of tectal membranes to axons originating
from the nasal region of the retina, as opposed to axons of temporal
origin, was observed. The adhesion of tectal membranes to nasal
axons reflects a discontinuous step of adhesiveness at the nasal-
temporal dimension of the retina with a sharp boundary at the center
of the retina (Fig. 6). This spatial difference in adhesion to
retinal axons was found only with membranes from the optic tectum.
In contrast to membranes from the tectum, membranes from fore-brain
or retina were not bound to nasal axons in a specific way. However, a slight overall adhesiveness to all axons was observed not
only with neural membranes but also with non-neural material such

as membranes from liver (Halfter et al., 1981).

The nasal-temporal polarity as revealed by membrane-binding in our in vitro system may be involved in the establishment of retino-tectal connections during in vivo development. Up to now, this has remained a speculation, which, however, recently has gained further support. Bonhoeffer and Huf (1981) have developed a technique allowing the interactions of axons with potential target tissue to be assayed in vitro quantitatively; graded preferences thus become detectable. Retinal explant strips, cut oriented in a naso-temporal direction, are grown on a monolayer of cells of type A. After having covered some distance, they are offered the choice between cell type A on which they grow and another cell type B as an alternative. The samples are observed microscopically under conditions allowing the quantitation of axons continuing to grow on cell type A and those preferring to swing to cell type B as a substrate for growth. Axon growth on the cell layers can be monitored easily after staining the retinal explants with the fluorescent vital stain rhodamine. When in a control experiment the two cell layers A and B between which the axons can choose are identical - both prepared from retina - an almost 50:50 ratio of axons growing on monolayer A or moving to monolayer B is counted showing the equivalence of both monolayers. With different monolayers, retina on layer A and tectum on layer B, different axonal preferences are found. Tectal cells are generally preferred to retinal cells, however, whereas 90% of nasal retinal axons prefer tectum to retina, only about 56% of the temporal axons prefer tectum, again showing a different response between nasal and temporal axons as described already for the membrane vesicle assay (see above). When tectal cells of different topological origin are offered to axons, temporal axons prefer cells from the anterior part of the tectum as compared with posterior tectal cells: In other words, adhesion is graded with respect to position on the tectum. In this assay, nasal axons do not show an equivalent preference for posterior tectum. However, if instead of monolayers of trypsin-treated cells, membrane vesicles made without proteolytic enzymes are used as a matrix for outgrowing axons, temporal and nasal axons show reciprocal preferences for anterior and posterior tectal membranes (Kern-Veits and Bonhoeffer, personal communication).

The preference of axons of temporal retina for tectal cells is obviously graded. The maximal adhesivity between nasal retinal axons and tectal cells decreases along the antero-posterior axis, although the gradient is rather slight. Identical results were obtained irrespective of whether the tecta had been innervated or not (Bonhoeffer and Huf, 1982). The differential preferences of topo-logically distinct tectal regions to retinal axons do not necessarily indicate a graded distribution of position-dependent tectal markers. The antero-posterior polarity which was found could also be due to developmental stage-dependent markers, because of the polarity of

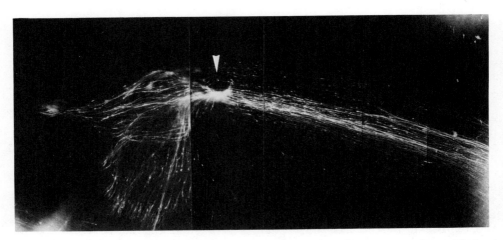

Figure 5. Vital-stained axons in a retina whole-mount after 30 h
in vitro; the staining of axons was achieved by local application
of rhodamine isothiocyanate at the periphery of the whole-mount.
Immediately after staining and before explantation the retina was
injured, at the point indicated by an arrow, close to the optic fissure (on the left, not visible). The axons originally grow in the
correct orientation to the optic nerve-head. Many of them cross
the lesion, others however, are mechanically deflected.

tectum development (Cowan et al., 1968; La Vail and Cowan, 1971).
Experiments using tectal cells of different age (embryonic day 6-9),
however, indicate that the higher adhesivity of anterior tectal
cells compared with posterior ones for axons from the temporal
region of the retina is indeed the result of tectal differences
depending on position rather than on age.

Both in the membrane adhesion assay and in choice experiments
with axons growing on different cell monolayers, no counterpart to
the nasotemporal gradient has been found in the dorso-ventral
direction as indicated by cell-cell adhesion assays (Gottlieb et
al., 1975; 1976) and by probing the distribution of specific antigens on the retina using monoclonal antibodies (Trissler et al.,
1981).

The experimental findings discussed above support the notion
that there are spatially distributed substances in both retina and
tectum. This supports the idea that spatial markers are involved in
generating neural maps, however, a definite proof would require the

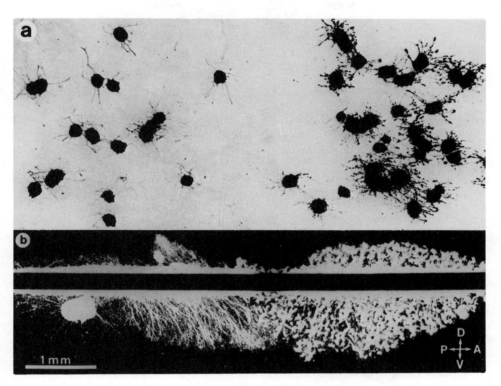

Figure 6.   Preferential adhesion of tectal membranes to nasal axons
of chick (E6) retinal explants.   (a) 300 x 300 µm explant pieces
from the temporal (left) and nasal (right) part of one retina were
cultured in the same dish and were incubated with tectal membranes.
After washing, much more membrane material was bound by axons from
nasal explants.   The specimens were stained with Sudan Black.   (b)
Adhesion of tectal membranes to axons of an explant cut in naso-
temporal direction (see Fig. 1).   Note the preferential adhesion of
membranes to nasal axons with a sharp boundary at the optic fissure
(darkfield-micrograph).   Nasal = anterior, Temporal = posterior.

identification of the compounds involved in cell-cell and/or axon-
cell recognition and a demonstration of their function in directing
axonal growth.

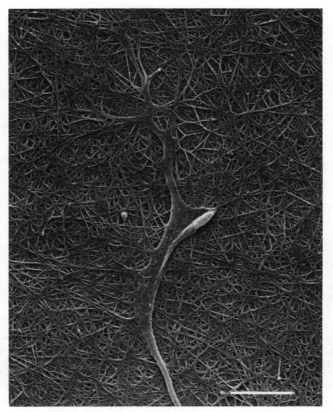

Figure 7.   Scanning electron micrograph of a retinal axon growth cone
on collagen substrate.   Note the intense intermingling of growth cone
microspikes with the collagen fibrils.   Bar: 5 μm.

        The identification of topological markers is certainly a diffi-
cult task for various reasons, the most trivial one being that only
small amounts of material are available for biochemical analysis.
This is especially so in retinal tissues, where the specificity of
recognition need only be expressed on the axon, that is on a small
and delicate portion of the cell surface.   To cope with this problem, we decided to develop an analytical technique sufficient in
resolution and sensitivity to handle the quantities available from
the embryo or from explant cultures.   For this purpose, a micro-gel
system has been elaborated for two-dimensional protein analysis at
high resolution (Neukirchen et al., 1982).

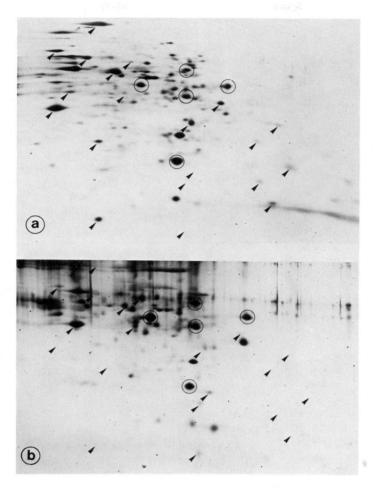

Figure 8. Comparison of retina proteins from explant cultures on two-dimensional microgels. After two days culturing of E6 retina strips, axons with growth cones were harvested by microdissection. (a) shows a gel containing mainly cell bodies, on (b) proteins from axons and growth cones are separated. A total of about 1 mg protein was applied to the gels (stamp size) which were stained with silver (Neukirchen et al., 1982). Major differences between the gels are marked with arrowheads; five corresponding spots are circled for orientation.

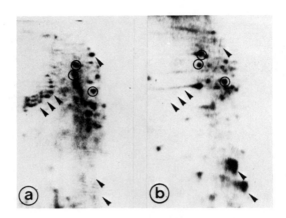

Figure 9. Comparison of proteins mainly from perikarya (a) and axons (b) on microgels. Autoradiographs of ^{35}S-methionine labelled proteins (a, 6000 cpm; b, 3000 cpm) were exposed for 20 h at -70°. Marks as in Fig. 8.

BIOCHEMICAL ANALYSIS ON A MICROSCALE: COMPARISON OF THE PROTEIN PATTERNS OF GROWTH CONES AND CELL BODIES WITH A TWO-DIMENSIONAL MICRO-GEL SYSTEM

For the analysis of small amounts of material, isoelectric focussing and SDS-polyacrylamide electrophoresis have been adjusted to microscale (Neuhoff, 1973; Bispink and Neuhoff, 1976). However, there are serious limits in resolution with either of these one-dimensional techniques. In combination, however, they yield high resolution of individual protein species from complex mixtures (O'Farrell, 1975; O'Farrell et al., 1977). With this method, proteins are separated according to independent parameters, the isoelectric point and the molecular weight, of a given protein. We scaled down this procedure, which up to now has been available only on a macroscale.

Gels are run in the first dimension - isoelectric focussing - in micro-capillaries with a total volume of about 10 µl to which 0.2 to 0.5 µl of sample solution were applied. The separation in the second dimension is achieved on slab gels of stamp size with a thickness of 0.1 to 0.2 mm. The separated proteins can be stained with Coomassie Blue and also with silver-staining essentially accord-

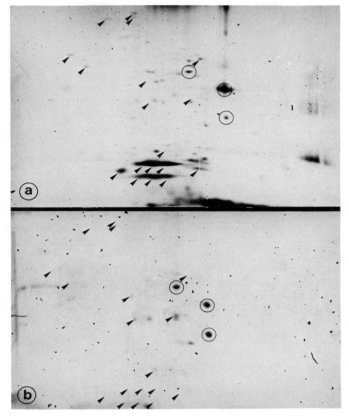

Figure 10.   Two-dimensional microgels mainly of perikarya (a) and
axons (b) after staining of glycoproteins with periodic acid/silver
(Dubray and Bezard, 1982). For orientation, several proteins found
on both gels are circled, differences between the gels are marked
with arrowheads.

ing to Oakley (1980).   Radio-labelled proteins can be detected by
autoradiography, and immunological techniques are applicable to the
microsystem.

The resolution of this system is at least equivalent to that
of conventional large size gels; several hundred spots are easily
resolved. With silver staining, three picograms of protein per
spot can be visualized; with ^{35}S-labelled proteins per count per mm[2]

can be detected by autoradiography after only 5 days exposure. The
reproducibility of the gels is very good since several gels can be
run in parallel.

The micro-gel system was used to initiate a biochemical search
for components involved in the exploration of the axonal environment.
It is quite clear that the growth cones (Fig. 7) on the axon tip
search the territory to be stepped on by the growing axon. Thus, it
is plausible to assume that growth cones might be enriched in compounds engaged in axonal recognition. Consequently, axonal tips
rich in growth cones were harvested from retinal explant cultures
(see above) by micromanipulation under the microscope and were
analyzed on micro-gels. Comparisons were made with the rest of
explants containing mainly perikarya from which axons and growth
cones had been harvested. The experiments were made with unlabelled material (Fig. 8), labelling with ^{35}S-methionine (Fig. 9) and
also after surface labelling of explants with ^{125}I using immobilized
lactoperoxidase or with isethionylacetimidate. Glycoproteins were
labelled using galactosyltransferase, and gels were also processed
with a new periodic acid silver staining to detect glycoproteins
(Dubray, 1982; Fig. 10). All experiments essentially gave one very
clear result: growth cones have a much simpler protein pattern as
compared with the rest of the tissue. This is true both for the
glycoproteins and for components exposed to the surface. This
finding is remarkable because a comparison between different tissues
(chick retina and tectum) or between different cell types of one
tissue (cells in different cell layers of the retina obtained by a
microdissection, Neukirchen, 1980) yield almost identical protein
patterns. Also the glycoprotein pattern of growth cones shows only
a small number of major components.

The relative simplicity found is encouraging for further
studies on the interaction of axons with target tissues. This is
difficult but not impossible, especially since very selective tools
such as monoclonal antibodies are now available (Henke, 1982).

ACKNOWLEDGEMENTS

We are much indebted to our colleagues Dr. F. Bonhoeffer,
Dr. A. Gierer, Dr. D.F. Newgreen, and B. Schlosshauer, for reading
of the manuscript, their criticisms and most helpful advice in
preparing the text. We are also greatly indebted to I. Baxivanelis
for her secretarial help and to B. Kern-Veits, W. Reckhaus, and
B. Schlosshauer for informing us of unpublished data.

REFERENCES

Bispink, G., and Neuhoff, V., 1976, Isoelektrische Fokussierung in
     Mikrogelen zur Fraktionierung komplexer Proteingemische in Nano-
     grammbereich, Hoppe-Seylers, Z. Physiol. Chem., 357:991-997.

Bonhoeffer, F., and Huf, J., 1982, In vitro experiments on axon
    guidance demonstrating an anterior-posterior gradient on the
    tectum, EMBO Journal, 1:427-431.
Claviez, M., 1981, Kultur embryonaler Hühnchen-Retina: Eigenschaften
    auswachsender Neuriten und ihre Wechselwirkung mit der Umgebung,
    Thesis, Universitat Tubingen.
Cowan, W.M., 1978, Aspects of neural development, Int. Rev. Physiol.
    Neurophysiol., 17:149-191.
Cowan, W.M., Martin, A.H., and Wenger, E., 1968, Mitotic patterns in
    the optic tectum of the chick during normal development and
    after early removal of the optic vesicle, J. Exp. Zool.,
    169:71-92.
Crossland, W.J., Cowan, W.M., and Rogers, L.A., 1975, Studies on the
    development of the chick optic tectum. IV. An autoradiographic
    study of the development of retino-tectal connections,
    Brain Res., 91:1-23.
Dubray, G., and Bezard, G., 1982, A highly sensitive periodic acid-
    silver stain for 1, 2-diol groups of glycoproteins and poly-
    saccharides in polyacrylamide gels, Analyt. Biochem.,
    119:325-329.
Fraser, S.E., 1980, A differential adhesion approach to the pattern-
    ing of nerve connections, Dev. Biol., 79:453-464.
Gierer, A., 1982, Model for the retino-tectal projection, Proc. Roy.
    Soc. B., in press.
Goldberg, S., 1974, Studies on the mechanics of development of the
    visual pathways in the chick embryo, Dev. Biol., 36:24-43.
Goldberg, S., 1977, Undirectional, bidirectional, and random growth
    of embryonic optic axons, Exp. Eye Res., 25:399-404.
Goldberg, S., and Coulombre, A.J., 1972, Topographical development
    of the nerve fiber layer in the chick retina. A whole mount
    study, J. Comp. Neurol., 146:507-517.
Gottlieb, D.J., and Glaser, L., 1975, A novel assay of neuronal
    cell adhesion, Biochem. Biophys. Res. Comm., 63:815-821.
Gottlieb, D.J., Rock, K., and Glaser, L., 1976, A gradient of
    adhesive specificity in developing avian retina, Proc. Nat.
    Acad. Sci. USA, 73:410-414.
Halfter, W., Claviez, M., and Schwarz, U., 1981, Preferential
    adhesion of tectal membranes to anterior embryonic chick
    retina neurites, Nature, 292:67-70.
Halfter, W., Newgreen, D.F., Sauter, J., and Schwarz, U., 1982,
    Oriented axon outgrowth from avian embryonic retinae in
    culture, Dev. Biol., in press.
Henke, S., 1982, Monoklonale Antikörper gegen Oberflachenkomponenten
    neuronaler Zellen, Thesis, Universitat Tubingen.
Hughes, W.F., and McLoon, S.C., 1979, Ganglion cell death during
    normal retinal development in the chick: Comparisons wtih cell
    death induced by early target field destructions, Exp. Neurol.,
    66:507-601.

Kahn, A.J., 1973, Ganglion cell formation in the chick neural retina, Brain Res., 63:285-290.

Kahn, A.J., 1974, An autoradiographic analysis of the time of appearance of neurons in the developing chick neural retina, Dev. Biol., 38:30-40.

Krayanek, S., and Goldberg, S., 1981, Oriented extracellular channels and axonal guidance in the embryonic chick retina, Dev. Biol., 84:41-50.

LaVail, J.H., and Cowan, W.M., 1971, The development of the chick optic tectum. II. Autoradiographic studies, Brain Res., 28:421-441.

Neuhoff, V. (ed.), 1973, in: Micromethods in Molecular Biology, Springer-Verlag, Heidelberg.

Neukirchen, R.O., 1980, Gel-Elektrophorese im Mikromasstab. Entwicklung und praktische Anwendung von ein- und zweidimensionaler Polyacrylamid-Gelelektrophorese zur Trennung von Proteinen im Nanogrammbereich, Thesis, Universität Tübingen.

Neukirchen, R.P., Schlosshauer, B., Baars, S., Jäckle, H., and Schwarz, U., 1982, Two-dimensional protein analysis of high resolution on a microscale, J. Biol. Chem., in press.

O'Farrell, P.H., 1975, High resolution two-dimensional electrophoresis of proteins, J. Biol. Chem., 250:4007-4021.

O'Farrell, P.Z., Goodman, H.M., and O'Farrell, P.H., 1977, High resolution two-dimensional electrophoresis of basic as well as acidic proteins, Cell, 12:1133-1142.

Rager, G., and von Oeynhausen, B., 1979, Ingrowth and ramification of retinal fibers in the developing optic tectum of the chick embryo, Exp. Brain Res., 35:213-227.

Silver, H., and Sidman, R.L., 1980, A mechanism for the guidance and topographic patterning of retinal ganglion cell axons, J. Comp. Neurol., 189:101-111.

Sperry, R.W., 1963, Chemoaffinity in the orderly growth of nerve fiber patterns and connections, Proc. Nat. Acad. Sci. USA., 50:703-710.

Trisler, G.D., Schneider, M.D., and Nirenberg, M., 1981, A topographic gradient of molecules in retina can be used to identify neuron position, Proc. Nat. Acad. Sci. USA., 78:2145-2149.

ORDERED NERVE CONNECTIONS: PATHWAYS AND MAPS

R.M. Gaze

National Institute for Medical Research
The Ridgeway, Mill Hill
London, England

The idea that orderly neuronal interconnections are based on chemoselective recognition between the cells and their processes was proposed by Cajal (1892) and given experimental support by the work of Langley (1895). In its present form the hypothesis of neuronal specificity, as it is now called, derives largely from the work of Sperry (1943; 1944; 1945; 1951; 1963; 1965) and it proposes that interconnecting populations of neurones each acquire positionally dependent chemoselectivity labels, or markers, early in development, and that properly ordered interconnections between the populations are based on selective affinities between the markers carried by one population and those carried by the other.

The hypothesis was derived from the study of regenerating nerve fibers; cat sympathetic neurones in Langley's experiments and amphibian optic nerve fibers in the work of Sperry. While this was the origin of the hypothesis, its intention was primarily to account for the initial development of ordered nerve connections during neurogenesis. Thus the implicit assumption was that the mechanisms involved in the establishment of neuronal maps were the same in development and in regeneration. This assumption has given rise to problems which have become more obtrusive recently, with the increasing awareness that there are major and significant differences between develment and regeneration. It is becoming more likely that different mechanisms are at work in the two situations; or at least that the emphasis is different.

There is very strong evidence that, in central nervous regeneration in amphibians and fish, a mechanism involving recognition

361

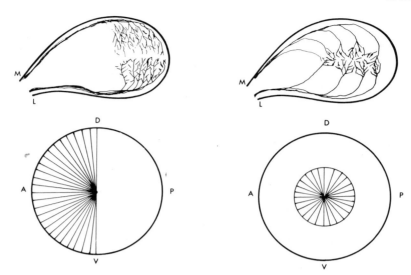

Fig. 1   Left: after interruption of the optic nerve and removal
of posterior retina in a goldfish, fibers from the remaining
anterior retina regenerate back past inappropriate rostral tectum
to reach their proper terminal zones in caudal tectum. Right:
central retinal fibers regenerate back to their proper termianl
zones in central tectum, passing inappropriate peripheral tectum on
the way. A, D, P, V: anterior, dorsal, posterior, ventral. M, L:
medial, lateral. After Attardi and Sperry, 1963.

and interaction between postional markers in the retina and on the
tectum is at work. The earliest good evidence for this was the
work of Attardi and Sperry (1963), who showed that optic nerve
fibers regenerating from a nasal half-retina in goldfish would grow
past empty rostral tectum to terminate in the appropriate caudal
part; similarly, fibers regenerating from the central region of the
retina would grow through the peripheral regions of the tectum to
terminate in the appropriate central part (Fig. 1).

Apart from this work of Attardi and Sperry, perhaps the most
convincing evidence for retino-tectal recognition comes from experiments in which pieces of tectum were translocated in the frog
(Jacobson and Levine, 1975) or in goldfish (Hope et al., 1976; Gaze
and Hope, 1982). In the latter cases the operation translocated
grafts between rostral and caudal parts of the same tectum (Fig.
2). Some months later, when the cut fibers had regenerated into
the grafts, or the optic nerve itself had regenerated if cut, electrophysiological mapping of the visuotectal projection showed that

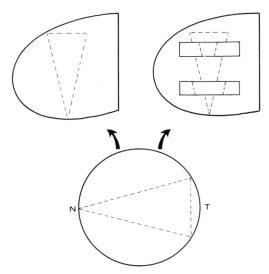

Fig. 2   Exchange of grafts between rostral and caudal tectum in
goldfish. The lower diagram represents the visual field of the
left eye; N, nasal; T, temporal. The upper two diagrams each represent a right optic tectum. On the left is the normal tectum,
with the interrupted triangle showing how the visual field is represented. On the right is a tectum carrying translocated grafts
(rectangles). Transposition of corresponding parts of the visual
field projection, as shown, would indicate the existence of a
target-recognition mechanism during regeneration of the optic.
fibers. See Hope et al., 1976.

there was translocation of parts of the visual field projection
corresponding to the translocated grafts (Fig. 3).

      In both types of experiment, that of Attardi and Sperry and
that involving graft-translocation, the result was that regenerating fibers made a choice of target when presented with various
possibilities. In each case the choice was "correct" and thus seems
to require a target-affinity mechanism (Gaze and Hope, 1976).

ROLE OF FIBER/FIBER INTERACTION

      In the above experiments it appears that recognition mechanisms
are at work in regeneration in these situations. However, even if
we confine our attention to regeneration, there are various

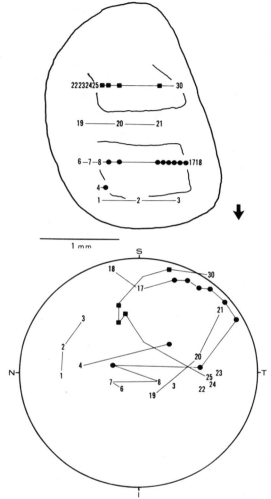

Fig. 3   Visuotectal map from a goldfish. The tectum carries
translocated grafts as indicated and the map shows corresponding
field translocation. Upper diagram represents the right optic
tectum. Numbers and symbols show electrode recording positions.
The filled circles represent postions in the rostral graft (translocated from caudal tectum) and the filled squares indicate positions in the caudal graft (translocated from rostral tectum). The
arrow points rostrally along the tectal midline. The lower diagram
represents the visual field of the left eye. N, nasal; S, superior;
T, temporal; I, inferior. The numbers and symbols represent optimal
stimulus positions corresponding to the tectal recording position.

experimental observations which show that target-affinity cannot be the only mechanism capable of producing an ordered map.

The earliest such observation was that of Gaze and Sharma (1970). These authors found that, if the caudal half of the optic-tectum was removed in adult goldfish, the fiber projection from the entire retina would eventually distribute itself, in a compressed but properly ordered fashion, over the residual rostral half-tectum (Fig. 4). This observation has been extensively confirmed in various laboratories and the converse observation has been made, that a surgically-formed half-retina in goldfish will, in due course, expand its fiber projection, in proper order, over the entire tectum (Horder, 1971; Yoon, 1972). The differences between the results in this latter case and those in the experiments of Attardi and Sperry (1963) may be shown to be a function of time; if one examines the fiber projection from the half-retina early in regeneration, the fibers reconstitute their original half-projection on the tectum, as shown by Attardi and Sperry; if one allows a considerably longer time to elapse before examining the fiber projection, this is found to have expanded across the tectum.

These experiments on expansion and compression of the retino-tectal projection indicate a major role for fiber/fiber interactions in the establishment of order in the final projections. For instance, when half the retina has been removed, the expansion of the projection from the remaining half-retina over the wrong half of the tectum can in no meaningful sense be associated with recognition between retinal and tectal sets of label. This is because, if labels do exist on the tectum, these labels on that other half of the tectum into which the fibers expand are appropriate to the missing half of the retina and not to the half retina which finally sends fibers to this part of the tectum. One could understand a form of expansion (without order) in terms merely of the concept of lebensraum for the fibers. However, the fact that when fibers do expand into extra territory like this, they do so in proper order amongst themselves, shows that the mechanisms maintaining this order involves in all probability fiber/fiber interaction rather than fiber/tectum inter-actions.

Field positions recorded from the rostral graft are translocated temporally (filled circles), while those from the caudal graft are translocated nasally (filled squares). After Gaze and Hope, 1972.

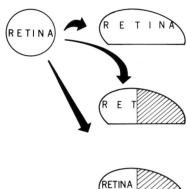

Fig. 4   Retinotectal compression. The retina (left of the diagram)
is shown projecting to the tectum (right of the diagram) under three
different conditions. The top diagram represents the normal retinotectal projection, covering the greater part of the tectum. The
middle diagram shows the situation soon after the optic fibers have
regenerated to the tectum, the caudal half of which has been removed.
There is a half-retinal projection to the half-tectum. The bottom
diagram shows the projection that is found after the lapse of several
weeks or months. The projection from the whole retina has now been
compressed, in proper order, over the residual half-tectum.

     Further evidence pointing to the active role that may be played
by the optic fibers themselves in establishing an ordered projection,
comes from the work of Schmidt (1978) on the projections formed by
half-retinae in goldfish. Firstly he showed (as had Attardi and
Sperry) that the initial projection from a half-retina formed a half-
map over the appropriate part of the tectum. Expansion of the map
took some months in fish of the size used. Once the projection had
spread, Schmidt caused the optic nerve to innervate the ipsilateral
tectum (connected also to the normal eye). Now the half-retina,
which had previously given an expanded map over its own tectum, gave
a normal half-map again, indicating that the retinal cell labels had
not changed. When the converse experiment was performed and the
optic nerve from a normal eye was fed onto a tectum carrying an
expanded half-retinal map, from the corresponding half of the retina
(Fig. 5). This clearly demonstrated that markers on the tectum had
changed in this experimental situation. Lastly, Schmidt found that,
if the tectum had been denervated of optic fibers for a period of
several months, the optic nerve from a half-retina then fed onto it
would form an expanded map right away, without the usual wait of
several months.

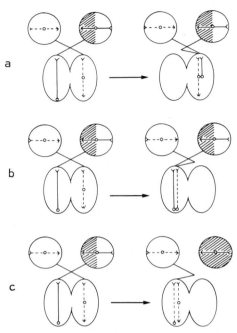

a

b

c

Fig. 5   Alteration of tectal positional markers by abnormal distributions of optic fibers in goldfish.   (a)   The diagram on the
left shows the normal projection from a left eye to the right
tectum. The nasal half of the right retina had been removed some
months previously and the projection from temporal retina has expanded over the whole of the left tectum.   The right-hand diagram shows
what happens when the fibers from the temporal half-retina are
diverted to the ipsilateral (right) tectum.   Here the fibers again
give an unexpanded half-map.   (b)   The left-hand diagram is as in
(a).   The right-hand diagram shows that if fibers from the normal
eye are now directed onto ipsilateral (left) tectum, which carries
an expanded half-map from the other eye, the normal eye now gives
an expanded half-map from the corresponding half of the retina.
(c) The left-hand diagram is as in (a).   If the fibers from the
normal eye are now directed onto the ipsilateral tectum as in the
right-hand diagram, and if, just before the fibers get there, the
previously-operated eye is removed, the normal eye then gives two
separate maps across the ipsilateral tectum.   One is an expanded
map from the half of the normal eye corresponding to the originally
operated other eye and the other map is complete.   After Schmidt,
1978.

These experiments of Schmidt thus indicate that retinal cell markers are stable in the face of an operation to form a half-retina, but that tectal markers may be altered by supplying the tectum with an abnormal distribution of fibers. Furthermore, the prolonged denervation experiment suggests that tectal markers are dependent, for their continued existence, on a continuing nerve supply.

These observations and interpretations raise the question of what may be the specificity-status of a developing, and as yet uninnervated tectum, before the optic fibers arrive. Experiments indicate that markers are put on the tectum by fibers. We do not know whether these markers are of the same kind as those that are postulated as controlling the normal development of the system. If they are, then we must ask how the fibers establish a correct map in the first place, before their markers are deposited on the tectum.

DEVELOPMENTAL OBSERVATIONS

The sequence of events that occurs during the normal development of the visual system in Xenopus suggests that some mechanism other than target-affinity is involved in the initial establishment of the retino-tectal map. The retina in Xenopus grows by the addition of rings of cells at the ciliary margin (Straznicky and Gaze (1971), whereas the tectum grows in a curvilinear fashion, from rostrolateral to caudomedial (Straznicky and Gaze, 1972). Despite these different modes of growth the retina and tectum start becoming interconnected early in the development of each, and from then on the visuotectal map maintains a normal internal order (Gaze et al.,1972; Gaze et al., 1974; Gaze et al., 1979). This implies that, during the extended development of the visual system in Xenopus, the retinotectal projection is continually shifting caudally across the tectum (Fig. 6). Any particular retinal ganglion cell forms connections with a particular part of the developing tectum early in larval life, and the same retinal cell projects to a different part of the tectum later on.

Under these circumstances we see that, if connections are formed by virtue of affinities between retinal cells (rather, their axons) and tectal cells, one or other set of labels must be continually altering during development; and this rapidly makes nonsense of the idea of localized positional labels in this situation. Normal development in the Xenopus visual system thus occurs in such a way as to suggest that localized target-affinity is not the mechanism at work. The same conclusion may be reached, and in an even more dramatic fashion, by consideration of what happens during the development of the projections from "compound eyes" in Xenopus.

Compound eyes in Xenopus (Gaze et al., 1963; Straznicky et al., 1974) are formed by operation on the embryo at or around stage 32

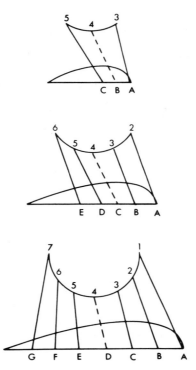

Fig. 6   Retinotectal relationships along the nasotemporal axis of
the retina and the rostrocaudal axis of the tectum, at various
stages (earliest at the top) during development in Xenopus.   The
retinal numbers and the tectal letters represent the cellular elements that have appeared at each stage.   The retina grows by addition of new cells at the ciliary margins, while the tectum grows
from rostral to caudal.   Most-temporal retina always projects to
most-rostral tectum (on the right of the diagram in each case) and
the whole projection thus moves caudally across the tectum during
development. After Gaze, 1974, British Medical Bulletin, 30:116-121.

(Nieuwkoop and Faber, 1956), before fibers have yet connected the
eye with the tectum.   To make a double-nasal (NN) eye the temporal
half of one eye is removed and replaced by the nasal half of an eye
taken from the opposite side of a donor embryo (Fig. 7).   Double-
temporal (TT) and double-ventral (VV) eyes may be made in comparable
fashion.   If the visuotectal projections from such compound eyes are
mapped electrophysiologically several months after metamorphosis, it
is found that the projection from each (similar) half of the retina
spreads out, in proper order, across the whole tectum, rather than
being restricted to the appropriate half-tectum as would be the case
for a projection from such a half-retina when forming part of a

normal eye (Fig. 8). This, which is the standard result with such compound eyes, prompts us to ask what may be happening to the retinal and tectal labels in these situations.

Before we can take our analysis much further, we must deal with one major problem. Before we can use the compound-eye experiment to tell us something about the nature of the tectum and its labels, we must be sure that we know what is the state of the compound eye itself, with respect to its positional labels. This particular question springs from the fact that the operation to form a compound eye is done in embryonic life, and it is at least conceivable that each half-eye has "regulated" in embryological terms, so as to give it the specificity-structure of a whole eye. If this were so we would automatically expect to get the type of projections from these eyes that we do in fact find; and we would be unable to use compound eyes for further analysis.

Fortunately this is not the case. Each half of a compound eye develops and maintains the markers characteristic of the particular half-eye making up the compound eye in question. The demonstration that this is so involves section of the nerve from the compound eye, close to the chiasma, shortly after metamorphosis. When this is done the nerve will regenerate, not merely back to its own contralateral tectum, but also up through the ipsilateral diencephalon to the ipsilateral tectum (Glastonbury and Straznicky, 1978). In this situation the fibers from the compound eye find themselves innervating a tectum which simultaneously carries the projection from the other, normal, eye. When this happens the projection from the compound eye, assessed autoradiographically, is found to be restricted to the appropriate half-tectum according to the nature of the compound eye (Gaze and Straznicky, 1980). Thus fibers from a TT eye are restricted to rostrolateral tectum, fibers from a VV eye are restricted to medial tectum and fibers from an NN eye innervate only caudomedial tectum (Fig. 9).

The fibers from each (similar) half of the compound eye are therefore recognizing something (in this regeneration experiment) which constrains them to terminate only in the appropriate half of the tectum. Thus each half of the compound eye still possesses (or expresses, functionally) only the markers characteristic of its component halves. Despite this, each compound eye regenerates at the same time a projection which covers (almost) the entire contralateral tectum (Fig. 9). The result from the ipsilateral tectum tells us that the eye carries only a half-complement of positional markers, while the result from the contralateral tectum (innervated by the compound eye) tell us something about this tectum has changed; it permits the half complement of retinal positions to spread its projection across the whole tectum.

Since we now know that the compound eye is an unregulated

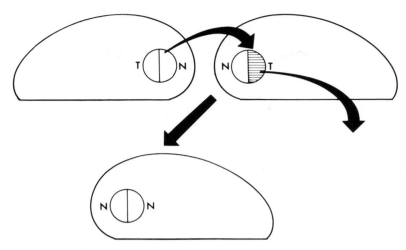

Fig. 7   The operation to make a double-nasal compound eye.

structure, in that it contains only a half-complement of positional
specificities, we can attempt to find out what is the nature of its
projection early in development, when the fibers first reach the
tectum. We might think (indeed, we did think, naively, and ignoring
what we already knew about shifting connections in normal development) that the early TT projection should be confined to the front
of the developing tectum, the early VV projection confined to
medial tectum and the early NN projection confined to caudal tectum.

     In the event we found that, at stage 50, (this being the earli-
est stage used for autoradiography), the TT fibers innervated rostrolateral tectum, VV fibers innervated medial tectum while NN fibers
innervated almost the entire available region of tectum. As the projections developed, the TT projection remained restricted to rostral
tectum until after metamorphosis, the VV projection also took
considerable time (though less) to spread over lateral tectum while
the NN projection at all times covered all available tectum, with a
decreased density of fibers in the most rostral part of the tectum,
at the tecto-diencephalic junction (Straznicky et al., 1981;
Steedman, 1981).

     This last type of projection, from the NN eye, is the one which
most obviously does not fit the idea of the matching of localized
retinal and tectal labels; the result would suggest that virtually
the whole of the tectum carried labels appropriate to nasal retina.

     While the developing NN projection is that which provides the
most obvious problems for localized target-affinity, the other two

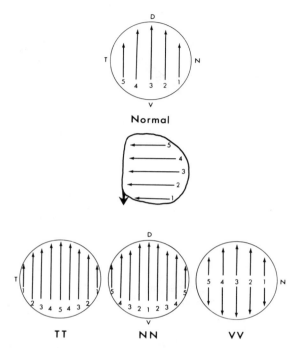

Fig. 8   Visuotectal projections from normal and compound eyes.
Upper diagram represents the visual field of the right eye.   Middle
diagram represents the dorsal surface of the left optic tectum.   The
numbered arrows on the tectum indicate rows of electrode recording
positions to which correspond the numbered positions in the visual
field charts.   The three lower diagrams represent the visuotectal
projections from TT, NN and VV eyes.

types of compound eye also do not fit this type of mechanism.   The
projection from a VV eye is initially confined to the medial tectum
and this (especially caudomedial tectum) is where the later stages
of tectal growth occur.   Eventually, however, the VV projection
spreads across the lateral region of the tectum, thus coming to
innervate older tectal tissue.   The projection from a TT eye is
initially confined to rostral tectum, but with time, comes to
spread over the greater part of the tectal surface.   In this case,
the "shift" of connections that occur as the system matures is considerably greater than that occurring in normal development, and
this poses even greater problems.

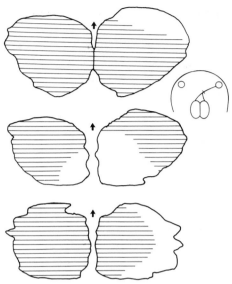

Fig. 9   The patterns of tectal innervation established by fibers
regenerating from double nasal, double temporal and double ventral
eyes in Xenopus. Right compound eyes were formed in embryos. Just
after metamorphosis the right optic nerve was allowed to regenerate
to both tecta. The diagrams represent reconstructions from serial
transverse sections through the tectum after labelling of the compound eye with tritiated proline. The hatched area represents the
distribution of proline in the tectum. Inset shows the experimental
arrangement. Top: Regeneration from an NN eye innervates the
whole of the contralateral tectum (left in the diagram) and all but
the most rostrolateral part of the ipsilateral tectum, which
carried simultaneously the projection from the normal eye.
Middle: Fibers regenerating from a double-temporal eye innervate the
greater part of the contralateral tectum but are confined to the
rostrolateral region of the ipsilateral tectum. Bottom: Fibers
regenerating from a double-ventral eye innervate the whole of the
contralateral tectum but are confined to the medial regions of the
ipsilateral tectum. In each case the heavy arrow points rostrally
along the tectal midline. From Gaze and Straznicky, 1980.

     These observations on the development of the projections from
normal and compound eyes seem to require that we postulate some
mechanism for the establishment of the projection, other than target-
affinity. The possibilities here seem limited only by the ingenuity

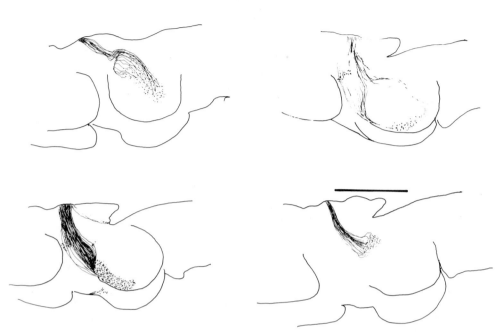

Fig. 10   The pathways of fibers from temporal, ventral, nasal and
dorsal regions of the retina in <u>Xenopus</u>.   The results of partial
retinal fills with HRP are illustrated in camera lucida drawings
from whole-mount preparations of the brain.   Top left: Temporal
fibers form a tight band running up the diencephalon and distribute
themselves in rostrolateral tectum.   Top right: Ventral fibers enter
the tectum through the medial brachium only and are distributed
across the medial aspect of the tectum.   Bottom left: Nasal fibers
are distributed across the entire extent of the optic tract and pass
to their caudomedial tectal destinations by running mostly through
the medial and lateral brachia of the optic tract.   Some fibers,
not shown in this diagram, pass directly to their terminations
across the dorsal surface of the tectum.   Bottom right: Dorsal
retinal fibers enter the tectum via the lateral brachium only and
are distributed only across the lateral tectum.   Bar - 1 mm for all
diagrams.   From Fawcett and Gaze, 1982.

of the experimenter, or theoretician.   Various classes of mechanisms
were considered by Gaze and Hope (1976); here I want to concentrate
on a hybrid mechanism towards which, it seem to me, the evidence is
converging.   The idea, which has been argued on other occasions (e.g.

Straznicky et al., 1981), is that, provided that fibers are fed onto
the tectum in fairly good retinotopic order, to provide an orientation for the map, the retinotectal projection can establish itself
in proper order across the tectum largely through fiber/fiber interaction.

It has been shown (Straznicky et al., 1979; Steedman, 1981;
Fawcett and Gaze, 1982) that the fibers from different parts of the
retina in a larval or young adult Xenopus normally approach the
tectum in a retinotopically-organized fashion. This has also been
shown to be so in the newt and in Rana (Fujisawa et al., 1981a and b).
Thus temporal retinal fibers stay closely together in the mid-region
of the optic tract and pass onto the rostral margin of the tectum
without forming brachia. Fibers from ventral retina approach the
tectum through the medial part of the tract and enter the tectum via
the medial brachium only. Fibers from dorsal retina approach the
tectum through the lateral part of the tract and pass via the lateral
brachium. Fibers from nasal retina, on the other hand, behave differently to the other three categories of fibers; nasal fibers approach
the tectum across the entire width of the diencephalic optic tract
(Fig. 10). They enter the tectum to reach their caudomedial destinations via both medial and lateral brachia, as well as (some few
fibers) passing directly across the top of the tectum. There are
thus clear cut differences in behavior between temporal, ventral
and dorsal fibers on the one hand and nasal fibers on the other.

As discussed above, the modes of growth of the Xenopus retina,
tectum and retinotectal projection are such that there must be a
continual shift of connections on the tectum itself, throughout
growth. However, the very fact that the optic pathway and the brain
itself continue to grow throughout larval life indicates that, once
the pathway is established, it is there permanently. Once the fiber
order in the optic tract has been established in the earlier stages
of development there is no way in which it can later be altered.
This is because the fibers in the tract are laid down successively
throughout the various stages of development (Gaze and Grant, 1978);
each batch of fibers, coming from the ciliary margin of the retina
at one particular stage, is separated from the previously grown
fibers, and from those arriving later, by intervening fibers of other
systems, many running at 90° to the optic fibers. There is thus
formed a sort of fiber-weaving which prevents any later sideways movement of the optic fibers, to vary the order amongst them. Thus the
order that we see in the tract in later life is that which has
existed from the beginning.

We therefore think we know two things. First, there is a proper
order in the optic tract from the start of visual development;
second, the fibers of the optic projection can, by interacting among
themselves, give rise to an appropriate order in the tectal map.
The obvious extension of these statements would be that these two

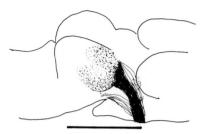

Fig. 11.   The fiber pathway from a double temporal compound eye in
Xenopus.   Magnification as in Fig. 11.   From Fawcett and Gaze, 1982.

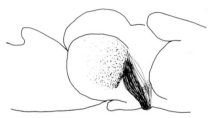

Fig. 12   The fiber pathway from a double ventral compound eye.
Magnification as in Fig. 11.   From Fawcett and Gaze, 1982.

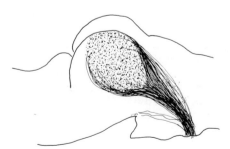

Fig. 13   The fiber pathway from a double nasal compound eye.
Magnification as in Fig. 11.   From Fawcett and Gaze, 1982.

factors, by themselves, are sufficient to account for the orderly
visual projection that we normally see.

To test this idea we need to disarrange the fibers in the optic
projection before they first reach the tectum during development.
In particular, we would like to feed the first incoming optic fibers
onto the tectum by an abnormal pathway, with and without a "normal"
arrangement amongst themselves.

The obvious way of feeding fibers onto the tectum from the
wrong direction would be by transplantation of an eye caudal to the
tectum. This has been done (Giogi and Van der Loos, 1978) but, up
to the present time, there is inadequate detailed information about
the mode of entry of fibers from these displaced eyes onto the
tectum, and whether or not there is any recognizable order in the
tectal projections so formed. These matters are being further
investigated at present. As for growing fibers onto the tectum
with disturbed internal fiber order in the pathway, this has been
attempted by a variety of compound-eye type experiments (Gaze et
al., 1963; Straznicky et al., 1974; Straznicky et al., 1981).

In the case of a compound eye of the classical NN, TT or VV
type, the fiber arrangements in the optic nerve as the fibers leave
the eye are of course abnormal in that the fibers are positioned as
coming from two similar half eyes facing each other in the whole-
eye structure. The question then is, how do fibers from compound
eyes behave as they approach the tectum in the optic tract? We
have recently used cobalt and HRP to investigate these matters
(Steedman, 1981; Fawcett and Gaze, 1982). It turns out that fibers
from a double temporal eye behave in a fashion reminiscent of fibers
from a temporal segment in a normal eye. That is, fibers from a
double temporal eye tend to bunch together towards the middle of
the region normally occupied by the tract, forming a compact narrow
tract which enters directly onto the front of the tectum without
forming brachia, and with terminal arborizations restricted to the
rostral part of the tectum (Fig. 11). Fibers from a double ventral
eye all behave as do fibers from the ventral part of a normal eye.
Double ventral fibers all enter the tectum via the medial part of
the optic tract and the medial brachium (see also Straznicky et
al., 1979). In such cases there are no fibers in the lateral part
of the tract or the lateral brachium at all and the eventual
filling of the whole of the tectum with terminal arborizations is
achieved by the fibers turning laterally once they have entered the
tectum from its medial aspect (Fig. 12). Fibers from double nasal
eyes tend to behave as do fibers from the nasal parts of the normal
eye. That is, double nasal fibers approach the tectum widespread
throughout the optic tract; they mostly advance towards their
terminal regions on the tectum via massive medial and lateral
brachia (Fig. 13). It is not feasible to make double dorsal eyes
(because of the damage to the ventral fissure occcasioned by such

operations) so we are not able to say what would happen to fibers
from such double dorsal eye were they able to approach the tectum.

These results suggest that the fibers from certain parts of
the retina locate themselves in the optic tract in an absolute
fashion. If the fibers are ventral retinal fibers and normally
would use the medial brachium, they do so even if the lateral
brachium is empty and there is plenty of room to expand. This
has to be partly because , as argued above, once the first fibers
have made their decision and entered the medial brachium those
same fibers cannot then change. If further fibers make a similar
decision to run medially in the tract, then all the fibers will
pile up medially and the existence of cross fibers forming a web
network will prevent the double ventral fibers from drifting
laterally to fill the rest of the tract. Similarly, fibers from a
double temporal eye behave as if they recognize absolutely the
position in the tract they should occupy. As for double nasal
fibers, we see that they behave similarly to ordinary nasal fibers
in that they appear to lack the localizing constraints that affect
the fibers from the rest of the retina.

How might these observations relate to the establishment of
retino-tectal projections by these and by normal eyes? As has been
shown previously (Steedman, 1981; Fawcett and Gaze, 1982), all temporal fibers approach the front of the tectum directly. We shall
assume (Straznicky et al., 1981) that when they reach the front of
the tectum these temporal fibers establish their first connections
there. Further temporal fibers arriving from, for instance, a double
temporal eye, also arrive at the front of the tectum, but they find
the ground already occupied. Before they can establish their own
connections at the front of the tectum they have to displace those
fibers that are already there. This they do, but it takes time; and
the result is that the eventual spreading of a double temporal projection across the whole of the tectum is a slow business and only
completed some considerable time after metamorphosis.

Similarly with ventral fibers. These, as we have seen, are
normally fed onto the tectum via the medial brachium. In normal
development these fibers thus innervate the tectum from its medial
edge and would meet with similar constraints in that further ventral
fibers being fed on after the first ones would find their place partly taken up by fibers which arrived earlier; not completely,
because the tectum is growing in the caudomedial direction so there
is a certain amount of extra tectum for them to connect with. But
if there are a lot of fibers arriving, they will again be constrained
by having the territory occupied; and before they can expand into
lateral tectum they will have to displace the previous ventral fibers
laterally. This idea is consistent with the observation that in
development the double ventral projection starts off distributed

across the medial aspect of the tectum and takes some time to spread to the most lateral part (Straznicky et al., 1981).

As for nasal fibers, from the start such fibers are fed onto the tectum via all possible pathways, particularly the two brachia. As the tectum is continually growing caudomedially, the new fibers coming in from nasal parts of the double nasal eye are continually being fed onto newly available tectum. This means that the developing double nasal projection will at all times cover the entire extent of the available tectum; and this indeed is what happens. In these preparations there appears to be a very restricted region rostrally, close by the bifurcation of the brachia of the tract, where nasal fibers leave a small "hole". This is the region that is of particular interest to the temporal fibers.

It may be seen that the result of these various arguments and suggestions is to move the problem of the establishment of order back one step, from the tectum to the tract. We still have to account for the formation of a retinotopically arranged fiber distribution in the tract, as it approaches the tectum. However this may be simpler than to account for order on the tectum, because position in the tract is fixed and does not shift with development.

If we postulate (Steedman, 1981; Fawcett and Gaze, 1982) that temporal fibers are more cohesive than other retinal fibers, thus giving them a competitive advantage in the innervation of rostral tectum; and if we in addition postulate the existence of some directional switch in the diencephalon for ventral vs. dorsal retinal fibers, this may be all that is needed over and above fiber/fiber terminal interactions, for the establishment of the tectal map during development. We need now to see whether we can find any evidence concerning these postulates.

REFERENCES

Attardi, D.G. and Sperry, R.W., 1963, Preferential selection of central pathways by regenerating optic fibres, Exp. Neurol., 7:46–64.

Cajal, S.R., 1892, The structure of the retina. English Translation, 1972, Charles C. Thomas, Springfield.

Fawcett, J.W. and Gaze, R.M., 1982, The retinotectal fiber pathways from normal and compound eyes in Xenopus, J. Embryol. exp. Morph., in press.

Fujisawa, H., Wakanabe, K., Tani, N. and Ibata, Y., 1981a, Retinotopic analyses of fiber pathways in amphibians. I. The adult newt, Cynops pyrrhogaster. Brain Res., 206:9–20.

Fujisawa, H., Wakanabe, K., Tani, N. and Ibata, Y., 1981b, Retinotopic analyses of fiber pathways in amphibians. II. The frog Rana nigromaculata. Brain Res., 206:21–26.

Gaze, R.M., Chung, S.-H. and Keating, M.J., 1972, Development of the
    retinotectal projection in Xenopus, Nature, 236:133-135.
Gaze, R.M. and Grant, P., 1978, The diencephalic course of regenera-
    ting retinotectal fibres in Xenopus tadpoles, J. Embryol. exp.
    Morph., 44:201-216.
Gaze, R.M. and Hope, R.A., 1976, The formation of continuously
    ordered mappings, Prog. Brain Res., 45:327-355.
Gaze, R.M. and Hope, R.A., 1982, The visuotectal projection following
    translocation of grafts within an optic tectum in the goldfish,
    J. Physiol. Lond., in press.
Gaze, R.M., Jacobson, M. and Székély, G., 1963, The retinotectal
    projection in Xenopus with compound eyes, J. Physiol. Lond.,
    165:484-499.
Gaze, R.M., Keating, M.J. and Chung, S.-H., 1974, The evolution of
    the retinotectal map during developing in Xenopus, Proc. Roy.
    Soc. Lond. B 185:301-330.
Gaze, R.M., Keating, M.J., Ostberg, A., and Chung, S.-H., 1979, The
    relationship between retinal and tectal growth in larval
    Xenopus: implications for the development of the retinotectal
    projection , J. Embryol. exp. Morph., 53:103-143.
Gaze, R.M. and Sharma, S.C., 1970, Axial differences in the
    reinnervation of the goldfish optic tectum by regenerating optic
    nerve fibres, Exp. Brain Res., 10:171-181.
Gaze, R.M. and Straznicky, C., 1980, Regeneration of optic nerve
    fibres from a compound eye to both tecta in Xenopus: evidence
    relating to the state of specification of the eye and the
    tectum, J. Embryol. exp. Morph., 60:125-140.
Giorgi, P.P. and Van der Loos, H., 1978, Axons from eyes grafted in
    Xenopus can grow into the spinal cord and reach the optic
    tectum, Nature, 275:746-748.
Glastonbury, J. and Straznicky, K., 1978, Aberrant ipsilateral
    retinotectal projection following optic nerve section in
    Xenopus, Neuroscience Letts., 7:67-72.
Hope, R.A., Hammond, B.J. and Gaze, R.M., 1976, The arrow model:
    retinotectal specificity and map formation in the goldfish
    visual system, Proc. Roy. Soc. Lond. B 194:447-466.
Horder, T.J., 1971, Retention by fish optic nerve fibres regenerating
    to new terminal sites in the tectum of "chemospecific" affinity
    for their original sites, J. Physiol. Lond., 216:53-55P.
Jacobson, M. and Levine, R.L., 1975, Stability of implanted
    duplicated tectal positional markers serving as targets for
    optic axons in adult frogs, Brain Res., 92:468-471.
Langley, J.N., 1895, A note on the regeneration of preganglion fibres
    in the cat sympathetic system, J. Physiol. Lond., 18:280-284.
Nieuwkoop, P.D. and Faber, J., 1956, Normal Table of Xenopus laevis,
    (Daudin), Amsterdam: North Holland.
Schmidt, J.T., 1978, Retinal fibers alter tectal positional markers
    during the expansion of the half retinal projection in goldfish,
    J. comp. Neurol., 177:279-300.

Sperry, R.W., 1943, Visuomotor coordination in the newt (Tritinus viridescens) after regeneration of the optic nerve, J. comp. Neurol., 79:33-55.

Sperry, R.W., 1944, Optic nerve regeneration with return of vision in aurans, J. Neurophysiol., 7:57-70.

Sperry, R.W., 1945, Restoration of vision after crossing of optic nerves and after contralateral transplantation of eye, J. Neurophysiol., 8:15-18.

Sperry, R.W., 1951, Mechanisms of neural maturation, In: Handbook of Experimental Psychology, S.S. Stevens (Ed.), Wiley, New York, pp. 236-280.

Sperry, R.W., 1963, Chemoaffinity in the orderly growth of nerve fiber patterns and connections, Proc. Nat. Acad. Sci. (U.S.A), 50:703-710.

Sperry, R.W., 1965, Embryogenesis of behavioural nerve ends (?) in Organogenesis, R.L. DeHann and Unspring, H. (Eds.), Holt, Rienehand and Winston, New York, pp. 161-186.

Steedman, J.G., 1981, Pattern formation in the visual pathways of Xenopus laevis., Ph.D. Thesis, London.

Straznicky, K. and Gaze, R.M., 1971, The growth of the retina in Xenopus laevis: an autoradiographic study, J. Embryol. exp. Morph., 26:67-79.

Straznicky, K. and Gaze, R.M., 1972, The development of the tectum in Xenopus laevis: an autoradiographic study, J. Embryol. exp. Morph., 28:87-115.

Straznicky, C., Gaze, R.M. and Horder, T.J., 1979, Selection of appropriate medial branch of the optic tract by fibres of ventral retinal origin during development and in regeneration: an autoradiograph study in Xenopus, J. Embryol. exp. Morph., 50:253-267.

Straznicky, K., Gaze, R.M. and Keating, M.J., 1974, The retinotectal projection from a double-ventral compound eye in Xenopus laevis, J. Embryol. exp. Morph., 31:123-137.

Straznicky, C., Gaze, R.M. and Keating, M.J., 1981, The development of the retinotectal projections from compound eyes in Xenopus, J. Embryol. exp. Morph., 62:13-35.

Yoon, M.G., 1972, Transposition of the visual projection from the nasal hemiretina onto the foreign rostral zone of the optic tectum in goldfish, Exp. Neurol., 37:451-462.

CHANGES IN THE CYTOSKELETON PROVIDE AN INDEX OF GROWTH ACTIVITY
AND CELL INTERACTIONS DURING NERVOUS SYSTEM REGENERATION AND
PLASTICITY

John Cronly-Dillon

Visual Sciences Laboratories
Department of Ophthalmic Optics
University of Manchester Institute of Science and Technology
Manchester, England

INTRODUCTION

The cytoskeleton of the neuron and axon consists primarily of
the three components, microtubules, microfilaments and neurofilaments: and recent evidence indicates that elements of the cytoskeleton play a significant role in mediating the active translocation
of materials along neurites (Schwartz, 1979). Cytoskeletal components such as tubulin and actin are therefore important for neurite
growth, and their involvement in synapse formation has also been
demonstrated (Jones and Matus, 1975; Lagnado et al., 1971). Consequently, it is not unreasonable to suppose that changes in cytoskeletal organization may coincide with many developmental changes
that affect a neuron's morphology.

From his classical observations on growing axons, Ramon y Cajal
(1919) deduced that the axon arises from the cell body during development; that growth and regeneration take place as a result of
materials supplied by the soma. Although it is well established that
there also exists a retrograde flow in axons, the tendency of those
studying the relationship of intracellular transport to neurite
growth has generally been to underestimate the possibility that local
feedback events within living tissue may regulate the anterograde
and retrograde flow of materials within growing neurites. Cajal
(1919)and Murray, et al. (1982) however, were well aware that local
influences within target tissue could affect the growth reactions of
developing neurites, and recently, Aguilar et al (1973), and Purves
and Lichtman (1980), have each proposed new schemes in which neurotrophic influences within target tissue participate in a local feed-

383

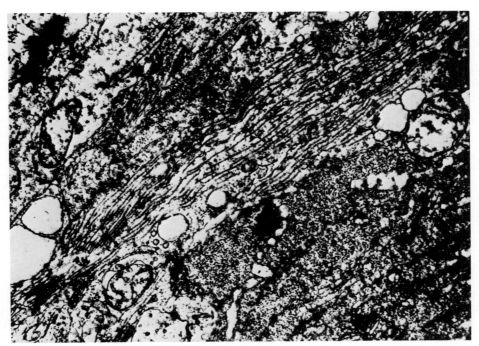

Figure 1. Electon micrograph of developing neurites in a Xenopus embryo, showing microtubules. (Courtesy John Dixon)

back control system to regulate the sprouting and terminal connectivity of ingrowing axons. The cytoskeleton is also the organelle traditionally associated with cell motility, and the trend of recent studies points to a presumed transmembrane connection between events linking the internal cytoskeleton with adhesive interactions of the cell surface (1982). Consequently, we may occasionally expect changes in the cytoskeleton and in cell growth activity to arise from adhesive interactions between nerve growth cones and cells in target tissue. Such changes in neural growth activity, arising from cell-cell adhesive interactions have indeed been been observed in the developing cerebellum (Berry et al, 1980). Cajal (1919) also suggested that most developing nerves establish more than the normal number of endings when they initially invade their targets, and he speculated that in some cases, a selection of endings proceeded on a functional basis. Similar proposals have been made for the function-

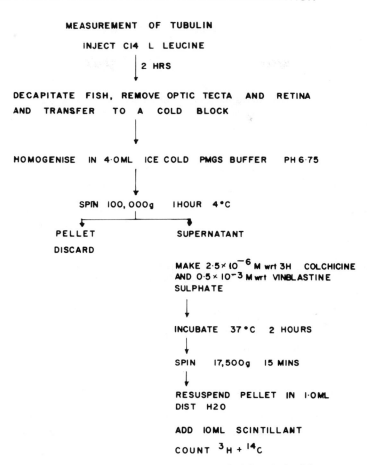

MEASUREMENT OF TUBULIN

INJECT CI4 L LEUCINE

↓ 2 HRS

DECAPITATE FISH, REMOVE OPTIC TECTA AND RETINA
AND TRANSFER TO A COLD BLOCK

↓

HOMOGENISE IN 4·0ML ICE COLD PMGS BUFFER PH 6·75

↓

SPIN 100,000g IHOUR 4°C

PELLET   SUPERNATANT
DISCARD

MAKE 2.5×10^{-6} M wrt 3H COLCHICINE
AND 0.5×10^{-3} M wrt VINBLASTINE
SULPHATE

↓

INCUBATE 37°C 2 HOURS

↓

SPIN 17,500g 15 MINS

↓

RESUSPEND PELLET IN I·0ML
DIST H2O

ADD 10ML SCINTILLANT

COUNT ^{3}H + ^{14}C

Figure 2. Method for measurement of soluble tubulin concentration
and incorporation of ^{14}C-radiolabelled-leucine into tubulin enriched
fraction in nervous tissue.

al modelling of the ipsilateral visual projection in developing
Xenopus embryos (Keating, 1977), and are supported by a recent
report that Tetrodotoxin blockade of nervous activity affects the
patterning of regenerating retinotectal connections in goldfish
(Meyer, 1982). Thus where nervous activity affects growth it is
also likely to affect the cell cytoskeleton. In the following we
describe a number of studies in which:

(i)   Changes in the synthesis of cytoskeletal components reveal
      growth regulating interactions between ingrowing optic
      axons and tectal cells during regeneration of the goldfish
      visual system.

(ii)   Synthesis of the cytoskeketal component <u>tubulin</u> in rat
       visual cortex is shown to be affected by functional
       activity in visual pathways during a critical period of
       visual cortical development.

(iii) A shift in **type** of cytoskeletal protein synthesized during
       development **seems** to be associated with different stages
       of neural growth and maturation.

(iv)   Colchicine blockade of tubulin polymerization is found to
       affect memory fixation and prevent the transfer of recent
       learning from short to long term memory.

GROWTH INTERACTIONS BETWEEN REGENERATING OPTIC AXONS AND TECTAL CELLS
IN GOLDFISH MODULATE TUBULIN SYNTHESIS DURING RETINOTECTAL PATTERN
FORMATION.

The visual system of fish and amphibia is remarkable in being
able to regenerate and re-establish a normal pattern of retinotectal
connections after damage to the optic nerve. The exact means by
which regenerating optic axons regain their terminal sites is still
unknown though it is generally accepted that target tissue exercises
some influence on the guidance of growing axons to their final des-
tination (Jacobson, 1978). In addition however, target tissue must
exercise some growth regulating influence on regenerating axons,
for when these contact their target neurones, growth and sprouting
generally cease. Our present study measures changes in the rates
of synthesis of soluble protein, and of a major cytoskeletal component (i.e. a soluble tubulin-enriched fraction) in retina and tectum
over a 7 week period during the course of optic nerve regeneration
and reinnervation of the tectum.

In our first experiment the optic nerves were crushed bilaterally close to the point of exit from the eye. At various times after
crushing the nerves, we injected ^{14}C-radiolabelled leucine into the
posterior chamber of each eye, and intracranially, into the subdural
space overlying the optic tectum. We did this 2 hours before killing
the fish and before removing the retinae and tectum to cold block
for biochemical assay. This enabled us to study the rate of incorporation of radiolabelled amino acid into nascent tubulin (and protein) in retina and tectum respectively. Vinblastine sulphate was
used to precipitate tubulin by a method adapted from Feit et al.,
(1971). (See Fig. 2.)

In the first week after nerve crush, tubulin synthesis rises
steadily in the retina but there is no change in the tectum (Fig. 3).
Between 1 and 1 1/2 weeks after nerve crush, there was a sudden rapid
rise in protein, and later, tubulin synthesis in the tectum, which
correlated with the time of arrival of regenerating optic axons at

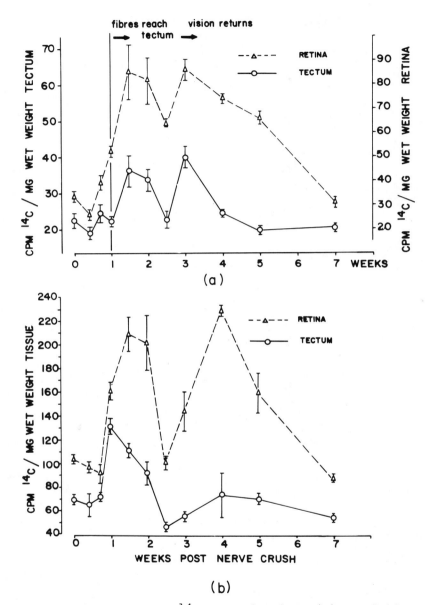

Figure 3. Incorporation of ^{14}C-L-Leucine into (a) a soluble tubulin enriched fraction and (b) total soluble protein, in goldfish retina and tectum at various times after the optic nerves have been crushed.

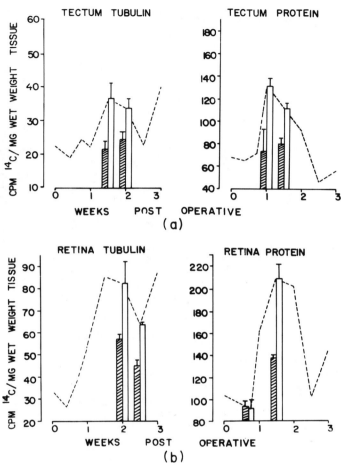

Figure 4. (a)   Preventing the ingrowth of optic fibers by eye removal abolishes the increase in synthesis of protein and tubulin in tectal cells at various times after eye ennucleation (shaded histograms) and after nerve crush (open histograms).   Broken line denotes control pattern of tectal protein/tubulin synthesis during first 2 1/2 weeks of regeneration of an optic nerve within the tectum. (b)   Reciprocal effect showing that removal of brain target area (tectum) of ingrowing optic fibers reduces the rate of synthesis of tubulin and total soluble protein in retina.   Shaded histogram denotes incorporation of radiolabelled leucine into retinal tubulin/ protein at various times after tectum removed and nerves crushed. Broken line, curve denotes the pattern occurring in retina during first 2 1/2 weeks of regeneration of an optic nerve with tectum in situ.

their target tissue. In addition, we found that during regeneration
of the retinotectal projection, the pattern of synthesis of soluble
protein and tubulin, in retina and tectum, were bimodal. This suggests that during reinnervation of the tectum, there are at least
two distinct bursts of growth activity occurring in retina and tectum.

In addition we carried out a number of experiments to determine:

(i)   if regenerating optic axons affect the growth activity of
      the tectum; and

(ii) if the tectum exerts a reciprocal influence on growth
      activity in regenerating optic axons and retina.

In one of these experiments we prevented optic fibers from growing into the tectum by surgically removing the eyes. We wished to
determine if this procedure affected the increase in tubulin and
protein synthesis normally present in the tectum at 1 1/2-2 weeks
following nerve crush. Figure 4 shows that preventing the ingrowth
of optic fibers by eye removal, abolishes the increase in tubulin
and protein synthesis in tectal cells.

We show also, that removing the principal brain target area
(tectum) of ingrowing optic fibers, reduces the rate of synthesis of
tubulin and total protein in the retina (Fig. 4). These results
support the idea that reciprocal growth regulating interactions take
place between ingrowing optic fibers and tectal cells during regeneration of the retinotectal projection.

Initial responses associated with locus specific differences of retinal neurites during tectal reinnervation

The modulating influence of the tectum on growth and protein
synthesis of the retina manifests itself even more strikingly when we
compare protein synthesis of a half-nasal (1/2N) versus a half-
temporal (1/2T) eye that is regenerating an optic nerve. Here we
surgically removed half the retina bilaterally leaving behind
either half-nasal or half-temporal retinae. We did this six weeks
before crushing the nerves to allow ample time for the eyes to heal.
We then proceeded as follows:

a)   In one group of 1/2T and 1/2N fish we surgically removed the
tectum at the time we crushed the nerves so as to eliminate any
possible modulatory influence of the tectum on the retina.

b)   In another group we crushed the nerves from our half eye
leaving the tectum in situ.

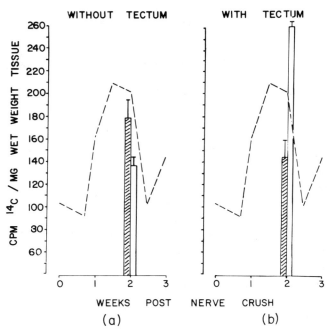

Figure 5. Incorporation of radiolabelled leucine (2 hr pulse) at 2 weeks post nerve crush in a <u>nasal</u> (open histogram) versus <u>temporal</u> (shaded histogram) hemiretina: (a) In the <u>absence</u> of a modulating influence of the tectum. (b) In the <u>presence</u> of the tectum.

    Protein synthesis in half nasal and half temporal retinae was then determined at 2 weeks after the optic nerves were crushed. (By permitting 2 weeks to elapse after crushing the nerves we allowed sufficient time for any intrinsic differences in rate of growth between half nasal and half temporal eyes to stabilize).

    Figure 6 shows that the tectum responds earlier to optic fibers regenerating from a 1/2T eye than those emanating from a 1/2N eye. <u>In the absence of the modulating influence of the tectum</u> we found that retinal protein synthesis in 1/2T eyes was significantly great- er than in 1/2N eyes at 2 weeks after nerve crush (Fig. 5a). Hence, <u>without the tectum</u> fibers from a 1/2T eye regenerate faster than those from a 1/2N eye. <u>With the tectum present</u>, we find that protein synthesis in 1/2N retinae now greatly exceeds that of 1/2T retinae at 2 weeks post nerve crush (Fig. 5b). This reverses the previous relationship found at 2 weeks when the tectum was absent. Figure 6 shows the profile of changes measured in the tectum and

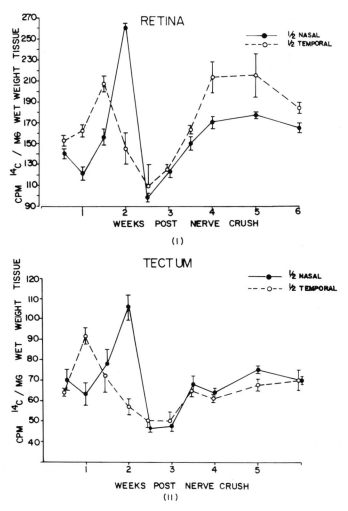

Figure 6   Incorporation of radiolabelled leucine (2 hr pulse) (i) in a nasal versus temporal hemiretina during optic nerve regeneration; and (ii) in a tectum being innervated by a nasal versus a temporal hemiretina.

retina at different times after nerve crush. Here, the initial peak retinal and tectal responses of the 1/2N group, although occurring later, were of significantly greater amplitude than for the 1/2T group. These results suggest that the growth of optic fibers that derive from different retinal locations are affected differently by

their interactions with the tectum, and this could be an important
factor in the retinotopic ordering of regenerating retinotectal connections. We suggest also that such differences displayed by 1/2N
and 1/2T groups, in their interaction with the tectum, may be related to differences in the strength of adhesion established by 1/2N
and 1/2T regenerating neurites with the tectal substratum.

It is known from in vitro studies that neurite outgrowth only
occurs in attached cells and that protein synthesis is considerably
greater in attached than in unattached cells. Indeed, no outgrowth
of axons occurs in the absence of attachment to a substratum
(Letourneau, 1982). Also, when the substratum exhibits an adhesive
gradient, growing axons advance by relinquishing one adhesive contact for others to which their filopodia adhere more firmly
(Letourneau, 1982). The possibility then, is that the greater the
attachment of regenerating axons to the substratum, the greater the
stimulus for nerve growth. Presumably this effect is mediated
through some transmembrane connection linking the adhesive contact
with the internal cytoskeleton (Solomon, 1982) Recently, it has been
reported for the chick embryo retina, that retinal neurites from
nasal retina are more adhesive, and bind more readily to tectal membrane fragments than those deriving from temporal retina (Halfter et
al. 1981). Hence the greater protein synthetic activity of goldfish
nasal optic fibers during the initial stage of interaction with the
tectum may be related to their greater adhesion with the tectal
substratum.

Correlation with morphological changes seen during tectal reinnervation

The pattern of biochemical changes observed in our present study
also correlate with certain morphological changes seen in the ultrastructural and light microscopic studies of optic nerve regeneration
in goldfish.

The first stage of tectal reinnervation, which lasts from 1 to
2 1/2 weeks post nerve crush, correlates with the time when regenerating optic fascicles are growing in the stratum opticum (S.O.) as
reported by Murray (1976)(see footnote). In the S.O., regenerating

---

Footnote: Although the conditions in Murray's experiment differ in
some respects from our own, in that the fish she used were larger,
and we crushed the optic nerve at a point adjacent to the eye
instead of cutting the tracts; both our estimated times of arrival
of regenerating optic axons at the tectum (7-11 days
postoperatively) and our estimate of the return of vision (3-4
weeks) were comparable in each of our respective studies.

optic fascicles contact NGF containing radial and other glial
elements, whose processes form 'channels' that supposedly guide the
regenerating fascicles with which they are closely associated. In
addition Murray (1976) observed that regenerating fascicles contain
a greater number of axonal profiles as they enter the S.O.; which is
consistent with the possibility that regenerating axons sprout in
response to some neurotrophic factor as they enter the tectum.
Hence the increase in retinal tubulin synthesis seen during the
initial stage of tectal reinnervation may be the result of some
neurotrophic growth promoting influence, exercised by radial and
other glia, on optic fascicles regenerating through the S.O.

The presence of NGF in the goldfish tectum (Benowitz and Sashoua,
1979) is suggestive of a putative role in regeneration and retinotectal pattern formation. Goldfish retinal neurites are sensitive to
NGF (Turner et al. 1980) and the latter is known to stimulate tubulin
synthesis (Fine and Bray, 1971) and promote neurite outgrowth. Also,
NGF has been found to affect cell adhesion (Schubert et al., 1978),
and it does so, supposedly, by promoting a redistribution, within the
plasma membrane of adhesive receptors. Part of the effect of NGF in
promoting tubulin synthesis and neurite outgrowth may therefore be
due to its enhancement of adhesion between growing axons and the
substratum with a consequent effect on both guidance and growth
activity of regenerating retinal neurites.

As for the tectum's response to reinnervation, Stevenson and
Yoon (1972) observed that radial glia within the tectum undergo
mitosis during optic reinnervation. Such radial glia contain microtubules, and the rise in tubulin synthesis exhibited by the tectum
during reinnervation may be partly associated with the mitotic
activity and morphogenesis of these newly generated radial glia.

Approximately 2 1/2 weeks after damage to the tract, regenerating optic axons from central retina leave the S.O. and enter the
stratum fibrosum et griseum superficiale (SFGS) where the majority
establish connections with tectal neurons. Murray (1976) also
observed that as these growing fascicles leave the S.O., they lose
their close apposition with radial glia. This event correlates with
the decline in retinal and tectal tubulin and protein synthesis
(Fig. 3) seen at this time and may be associated with the loss of
attachment to the radial glia as regenerating optic fascicles enter
the SFGS.

Synaptogenesis within the SFGS inhibits growth activity

Beyond 2 1/2 weeks post nerve crush, there is a renewed burst of
retinal growth activity that seems to be associated with some new
growth stimulus in the SFGS. As vision returns at around 3-4 postoperatively there is increasing morphological indication of synapse
formation and maturation within the SFGS (Murray, 1976) which is cor-

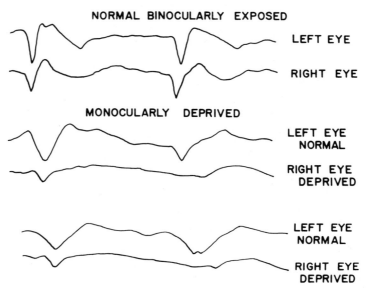

Figure 7. IPSILATERAL RESPONSES - Visual evoked potentials to a
reversing contrast stimulus, recorded using silver/silver chloride
surface electrodes. Top trace shows ipsilateral responses on
stimulation to the left and right eyes of a normal, binocularly
exposed rat. Bottom trace shows ipsilateral responses from
monocularly deprived rats and illustrate the diminished response
resulting from stimulation through the deprived (right) eye.
(Courtesy of Carole Stafford)

related with a subsequent decline in retinal tubulin synthesis
(Fig. 3). The situation found during the later stages of tectal
reinnervation may not be dissimilar to that found during reinnervation of adult skeletal muscle where denervation causes hypersensitivity and increased ACh receptor synthesis; while reinnervation on
the other hand, inhibits receptor synthesis and causes receptor
clustering (Lomo and Westgaard, 1975). Also, in muscle, denervation
hypersensitivity and the appearance of extrajunctional receptors is
apparently associated with some growth stimulus that affects motor
terminal sprouting (Pestronk and Drachman, 1978). The goldfish
visual system has recently been found to contain a significant population of cholinergic synapses (Oswald et al., 1980). Alpha-
bungarotoxin treatment of the optic tectum affects the cholinergic
receptors of retinotectal synapses and causes sprouting of adjacent
visual afferent terminals (Freeman, 1977). As in muscle, the cholinergic receptors of retinotectal synapses seem to exercise some regulatory role on the growth of nerve terminals (Freeman, 1977), and

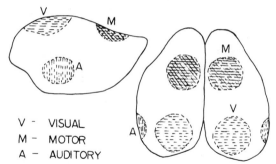

Figure 8. RAT CEREBRAL CORTEX - Position and extent of areas removed. Regions of rat cerebral cortex used in our studies on critical period plasticity.

this could be the source of our second nerve growth stimulus as regenerating axons enter the SFGS. Likewise, synaptogenesis in the SFGS may be associated with the inhibition of the growth stimulus as mirrored by the decline in retinal and tectal protein and tubulin synthesis as retinotectal synapses form and mature.

Differences in response of nasal and temporal hemi-retina during later stages of tectal reinnervation

In the course of the second stage of optic fiber ingrowth into the tectum, which begins approximately 2 1/2 weeks after nerve crush, the pattern of protein synthesis in nasal and temporal hemi-retina differs significantly from that seen during the first stage; and this requires some explanation.

After 2 1/2 weeks, the initial difference in phase between the two experimental groups disappears, and the pattern of response for both nasal and temporal groups thereafter display the same time course and appear to be synchronous (Fig. 6). In addition, the maximum amplitude for the response of temporal hemi-retina is now significantly greater than that for a nasal hemi-retina, whereas the reverse was true during the first stage of ingrowth into the tectum (Figs. 5 and 6).

One possible explanation for this difference may have to do with the particular functional significance represented by the region of the visual field served by temporal hemi-retina. Indeed, it is this portion of the retinal mosaic which receives its input from visual stimuli situated in front of the fish, and therefore represents that part of the field requiring the most detailed analysis in the fish's exploration of its visual environment. By contrast,

nasal retina receives its input largely from the sides and back of
the fish, and is more likely to be concerned with a coarser analysis
of the visual environment, such as the detection of sudden movement,
signalling the possible presence of a predator. Such locus specific
differences, if they exist, do not appear to be reflected in the distribution of ganglion cell types in the retina, but instead may
depend on differences in central connectivity, and in particular,
on differences in the abundance and variety of connections established with functionally different neuronal types in the tectum.
In such a case, one might expect that the pattern of connectivity
established by fibers from temporal retina within the tectum, should
be more elaborate than those formed by fibers from nasal hemi-
retina. If the former's connectivity and ramification within the
SFGS are more numerous or elaborate than those for the nasal retinal
fibers, this should be mirrored in the responses to the growth
stimulus within the SFGS. That displayed by a temporal hemi-retina
should be correspondingly greater during the second stage of tectal
reinnervation than for a nasal counterpart. Final confirmation of
this tentative interpretation must however await further anatomical
studies on goldfish optic tectum to reveal possible differences in
central connectivity established by each half-eye.

Our finding that there is enhanced labelling of tubulin in goldfish retina following optic nerve axotomy has recently been confirmed
by M. Schwartz (1982). In addition, she also found an increase in
microtubule associated protein during nerve regeneration and suggested
that these proteins, together with tubulin, play a regulatory role in
optic nerve regeneration by participating in the formation of the new
axonal matrix. Finally, our results on the regenerating visual system
indicate:

i)   First, that important growth regulating interactions take place
      reciprocally between ingrowing optic axons and tectal cells
      during regeneration of the retinotectal projection.

ii)   Secondly, our findings are consistent with the view that neuro-
      trophic influences within target tissue provide a local feedback
      control which regulates the growth responses and terminal con-
      nectivity of ingrowing optic axons. Consequently, regeneration
      of the retinotectal system seems to be a multiple stage process
      that involves the local control of fiber growth as well as the
      recognition of appropriate synaptic targets.

CRITICAL PERIOD PLASTICITY

In our studies on regeneration of the goldfish visual system,
we only examined the behavior of one cytoskeketal component, namely
tubulin. We now have evidence from another species, that different
components of the cytoskeleton may be associated with different stages
of growth and morphogenesis, and that one of these in particular,

i.e. tubulin, may be important in mediating neural plasticity.

In some species, restriction of visual experience during a certain critical period of early postnatal life can affect the normal functional development of visual cortical cells. This has now been confirmed for Man (Freeman et al., 1972), monkey (Hubel et al., 1977), cat (Wiesel and Hubel, 1965), mice (Drager, 1975), and recently by Carole Stafford in our laboratory, for the hooded rat (see figure 7). While a great deal of effort has been devoted to the task of defining the morphological and functional changes in the nervous system that result from visual deprivation, there has been surprisingly little attempt to identify corresponding changes in the biochemical and molecular organization of developing visual cortical cells during the maturationally sensitive period; yet it is clear that intracellular events must orchestrate and reflect the developmental program which determines the ontogenetic sequence and maturation of the brain's functional characteristics. For instance, intracellular events which affect the number or nature of molecules available for incorporation into a synaptic membrane may affect synaptic transmission and thereby change a cell's functional properties. It therefore becomes relevant to consider also those intracellular systems which regulate the flow and differential distribution of materials needed for growth and maintenance of neurites and synaptic contacts.

Accordingly, we have studied changes in concentration and synthesis of the cytoskeletal components, tubulin and actin, occurring in functionally different regions of the rat cerebral cortex during postnatal brain development (Fig. 8). In addition, we examined the effects of visual deprivation during early postnatal life on the cellular pool of these components in the visual cortex (Cronly-Dillon and Perry, 1975; Perry and Cronly-Dillon, 1978; Cronly-Dillon and Perry, 1979).

Rats were killed by decapitation at various times after birth and a plug of tissue removed with a 'cork borer' instrument, from area 17 of the visual cortex in each hemisphere. Other assays were also carried out on samples of whole cortex, and plugs of tissue removed from motor and auditory cortex. Tritiated colchicine was used to assay tubulin and ^{14}C-radiolabelled-L-leucine injected into the brain ventricles 2 hours before death was used to study the rate of tubulin synthesis at different postnatal ages. The measurement of soluble tubulin and its rate of synthesis was determined by a double labelling method adapted from a method described by Feit et al. (1971,)(Perry and Cronly-Dillon, 1978) and was essentially the same as that used in our studies on goldfish regeneration.

Tubulin synthesis in visual cortex of normal light reared rats
---

We found that the peaks in tubulin synthesis for visual, motor and auditory (not shown) cortex occurred at different times in develop-

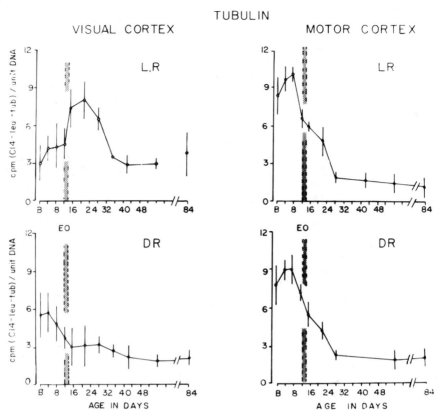

Figure 9.   Incorporation of ^{14}C-L-Leucine into tubulin in developing:
A. visual cortex of normal light-reared rats; B. motor cortex of
normal light-reared rats; C. visual cortex of dark-reared rats;
D. motor cortex of dark-reared rats.   Results normalized with respect
to DNA.   E.O., eye opening; LR, light-reared; DR, dark-reared.

ment, which may indicate that these functional regions of the rat
cerebral cortex mature at different times (Figure 9).   We also found
that rats reared under normal illumination and with no restriction of
visual experience display a transient increase in rate of synthesis
of the tubulin enriched fraction in visual cortex following eye opening.   This elevated level of tubulin synthesis lasted until about the
35th day postnatally, whereupon the curve dropped to approximately
the level it had attained at birth, and thereafter appeared to maintain this level into adult life (Figures 9,10).   Figure 10 shows

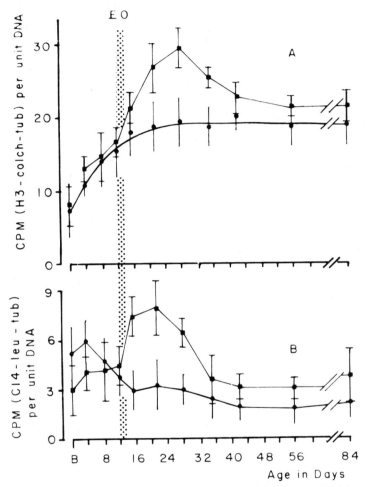

Figure 10. A: Changes in concentration of soluble tubulin in visual cortex of normal light-reared rats (squares) and dark-reared rats (filled circles) measuring using ^{3}H colchicine bound to tubulin precipitated with vinblastine sulphate. B: Changes in rate of synthesis of soluble tubulin in visual cortex of normal, light-reared rats (squares) and dark-reared rats (circles). The relative rates were determined by measuring the amount of ^{14}C-L-leucine (incorporated in the 2 hrs prior to death) in tubulin precipitated with vinblastine sulphate. Each point is normalized with respect to the amount of DNA per unit wet weight of tissue (determined for each postnatal age). E.O. represents time of eye opening.

the corresponding changes in tubulin concentration in visual cortex
in relation to eye opening.

What functional significance may we attribute to this pattern of
growth activity in the visual cortex? From a physiological stand-
point, the consequences to a nerve cell of having a sudden and large
increase in the size of its available pool of tubulin may be that
it enables the cell to maintain an uncommonly large number of connections and nerve processes during the critical period. This interpretation seems to be borne out by anatomical studies in which
it was found that the most sensitive period in the development of
the visual cortex occurs when the number of synaptic connections is
greatest. At the end of the critical period, many synapses drop out
and the number of connections is reduced (Cragg, 1975). The significant factor to note in relation to our own studies is that the
drop in the level of tubulin at the end of the critical period is
likely to cause a reduction in the number of microtubules within
cells of the visual cortex. Consequently, many nerve connections
drop out because there are now insufficient microtubules within each
cell to keep all connections supplied with the materials essential
for their maintenance. As a result, different connections are forced
to compete with one another for the limited supply of tubulin, neurotrophic factors and other cytoskeletal components that are needed
for their maintenance and stabilization. The function of experience
in determining brain connectivity is seen in part as selecting for
survival only those connections that are used, and which attract to
them the materials needed for their stabilization.

Effect of visual experience

Perry and I (1978, 1979) have examined the effects of visual experience in regulating growth activity. We found that the burst in
tubulin synthesis in the visual cortex which normally follows eye
opening was absent if the rats were raised from birth in total darkness. The effect of visual experience was also specific to the visual
cortex and did not occur for the motor cortex (Figure 9). Although
tubulin synthesis in visually deprived rats was greatly reduced we
found it could still be triggered again by visual experience provided
the animal was brought out into the light within the critical period
but not if visual experience were delayed beyond this time (Figure
11). This observation is relevant, in that neurophysiologists define
the visual critical period as that developmental interval when
exposure to appropriate visual experience may still reverse the
deleterious effects produced by previous visual deprivation.

Competitive interactions in monocularly deprived animals

A possible relationship between bioelectric activity and microtubule activation is suggested by the results of Kerkut et al.(1967)
who showed that axonal transport in a motor nerve was enhanced in

proportion to the increase in discharge of the nerve. Consequently
nervous activity may enhance the transport of neurotrophic substances
and materials needed for nerve growth and synapse stabilization.
Experimental manipulation of visual experience has revealed that
binocular suppression of visual input is less deleterious than monocular deprivation during the critical period (Wiesel and Hubel,
1965). A possible explanation of this finding is that active
terminals may receive a greater supply of neurotrophic substances
which gives them a growth advantage over inactive terminals in the
competition for terminal space.

Recently, Changeux and Danchin (1976) have reviewed and discussed
the evidence which suggests that the late phase of synapse maturation,
i.e. that which is associated with the regression of multiple innervation and the selective stabilization of certain synapses, is coupled
to neuronal activity. In adult denervated muscle (Lomo and Westgaard,
1975) and in developing non-innervated embryonic myotubes (Cohen and
Fishbach, 1973), direct electrical stimulation abolishes hypersensitivity in the extrajunctional areas. The result depends critically
on the amount and pattern of the stimuli and suggests that optimal
stimulation blocks receptor synthesis (Lomo and Westgaard, 1975).
Thus at the cellular level, certain patterns of neural and synaptic
activity may be required to activate or shut off the synthesis of
specific intra-cellular substances needed by the cell to complete its
final maturation. The possibility then, is that during the critical
period of visual brain development, genes that control cell growth
may be switched on by visual experience. Indeed, several instances
are already known where neuroelectric activity at synaptic junctions
affect the action of genes. In the autonomic nervous system, it has
been shown that activity of the enzyme, adrenal tyrosine hydroxylase
is increased by nervous activity (Thoenen and Otten, 1977). Thoenen's
(1977) studies also provide evidence that the triggering of a gene
system that regulates the synthesis of noradrenalin may be brought
about by nervous action. Alternatively, the effect of neural activity
may be to modulate translation. Clearly then, if during the critical
period for a particular region of the brain, major changes in macromolecular synthesis associated with cell growth, are triggered by
nervous action, this could in part account for the alteration in the
morphology and function of nerve cells that result from deprivation
of the appropriate sensory experience in early postnatal life.

Changes in actin concentration during postnatal development of
visual cortex

Components of the cytoskeleton such as actin, tubulin and neurofilament protein may be indicative of specific stages of growth and
maturation in the life of a neurone (Hoffman and Lask, 1980). Briefly, tubulin is mainly found in dendrites and the smaller myelinated
axons whilst neurofilament protein only predominates in large mature
neurones and their large myelinated axons.

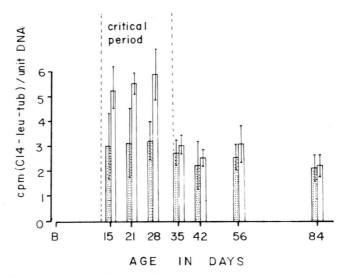

Figure 11. Sensitivity of tubulin response to visual stimulation of developing visual cortex in relation to postnatal age. Rats were reared in total darkness from birth for various lengths of time and then exposed to a normally illuminated visual environment for 24 hrs at different ages (unfilled histograms). These are compared with corresponding values for rats reared continuously in the dark (stippled histograms).

        After tubulin, actin is the second most abundant cytoskeletal protein found in brain. Reliable estimates of actin concentration in the brains of embryonic and adult chickens were obtained by Pardee and Bamberg (1979). They found that actin constitutes 8-10% of their soluble protein fractions in embryonic brain. This value declined to 6% in the adult. Chang and Goldman (1973) used heavy meromyosin labelling to show that the pattern of actin distribution in glycerinated nerve cells followed the location of microfilaments in undisturbed cells. A layer of actin beneath the plasma membrane was revealed which was more pronounced where the nerve cell body contacted the substratum. The axon itself contained very few micro-filaments but concentrations were observed at sites of filopodial projections. Recently, using fluorescence labelled antibodies directed against tubulin and actin Spooner and Halliday (1981) de-scribed 'hot spots' of intense anti-actin fluorescence in growth cones, with little actin in neurites. Also inhibition of the motile activity of the growth cone follows treatment with cytochalasin B and results in a concomitant change in the neuronal microfilament network (Wessells et al., 1971). The important and distinct roles of the microtubules and microfilaments are underlined by the fact that microtubule disruption with colchicine causes axonal collapse in the presence of and apparently opposed by a functional growth cone.

Another suggestion regarding the function of actin in the neurone is that it mediates synaptic activity in the mature nervous system. Actin like filaments have been identified within synapses using heavy meromyosin staining under the electron microscope while similar filaments were not present in other regions of the neurone although a careful search was made (Metuzals and Mushynski, 1974). Biochemical work has also identified an actomyosin-like protein in synaptosomes (Berl et al., 1973). Thus in view of the high levels of actin in the neurone and its special function in neural development it was decided to investigate this protein. The work has been carried out in our laboratory by Stephen Trowel (1983, 1982) who examined changes in the pool of actin in rat visual cortex during postnatal brain development and studied the effect of visual deprivation on the concentration of this cytoskeletal component in nervous tissue.

The method used for measuring actin concentration was derived from a method described by Bliksted et al. (1978), and is based on the finding that actin exerts an inhibitory action on the activity of DNase in its degradation of DNA. Therefore, using a standard amount of DNA and DNase, it was possible to compare the extent of inhibition produced by various homogenates from brain and thereby derive the actin concentration, as expressed as a percentage of brain protein, for different regions of cerebral cortex.

Figures 12 and 13 show the developmental profile for actin concentration measured in different regions of the cerebral cortex in both light- and dark-reared rats. Comparing these findings with the corresponding profile for tubulin it was found:

(i)   that unlike tubulin, there appears to be no significant difference in the developmental profile for actin in different regions of cerebral cortex. In particular, the developmental profile, for both visual (area 17) and motor cortex appear to be identical (Fig. 12).

(ii)   the peak in actin concentration in either visual or motor cortex occurs earlier than the peak in tubulin concentration in these areas (Fig. 12).

(iii) unlike tubulin, dark rearing appears to have no effect on the developmental profile for actin concentration in rat visual cortex (Fig. 13).

Actin requirement relative to other proteins is maximal at three days of age and has declined to a steady plateau by thirty days of age. While apical shafts are present on many neurones on postnatal

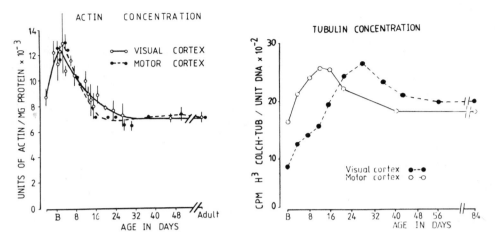

Figure 12. Comparison of the changes in (a) total actin concentration in two functionally distinct regions of rat neocortex (one unit
of actin is the amount which inhibits DNase activity by 1% in the
standard assay). (b) Soluble tubulin concentration in the same
cortical regions.

day 1, Juraska and Fifkova (1979) report that "tremendous" dendritic
growth occurs between the third and tenth day postnatally. This
finding has been confirmed and extended by Miller and Peters (1981)
who could only find dendritic filopodia and growth cones in the visual
cortex of the rat between day 3 and day 12 postnatally.

    One interpretation of the early peak in actin concentration is
that it coincides with the time of initiation of neurites during postnatal development of the visual cortex and may represent a special
requirement for growth cone actin which is subsequently diluted out by
tubulin and other proteins during the elongation and maturation phase.
It seems that actin is required in most abundance in early development
of the cortex before visually driven plasticity is relevant. This
contrasts with the lability of tubulin to visual deprivation and
supports the view that a shift in types of cytoskeletal protein may
define the start and end of neural plasticity. This accords with the
hypothesis advanced by Hoffman and Lasek (1980). They see high numbers
of microtubules as possibly indicating an enhanced sprouting potential,
which in their estimation is synonomous with plasticity. They also
suggest that the increasing numbers of neurofilaments which build up
in the neurones of the central nervous system lead to the progressive

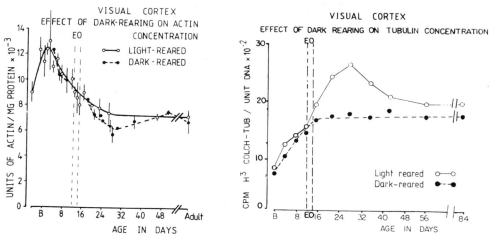

Figure 13. Effect of dark-rearing on: (a) the change in total actin concentration with age in the primary visual cortex for rats reared on a normal light-dark cycle (open circles) or brought up in total darkness (filled circles). (b) corresponding change in soluble tubulin concentration in visual cortex of normal light-reared and dark-reared rats.

loss of plasticity of all forms. This indeed is the sort of cytoske-letal change which might end the various critical periods including that of visual plasticity. Actin on the other hand seems to be the cytoskeletal protein that is predominantly associated with the pre-plastic phase and this is supported by the finding that there is little or no difference between regions of the cortex in respect of their actin profile. On the other hand tubulin may respond to modulation at different times depending on the particular region and stage of brain development.

THE POSSIBLE INVOLVEMENT OF TUBULIN IN MEMORY FIXATION

     In the preceding studies, we monitored changes in the concentra-tion and synthesis of tubulin in nervous tissue and observed how this changed during critical period plasticity. Another approach is to block the action of certain cytoskeletal components by the use of specific drugs and to observe how plasticity of the system is affected by such treatment (Cronly-Dillon et al., 1974).

Colchicine which binds specifically to tubulin interferes with tubulin polymerization and is known to interfere with axonal elongation during nerve growth or regeneration. It was therefore pertinent to enquire if colchicine would also interfere with the plasticity manifested in learning and memory. If we assume that some form of synapse modification is involved in memory fixation the question becomes even more relevant. Firstly because maintenance of the synapse depends on fast axonal transport which in turn relies on microtubules and the ability of tubulin to polymerize. Secondly, because tubulin is a significant constituent of the postsynaptic lattice network and is thought to be one of the components involved in the stabilization of synaptic receptors in the postsynaptic membrane (Jones and Matus, 1975).

Goldfish were therefore trained in a shock avoidance situation to discriminate between two illuminated panels of different color situated at opposite ends of a training tank. The fish were required to swim to the side of the tank illuminated with the positive color within a certain time interval, to avoid a mild electric shock. We found that they learned this task extremely readily. Individual fish were scored on the basis of the number of correct responses, in consecutive blocks of ten trials. Also initial training never exceeded one hour duration, and all fish that failed to attain a score of 14/20 correct responses during initial training were excluded from the experiment. Each fish was then retrained 36 to 48 hours after initial training to determine if it displayed any significant improvement in performance to reach criterion as compared to initial training. In our experiments, all injections were given intracranially into the subdural space overlying the optic tectum.

First we examined the behavior of a control group of fish into which we injected a neutral (saline) solution into the cavity overlying the brain. This was done immediately after the fish had been trained and had learned the discrimination to the set criterion. When tested two days later we found that they immediately scored highly in their performance of the task; clearly therefore these fish had successfully transferred the learning into long-term memory and were able to recall the information they had learned two days previously. If instead of the neutral saline, we gave an injection of colchicine immediately after the first training session, the fish displayed complete retrograde amnesia when tested two days later. The loss of memory however did not impair short term storage or the ability of the fish to relearn the discrimination. In a third experiment we gave the colchicine injection 1 3/4 hours after the initial training. When tested two days later, these fish displayed considerable retention for the discrimination. Consequently, by the time these fish received the colchicine injection, the memory had already been transferred into a structurally stable form and was no longer accessible to the disruptive influence of the drug. Finally, we injected the colchicine solution 1 1/4 hours before we started

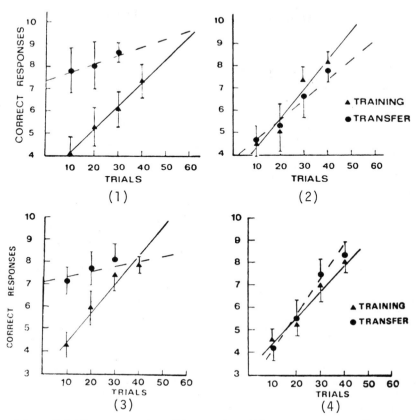

Figure 14. Solid regression lines show the group's performance
during initial training, while the broken lines relate to performance during transfer retraining. Solid circles and triangles each
give mean score for 15 fish. Vertical bars denote standard devia-
tions. (1) Control Group: These fish received 50μl saline injected
into the cranial cavity overlying the optic tectum, immediately after
initial training. The fish were then retrained forty-eight hours
later and displayed considerable retention for the originally learned task. (2) Colchicine Group I: These fish received an intracranial
saline injection which contained 12.5μg colchicine immediately after
initial training. When retrained forty-eight hours later they
displayed complete retrograde amnesia for the task which had to be
relearned. (3) Colchicine Group II: These fish received the same
dose of colchicine intracranially except that this was administered
1 1/4 hours after completion of initial training. When retrained

(continued)

training the fish. Colchicine was therefore present in the brain throughout the initial training period, and we found no indication that this drug interfered with short term memory required for learning, or with cell processes involved in the initial acquisition of the discrimination. When tested two days later however, these fish showed complete retrograde amnesia and had to relearn the discrimination again as if they had never before encountered the task. Further control experiments also established that the effect of colchicine on memory fixation was not associated with either a depression of neuroelectric activity or of inhibition of total protein synthesis in brain (Cronly-Dillon et al., 1974).

Our studies suggest that colchicine can prevent a recently acquired memory from being transferred into a structurally stable form. One possibility is that colchicine, which binds to tubulin, may interfere with tubulin polymerization at synaptic membrane sites, and thereby prevent tubulin from stabilizing a structural change at the synaptic connections between cells that is brought about by learning. Figure 15 illustrates a hypothetical scheme on how this may occur. The plasma membrane adjacent to the modifiable synapse is presumed to contain a number of extrajunctional receptors that are free to migrate in the plane of the membrane, and are induced to cluster at the postsynaptic site when the nerve terminal is active. While these extrajunctional receptors are in this clustered configuration the efficiency of the synapse that has been activated during learning is enhanced. These extrajunctional receptors are linked to actin and tubulin molecules. Memory fixation occurs when the extrajunctional receptors which have migrated and clustered at the active synapse become stabilized by the 'crosslinking' of their cytoskeletal components with others in the postsynaptic lattice. This reaction is presumed to occur in response to a NOW FIX signal that produces the requisite crosslinking of cytoskeletal component which leads to stabilization of the receptors within the postsynaptic lattice. In the absence of this stabilizing signal, extrajunctional receptors are free to diffuse away from the postsynaptic site once activity in terminals ceases. Thus the efficiency of the synapse may be temporarily enhanced by repeated use during learning, but unless the change that has occurred at the synapse is stabilized, the memory does not endure. The disruptive action of colchicine on

---

Fig. 14 (continued)

forty-eight hours later the fish displayed considerable retention for the originally learned task. (4) Colchicine Group III: These fish received the intracranial injection of colchicine 1 1/4 hours before they were trained. This apparently did not interfere with their ability to acquire the task. However when retested two days later there was considerable loss of memory for that task.

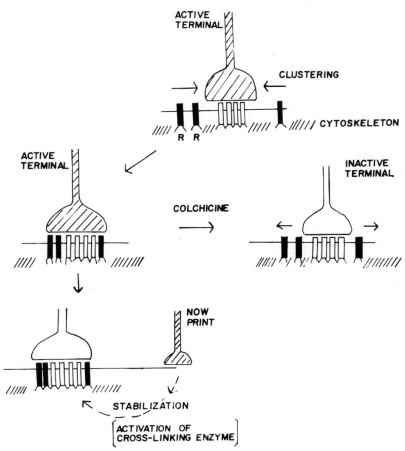

Figure 15. In this hypothetical scheme, activity in the presynaptic
terminal causes 'clustering' of extrajunctional receptors (here represented in black) to the junctional site. Receptors are associated
with cytoskeletal components. In the 'clustered' configuration the
'efficiency' of the synapse is enhanced. Memory fixation occurs as
the result of a NOW PRINT signal which causes the cross-linking of
cytoskeletal components associated with receptors and so stabilizes
the 'cluster' at the junctional site. Colchicine interferes with
this cross-linking event and when activity in the terminal ceases,
extrajunctional receptors diffuse away from the junctional site.

memory fixation may perhaps be attributed to its interference with the cross linking and stabilization of cytoskeletal components in the postsynaptic lattice. The model also suggests that colchicine should not interfere with the processes of short term memory that are involved in the acquisition phase of learning.

Another possibility is that by blocking the formation of microtubules, colchicine may inhibit the transport of materials in nerve cell processes which are needed to bring about a structural change at the points of synaptic connection between nerve cells. In this respect, it is interesting that a converse effect has been reported. Heavy water, deuterium oxide, is known to stabilize microtubules, and it apparently does so by substituting deuterium for hydrogen in these structures. Heavy water facilitates learning in goldfish (Lehr et al., 1970), and also accelerates nerve growth in isolated nerve tissues (Murray and Benitez, 1968), again possibly by stabilizing microtubules and thereby enhancing the flow of materials along nerve cell processes. It seems clear that microtubules and tubulin polymerization are in some way implicated in mediating some of the growth and structural changes that are involved in the establishment of long term memory.

In conclusion, our experiments have shown that the cytoskeleton is intimately associated with cell interactions that control the growth activity and behavior of growing axons during the patterning of nerve connections in development and regeneration. Secondly, that a shift in the type of cytoskeletal protein may define different stages of growth and morphogenesis of nervous tissue, and that changes in cytoskeletal organization associated with critical period plasticity in the visual cortex are influenced by nervous activity. Thirdly, that the cytoskeleton and its components may be implicated in the stabilization and fixation of learned responses. In general then, what these studies illustrate is that the cytoskeleton may provide a useful starting point for the molecular dissection of cell mechanisms involved in the formation and plasticity of brain circuits.

Acknowledgements: I thank Carole Stafford and Stephen Trowell for their critical reading of the manuscript and the Science Research Council and Wellcome Trust for financial support.

REFERENCES

Aguilar, C.E., Bisby, M.A., Cooper, E. and Diamond, J. (1973) Evidence that axonal transport of trophic factors is involved in the regulation of peripheral nerve fields in salamanders. J. Physiol. (Lond.) 234, 449-464.

Benowitz, L.I. and Shashoua, V.E. (1979) Immunoreactive sites for nerve growth factor in the goldfish. Brain Res. 172, 561-565.

Berl, S. Puszkin, S. and Nicklas, W.K. (1973) Actomyosin-like protein in brain. Science 179, 441-445.

Berry, M., McConnell, P., Sievers, P. and Ansar, A. (1980) Factors influencing the growth of cerebellar neural networks in "Studies of normal and abnormal development of the nervous system" (eds. Lierse, Hamburg and Beck) S. Karger, publ. Basel, Switzerland.

Bliksted, I., Markey, F., Carlsson, L., Persson, J. and Lindberg, U. (1978) Selective assay of monomeric and filamentous actin in cell extracts using inhibition of Deoxyribonuclease I. Cell 15, 935-943.

Chang, C. and Goldman, R.D. (1973) The localization of actin-like fibres in cultured neuroblastoma cells as revealed by heavy meromyosin binding. J. Cell Biol. 57, 867-874.

Changeux, J.P. and Danchin, A. (1976) Selective stabilization of developing synapses as a mechanism for the specification of neuronal networks. Nature 264, 705-712.

Cohen, S.A. and Fishbach, G.D. (1973) Regulation of muscle acetyl-choline sensitivity by muscle activity in cell culture. Science 181, 76-78.

Cragg, B.G. (1975) The development of synapses in kitten visual cortex during visual deprivation. Exptl. Neurol. 46, 445-451.

Cronly-Dillon, J., Carden, D. and Birks, C. (1974) The possible involvement of brain microtubules in memory fixation. J. Exp. Biol. 61, 443-454.

Cronly-Dillon, J. and Perry, G.W. (1975) Synthesis of microtubule protein in rat visual cortex during early post-natal life in relation to eye opening. J. Physiol. (Lond.) 252, 27-28P.

Cronly-Dillon, J. and Perry, G.W. (1979) Effect of visual experience on tubulin synthesis during a critical period of visual cortex development in the hooded rat. J. Physiol. (Lond.) 293, 469-484.

Dräger, U.C. (1975) Extent of plasticity of connections in visual cortex and tectum of normal and retinal-dystrophic mice. Assoc. for Res. in Vision & Ophthalmology, Sarasota, Florida. p. 64.

Feit, H., Dutton, G.R., Barondes, S.H. and Shelanski, M. (1971) Microtubule protein identification in and transport to nerve endings. J. Cell Biol. 51, 138-147.

Fine, R. and Bray, D. (1971) Actin in growing nerve cells. Nature New Biol. 234, 319-330.

Freeman, J.A. (1977) Possible regulatory function of acetylcholine receptor in maintenance of retinotectal synapses. Nature 269, 218-222.

Freeman, R.D., Mitchell, D.E., Millodot, M. (1972) A neural effect of partial visual deprivation in humans. Science 175, 1384-1386.

Halfter, W., Claviez, M. and Schwarz, U. (1981) Preferential adhesion of tectal membranes to anterior embryonic chick retina neurites. Nature 292, 67-70.

Hoffman, F. and Lask, R.J. (1980) Axonal transport of the cytoskeleton
     in regenerating motor neurons: constancy and change. Brain Res.
     202, 317-333.
Hubel, D.H., Wiesel, T.N. and LeVay, S. (1977) Plasticity of ocular
     dominance columns in monkey striate cortex. Phil. Trans. Roy.
     Soc. Lond. B. 278, 377-409.
Jacobson, M. (1978) Developmental Neurobiology. Plenum Press. N.Y.
Jones, D.H. and Matus, A.I. (1975) Changes in protein content of
     developing brain synaptic membranes, mitochondria and myelin.
     Neurosci. Letters 1, 153-158.
Juraska, J.M. and Fifkova, E. (1979) A Golgi study of the early post-
     natal development of the visual system of the hooded rat. J.
     Comp. Neurol. 183, 247-256.
Keating, M.J. (1977) Evidence for plasticity of intertectal neuronal
     connections in adult xenopus. Phil. Trans. R. Soc. Lond. B
     278, 277-294.
Kerkut, J., Shapira, A. and Walker, R.J. (1967) The transport of
     ^{14}C-labelled material from CNS to and from muscle along a nerve
     trunk. Comp. Biochem. Physiol. 23, 729-748.
Lagnado, J.R., Lyons, C. and Wickremasinghe, G. (1971) The subcellu-
     lar distribution of colchicine binding protein. F.E.B.S.
     Letters. 15, 254.
Lehr, E., Werner, M. and Wenzel, G. (1970) Zur biochemie des
     gedachtnisser I. Einfluss von schwerem wasser auf des
     gedactnisses von Fischen. Naturwissenschaften 57, 521-524.
Letourneau, P.C. (1982) 'Nerve Fibre Growth and Extrinsic Factors' in
     Neuronal Development. (ed. Nicholas C. Spitzer) Plenum Press.
     N.Y.
Lomo, T. and Westgaard, R.H. (1975) Further studies on the control of
     ACh sensitivity by muscle activity in the rat. J. Physiol. 252,
     603-626.
Metuzals, J. and Mushynski, W.E. (1974) Electron microscope and
     experimental investigations of the neural filamentous network of
     Dieter's neurons. J. Cell Biol. 61, 701-722.
Meyer, R.L. (1982) Tetrodotoxin blocks the formation of ocular
     dominance columns and refined retinotopography in Goldfish.
     Soc. Neurosci. Abst. 8, 12th Ann. Meeting, Minneapolis, 121, 8
     (Plenum Press).
Miller, M. and Peters, A. (1981) Maturation of Rat Visual Cortex II.
     A combined Golgi-electron microscope study of pyramidal neurons.
     J. Comp. Neurol. 203, 555-573.
Murray, J.R. and Benitez, H. (1968) Action of heavy water (D$_2$O) on
     growth and development of isolated nervous tissue. In "Growth of
     the Nervous System" (ed. G.E.W. Wolstenholme & M. O'Connor).
     London: J & A Churchill Ltd.
Murray, M. (1976) Regeneration of retinal axons into the Goldfish
     optic tectum. J. Comp. Neurol. 168, 175-195.
Murray, M., Sharma, S. and Edwards, M.A. (1982) Target regulation of
     synaptic number in the compressed retinotectal projection of
     Goldfish. J. Comp. Neurol. 209, 374-385.

Oswald, R.E., Schmidt, J.T., Norden, J. and Freeman, J.A. (1980) Localization of bungarotoxin binding sites to the goldfish retinotectal projection. Brain Res. 187, 113-127.

Pardee, J.D. and Bamburg, J.R. (1979) Actin from embryonic chick brain. Isolation in high yield and comparison of biochemical properties with chicken muscle actin. Biochemistry (U.S.A.), 18, 2245-2252.

Perry, G.W. and Cronly-Dillon, J. (1978) Tubulin synthesis during a critical period in visual cortex development. Brain Res. 142, 374-378.

Pestronk, A. and Drachman, D.B. (1978) Motor nerve sprouting and Acetylocholine receptors. Science 199, 1223-1225.

Purves, D. and Lichtman, J.W. (1980) Elimination of synapses in the developing nervous system. Science 210, 153-157.

Ramon y Cajal (1919) Lab. Invest. Biol. Univ. Madrid in Studies in vertebrate neurogenesis, L. Guth (transl.)

Schubert, D., Lacorbiere, M., Whitlock and Stallcup, W. (1978) Alterations in the surface properties of cells responsive to nerve growth factor. Nature 273, 718-723.

Schwartz,. H. (1979) Axonal transport components, mechanism and specificity. Ann. Rev. Neurosci. 2, 467-504.

Schwartz, M. (1982) Enhanced labelling of microtubule-associated TAU factors and β-tubulin in Goldfish retina during optic nerve regeneration. Soc. Neurosci. Abstr. 8, 262.

Solomon (1982) 'Cell interactions and the cytoskeleton'. In "Neuronal Glia interrelationships". (ed. T. Sears) Springer-Verlag, Berlin.

Spooner, B.S., and Holladay, C.R. (1981) Distribution of tubulin and actin in neurites and growth cones of differentiating nerve cells. Cell Motility 1, 167-178.

Stevenson, J.A. and Yoon, M.G. (1972) Morphology of radial glia, ependymal cells and periventricular neurons. J. Comp. Neurol. 205, 128-138.

Thoenen, H. and Otten, U. (1977) Molecular events in trans-synaptic regulation of the synthesis of macromolecules. In "Essays in Neuro-chemistry & Neuropathology" Vol. I. (eds. Youdin, Louvenberg, Sharman, Lagnado) Wiley, London.

Trowell, S.C. (1982) Changes in brain actin during postnatal development of the hooded rat. MSc thesis.

Trowell, S.C. (1983) Changes in actin during postnatal brain development in the hooded rat. J. Physiol. (in press).

Turner, J.E., Delaney, R.K. and Johnson, J.E. (1980) Retinal ganglion cell response to nerve growth factor in the regenerating and intact visual system of the goldfish Carassius auratus. Brain Res. 197, 319-330.

Wessells, N.K., Spooner, B.S, Ash, J.F., Bradley, M.O., Laduena, M.A., Taylor, E.L., Wrenn, J.T. and Yamada, K.M. (1971) Microfilaments in cellular and developmental processes. Science 171, 135-143.

Wiesel, T.N. and Hubel, D.H. (1965) Comparison of the effects of unilateral and bilateral eye closure on cortical unit responses in kittens. J. Neurophysiol. 28, 1029-1040.

LECTURERS AND PARTICIPANTS

ACHESON, A., Department of Neurochemistry, Max-Planck Institute of Psychiatry, 8033 Martinsried, West Germany.

BARBOSA, M., Department of Anatomy, Porto School of Medicine, Porto, Portugal.

BIZET, M., Laboratoire de Zoologie et Biologie, Universite Scientifique et Medicale, Grenoble, France.

BRECHA, N., CURE V.A. Center/Wadsworth, Los Angeles, California USA.

CAMPOS-ORTEGA, J., Ludwig University, Institute fur Biologie III, Freiburg D-7800, West Germany.

CARVALHO, A., Department of Zoology, University of Coimbra, Coimbra, Portugal.

CARVALHO, C., Department of Zoology, University of Coimbra, Coimbra, Portugal.

CAVINESS, V., Shriver Center, 200 Trapelo Road, Waltham, Mass. 02154, USA.

COIMBRA, A., Institute of Histology and Embryology, Porto School of Medicine, Porto, Portugal.

DA SILVA, A., Department of Anatomy, Porto School of Medicine, Porto, Portugal.

DA SILVA, C., Children's Hospital, Department of Neuroscience, Boston, Mass. USA.

DIAMOND, J., Department of Neurosciences, McMaster University, 1200 Main Street W., Hamilton, Ontario, Canada L8N 3ZS.

DI GREGORIO, F., Fidia Research Research Lab, 3/A 35031 Abano Terme (PD) Italy.

EBENDAL, T., Institute of Zoology, Uppsala University, Box 561, S-75122 Uppsala, Sweden.

FERNANDES, C., Department of Anatomy, Porto School of Medicine, Porto, Portugal.

FOERSTER, A., Department of Neurosciences, McMaster University, Hamilton, Ontario, Canada L8N 3ZS.

FOSSE, V., Norwegian Defence Research Establishment, Division of Toxicology, N-2007, Kjeller, Norway.

FRALEY, S., Department of Ophthalmology, New York Medical College, Valhalla, NY 10595, USA.

FREDENS, K., Institute of Anatomy B, University of Aarhus, Aarhus, Denmark.

GAARSKJAER, F., Institute of Anatomy B, University of Aarhus, Aarhus, Denmark.

GAZE, R.M., Medical Research Council, Mill Hill, London, NW7 1AA, England.

GNAHN, H., Max-Planck Institute of Psychiatry, Department of Neurochemistry, 8033 Martinsried, West Germany.

GOFFINET, A., University Catholoque de Louvain, B-1970 Wezembeek-Oppem, Belgium.

HABETS, A., Netherlands Institute for Brain Research, Ijdijk 28, 1095 KJ Amsterdam, The Netherlands.

HARTENSTEIN, V., Leo-Wohlebstrasse 8, 78 Freiburg, West Germany.

INGOGLIA, N., Department of Physiology, New Jersey College of Medicine and Dentistry, Newark, NJ, USA.

JOOS, S., Institute fur Biologie III, 78 Freiburg, West Germany.

KIRSTJANSSON, G., Department of Pharmacology, Uppsala University, Sweden.

LANCA, A., Institute of Histology and Embryology, Faculty of Medicine, University of Coimbra, Coimbra, Portugal.

LE DOUARIN, N., Institute of Embryology CNRS, 94130 Nogent-Sur-Marne, France.

LEVI-MONTALCINI, R., Laboratory of Cell Biology, via G. Ramagnosi 18/A, CNR-Rome, Italy 001961.

LIMA, D., Department of Anatomy, Porto School of Medicine, Porto, Portugal.

LOWE, I., Department of Pharmacology, University of Pittsburgh, Pittsburgh, PA, USA.

LUND, J., Department of Ophthalmology, Medical University of South Carolina, Charleston, SC 29403, USA.

LUND, R., Department of Anatomy, Medical University of South Carolina, Charleston, SC 29403, USA.

MANSFIELD, D., Department of Anatomy, Cambridge University, Cambridge, England.

MARCHISIO, P., Faculty of Medicine and Surgery, University of Torino, Instituto di Istologia ed Embryologia Generale, Torino, Italy.

MC HANWELL, S., L'Institute d'Embryologie du CNRS et du College de France, Nogent-Sur-Marne, France.

MC LOON, L., Department of Anatomy, Medical University of South Carolina, Charleston, SC 29403, USA.

MC LOON, S., Department of Anatomy, Medical University of South Carolina, Charleston, SC 29403, USA.

MISHRA, P., Department of Anatomy, All-India Institute of Medical Sciences, New Delhi, India.

NOWAKOWSKI, R., Department of Anatomy, University of Mississippi Medical Center, Jackson, Miss., USA.

OPPENHEIM, R., Research Section, North Carolina Division of Mental Health, University of North Carolina, Raleigh, NC 27611, USA.

PEARLMAN, A., Department of Physiology and Biophysics, Washington University, 660 S. Euclid Avenue, St. Louis, MO 63110, USA.

RAKIC, P., School of Medicine, Yale University, New Haven, CT 06510, USA.

SCHWARZ, U., Max-Planck Institute fur Virusforschung, Abteilung Biochemie, D-7400 Tubingen Spemannstrasse, 35/11 West Germany.

SHARMA, S., Department of Ophthalmology, New York Medical College, Valhalla, NY 10595, USA.

SOTELO, C., INSERM, U-106, 42 Rue Desbassayns de Richemont, 92150 Suresnes, France.

STENT, G., Department of Molecular Biology, University of California at Berkeley, Berkeley, CA 94720, USA.

TAVARES, M., Department of Anatomy, Porto School of Medicine, Porto, Portugal.

TAYLOR, J., Medical Research Council, Mill Hill, London NW7 1AA, England.

THOENEN, H., Max-Planck Institute for Phychistrie, Abteilung Neurochemie, 8033 Martinsried bei Munchen, West Germany.

VAN HUIZEN, F., Netherlands Institute for Brain Research, Ijdijk 28, 1095 KJ Amsterdam, The Netherlands.

WEST, M., Institute of Anatomy, University of Aarhus, Aarhus, Denmark.

INDEX